RCGP Guide to
The Management

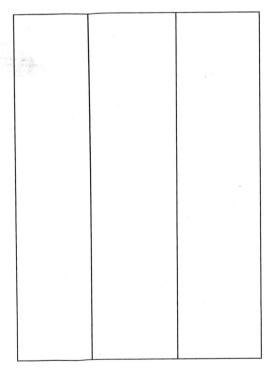

EDITED BY
Clare Gerada

RCGP Guide to
The Management
of Substance Misuse
in Primary Care

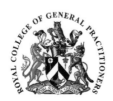

The Royal College of General Practitioners was founded
in 1952 with this object:

*'To encourage, foster and maintain the highest possible
standards in general practice and for that purpose to take or
join with others in taking steps consistent with the charitable
nature of that object which may assist towards the same.'*

Among its responsibilities under its Royal Charter
the College is entitled to:

*'Diffuse information on all matters affecting general
practice and issue such publications as may assist the
object of the College.'*

British Library Cataloguing-in-Publication Data
A catalogue record for this book is available from the British Library

© Royal College of General Practitioners, 2005
Published by the Royal College of General Practitioners 2005
14 Princes Gate, Hyde Park, London SW7 1PU

DISCLAIMER
This publication is intended for the use of medical practitioners in the UK and not
for patients. The authors, editors and publishers have taken care to ensure that the
information contained in this book is correct to the best of their knowledge, at the time
of publication. Whilst efforts have been made to ensure the accuracy of the information
presented, particularly that related to the prescription of drugs, the authors, editors
and Publisher cannot accept liability for information that is subsequently shown to
be wrong. Readers are advised to check that the information, especially that related
to drug usage, complies with information contained in the British National Formulary,
or equivalent, or manufacturers' datasheets, and that it complies with the latest
legislation and standards of practice.

Designed and typeset by Typographic Design Unit, Newcastle-upon-Tyne

Printed by Bell & Bain Ltd, Glasgow

Indexed by Carol Ball

ISBN: 0 85084 297 2

Contents

Foreword

The management of substance misuse in the primary care setting has undergone substantial change over the last few years. Much of this change can be attributed to the establishment of the RCGP Certificate in the Management of Substance Misuse. Previously, GPs and other clinicians struggled to gain access to adequate training to support them in delivering services in this area. Moreover, there was a view in some parts of the profession that this work was not something that GPs and primary health care teams should be involved with. Politicians and policy makers were likewise not convinced that GPs and practices were capable of taking on this issue and delivering services. The success of the RCGP Certificate has demonstrated that GPs and other primary care professionals do care about the health problems experienced by users and that significant numbers want to be trained and accredited to provide dedicated services.

Clare Gerada has championed the cause of primary care management of substance misuse, both within the Department of Health and within the Royal College of General Practitioners. She has been instrumental in designing and delivering the RCGP Certificate and much of the success of the programme can be directly attributed to her leadership. This book has been produced to disseminate some of the material used in the Certificate programme to a wider readership and we hope that this will further enhance standards of management in this field. The College exists to develop and maintain the highest possible standards in general practice and therefore on behalf of RCGP Council I would like to state how proud we are of the Certificate in the Management of Substance Misuse. I hope that all who use this book find the material interesting and relevant to their day-to-day clinical work.

Dr Maureen Baker CBE, DM, FRCGP
Honorary Secretary,
Royal College of General Practitioners.

Acknowledgements

Dorett Woodfine for her patience. My husband Simon and children Alex and Ben for not objecting to the occasional late meal. To my partners at the Hurley Clinic for allowing me the time away to write the book.

Finally, to those from the RCGP Substance Misuse Unit for all their hard work and commitment.

Introduction

General practitioners, primary care nurses, and pharmacists are increasingly becoming involved in the management of substance misusers.

This book is for those who wish to delve beyond the basics of the subject. It aims to provide health professionals with both the evidence for, and the practicalities of, a range of treatment interventions for opioid, stimulant, tobacco, and alcohol users and provides an analysis of the roles that nurses, general practitioners, and pharmacists can play.

The book contains a guide for treating drug users taking into account the nature of drug misuse and special considerations such as young people, pregnant users, and the homeless.

Throughout the book there is an emphasis on evidence-based treatment and details of potential breakthroughs and developing treatments as they are tried and tested.

Drug misuse and dependence covers a vast area and this book makes no apologies in leaving gaps. The reader is guided to additional reading to cover these gaps. For those who have taken the Royal College of General Practitioners certificate course, this book will provide an accompaniment to what has been learnt in masterclasses and should expand their knowledge in all areas of the field. It is hoped that those dipping their toes into this area will be stimulated to take their learning further.

About the authors

Clare Gerada MBE, FRCGP, MRCPsych

Dr Clare Gerada has been a GP for 14 years in a large inner city practice, where she set up and continues to run the CLAS (Consultancy Liaison Addiction Service) Team. Prior to this she was a psychiatrist, having trained at the Maudsley Hospital, and developed an interest in community management of substance misuse.

She is the director and lead for the RCGP Substance Misuse Unit and was the previous Senior Policy Officer for drugs and alcohol. She was responsible, amongst other things, for pulling together the 1999 National Clinical Guidelines for Substance Misuse.

She is currently the Director of the National Clinical Governance Support Team.

Alex Laffan

Alex Laffan attended Haberdashers' Aske's Boys School before helping research and write this book during his gap year. He is now studying for a degree in modern history at Exeter College, Oxford. As well as working on this book, Alex also spent part of his year out as a parliamentary researcher for Don Foster MP and later travelled in Australia, New Zealand, Thailand and Vietnam with friends.

Dave Roberts

After receiving a degree in psychology from York University and two years of lecturing in the same subject, Dave joined the Prescribing Research Unit in 1990. In 1996 it became the Prescribing Support Unit and Dave became the manager at its inception.

Linda Harris MBBS, DAGP

Dr Linda Harris worked for 10 years as a GP principal during which time she developed a special interest in substance misuse and mental health.

As Clinical Director of the Wakefield Integrated Substance Misuse Services she has a key role in the commissioning and provision of whole system treatment and care for substance misusing patients across the two PCTs.

Linda is Deputy Director of the RCGP National Drug Misuse Training Team where she leads on alcohol and professional development. She continues as a member of the Professional Executive Committee of Wakefield West PCT and occasionally works as a consultant to the Sainsbury's Centre for Mental Health.

David Harding-Price RMN, Dip SP&C (Open), DADN, ENB998, ENB 934 Award of Merit RCN, Churchill Fellowship

David's nursing career has taken him around the world. He is currently the Nurse Lead for the National Substance Misuse Training Programme where he developed the nursing elements of the Royal College of General Practitioners' drugs training course and an internet training package in drug misuse. He has worked in primary care for over 20 years in both mental health and substance misuse. David is Chairman of the Royal College of Nursing Mental Health Practice Forum and a Director of the UK Alcohol Forum. His links with the voluntary sector lie both locally and nationally. He is a panellist on the Nurses and Midwives Council and has been a Healthcare Commission investigations team member.

Jane Haywood RGN, Dip Drug Dependence, MSc in Clinical and Public Health Aspects of Addiction, Extended and Supplementary Nurse Prescriber

Jane Heywood is Team Leader of the Consultancy Liaison Addiction Service (CLAS), which is a nurse lead-primary care based team, supporting GPs and primary care staff in the treatment and management of patients with substance misuse problems.

Jane has over 11 years experience of working with drug users in various settings: from street outreach to detox and rehab. She has been working in primary care for 7 years and is particularly interested in engaging and maintaining treatment for those who are hard to reach and have complex needs.

Diana Kay Roberts MRPharms, FRPharms

Diana Roberts qualified in pharmacy from the University of Sunderland in 1960. After spending her pre-registration year at Middlesborough General Hospital she registered as a pharmacist (MRPharmS) in 1961. She was designated a Fellow (FRPharmS) by the Royal Pharmaceutical Society in 1989 and gained her Master of Philosophy Degree from University of Wales, Cardiff in 1992.

Her career has spanned hospital and community pharmacy practice as well as the civil service. She is lead pharmacist on the RCGP Drug Misuse Training Programme. Until the end of July 2003 she was Area Pharmacy Specialist in Drug Misuse for Greater Glasgow Primary Care NHS Trust. She is currently co-ordinator of the Greater Glasgow Pharmacy Needle Exchange Scheme; (Scottish) National Pharmacy Specialist – Drug Misuse; member of the UK Government's Advisory Council on the Misuse of Drugs; member of the Scottish Advisory Committee on Drug Misuse and chairman of its Psychostimulants Working Group; member of the Scottish Needle Exchange Workers Forum; founder member and chairman of PharMAG (an international advisory group for those with an interest in the pharmaceutical care of drug misusers). Diana has undertaken a number of substance misuse related research projects and in 2002 was rewarded with two of the grants from the research competition held by the Scottish Executive's Effective Interventions Unit. She is currently involved in substance misuse research projects being undertaken in universities in Scotland and England.

Janie Sheridan BA, BPharm, PhD, MRPharms, MPS(NZ)

Associate Professor Janie Sheridan is a qualified pharmacist and has a PhD from the University of London. Janie worked at the National Addiction Centre, Institute of Psychiatry in London until 2002, researching in the field of substance misuse, and specialising in researching and evaluating healthcare services for problem drug users and methadone prescribing patterns. Her main focus has been on community pharmacists and their role in caring for problem drug users. Her recent research has investigated the changing role of general practitioners who work with opiate dependent patients. She is currently involved in exploring methadone prescribing patterns and investigating the use of methamphatemine in New Zealand, where she now lives. Janie has recently published a book, *Drug Misuse and Community Pharmacy*, which she co-edited with Professor John Strang.

Jenny Keen BA, MSc, MBBS, MRCGP, DRCOG

Dr Jenny Keen is a GP with a special interest in drug dependence, and clinical director of the Primary Care Clinic for Drug Dependence in Sheffield. She holds a clinical research fellowship at the Institute of General Practice and Primary Care, University of Sheffield and has published a number of research papers in the fields of methadone maintenance, harm reduction and safe prescribing for drug users in primary care.

She is also involved in medical training at all levels in the drugs field, in particular the development of the new RCGP training programme for general practitioners working with drug users.

Chris Ford FRCGP, MRCP

Dr Chris Ford has been a GP in London for 18 years and works with a large number of drug users in general practice and enjoys this work. She is a member of the RCGP Sex, Drugs and HIV Task Group and is the GP Adviser for Substance Misuse in General Practice (SMMGP).

She is a member of the RCGP National Expert Advisory Group and the RCGP London Regional Clinical Lead for drugs. She is the chair of the Alliance, a drug-user-led organisation.

Hans-Christian Raabe MRCP, MRCGP, DRCOG

Dr Hans-Christian Raabe is a GP in Leigh, Lancashire in a three-doctor practice. Leigh has a significant drug problem and Dr Raabe has become increasingly concerned about the dangers of cannabis use, through his work as a GP and that which brings him into contact with homeless people.

Last year, he completed the RCGP training course in substance misuse. He has been involved in organising several parliamentary meetings on drugs, especially cannabis, in both Houses of Parliament.

Deborah Arnott

Deborah Arnott has been the Director of Action on Smoking and Health (ASH), one of the UK's leading campaigning charities, since May 2003. She has been a key contributor to both the Wanless review of effective delivery of public health published in February 2004 and the consultation process for the White Paper on Public Health. Previously as Head of Consumer Education for the Financial Services Authority (FSA), Arnott set up the FSA's consumer education function from scratch and while there was successful in lobbying to get financial education into the school curriculum.

Emer Coffey MSc (PHDC) MICGP

Dr Emer Coffey trained as a GP after graduating from Trinity College in Dublin in 1992. She has worked with drug treatment services in Ireland and overseas with Medecins Sans Frontieres (MSF) in Ghana, Afghanistan and Sudan. In 1998, she obtained an MSc in Public Health for Developing Countries at the London School of Tropical Medicine and is currently training as a Specialist Registrar in Public Health in the North West. In 2003, she worked with a multidisciplinary team in Merseyside to improve the local hepatitis B vaccination system for drug users.

David Young MBBS

Dr David Young is Clinical Director of the Drug and Alcohol Directorate for East and Central Cheshire for the Cheshire and Wirral Partnership Trust. He trained at Guy's Hospital, London and qualified in 1974. From 1977 to 1978 he worked as Medical Officer at Parammatta Psychiatric Centre in Sydney, Australia, where he first encountered working with people with substance misuse problems. On his return to England he started in general practice in Macclesfield in January 1979 and worked as a full-time principal in general practice until April 2001 when he joined the Cheshire and Wirral Partnership Trust initially as Lead Clinician for East Cheshire Community Drug Team and then as Clinical Director. In 1985 he chaired the local drug advisory committee in Macclesfield which was responsible for setting up the Barnabas Drug Problem Centre in Macclesfield. In January 2003 he was appointed by the Royal College of General Practitioners as Regional Primary Care Lead for the North West of England, this post he job shares with Dr Janikiewicz.

Gordon R Morse MB ChB, MRCGP, DRCOG

His current appointments include being a single handed GP principal in rural Wiltshire, a GP Trainer, and Honorary Lecturer in General Practice at Southampton University Medical School. Since 1995 he has also been Medical Consultant to Clouds House, one of the UK's longest established residential treatment centres for chemical dependency. At Clouds he has been responsible for the detoxification and medical care of more than 4000 chemically addicted patients. He is also Trust Specialist to the West Wiltshire Specialist Drug and Alcohol Service, and Consultant Lead in the Isle of Wight Specialist Drug and Alcohol service, is Medical Adviser to the National Association for Children of Alcoholics and is serving on the Wiltshire Shared Care Monitoring Group and has been involved in generalist substance misuse training throughout Wiltshire. In 2002 he was appointed to the position of RCGP Regional Substance Misuse Training Lead for the South West of England. He is Clinical Director to Drug Treatment Ltd as well as a Mentor for the training course for the GP Certificate in Addiction, and has been Lead GP in Mental Health and Addiction services to the South Wilts PCT.

Gordon has been closely involved with the RCGP Substance Misuse Management in General Practice group since it started and has been delegate or speaker at all the national conferences to date. He spoke at the RCGP national conference 2001 on *Developing a Core Curriculum for Certificate Training – What we Need to Know*, and in 2004 on *The Holy Grail of Abstinence*. He is also a founder member of the International Society for Addiction Medicine and has designed and chaired various conferences including *Innovations and Insights in Drug Abuse* at the Maudsley Hospital in 2001. He is author of *Detoxification* (Quay Books), a reference on medically assisted withdrawal from addiction in the residential setting and in 2004 contributed the chapter on detoxification to the revised *Caring for Substance Misusers in General Practice – a Harm Minimisation Approach*.

Beate Becker MB, JCPTGP, DFFP

Having graduated in Germany, Dr Beate Becker came to the UK as a pre-registration house officer and stayed on to complete a Vocational Training Scheme in Norwich. Her interest in the subject of young peoples' substance misuse was initiated by spending time at the local substance misuse clinic as part of her psychiatric attachment. She works as a part-time salaried GP in a socially deprived area of Norwich with support of a shared-care substance misuse service attached to the Practice.

Daphne Rumball MB ChB, FRCPsych, DRCOG

Dr Rumball is a Consultant Psychiatrist and Lead Clinician in the Alcohol and Drug Service, Norfolk and Waveney Mental Health Partnership (NHS) Trust, as well as Honorary Senior Lecturer at the School of Medicine, Health Policy and Practice, University of East Anglia (UEA). She has worked with young people's substance misuse services in a collaborative way for many years and helped develop a Tier 3 alcohol and drug treatment service in Norfolk. Her role now includes regular consultation with the team as well as direct clinical care of young people.

Her writing in the addictions field has included contributions to the Gaskell (RCPsych) publication *Young People and Substance Misuse* (2004).

She has an enduring interest in training professionals in the basic and specialist skills of addictions psychiatry, trains psychiatric and GP trainees and undertakes developmental work in the medical school at UEA.

Sharon Dawe MA, PhD

Sharon Dawe is an Associate Professor in Clinical Psychology at Griffith University. She was trained as a clinical psychologist and then undertook a PhD at the Institute of Psychiatry, University of London. Professor Dawe has a long-standing research interest in substance misuse and severe mental illness. She has been successful in developing the Parents Under Pressure (PUP) program with her colleague at the University of Queensland, Dr Paul Harnett, for 2–6-year-old children of drug-dependent mothers and has attracted NHMRC funding to move this work forward. She is currently extending this work in New South Wales through methadone clinics in both rural and urban settings and has also just received funding to train Queensland Health Staff across 20 methadone clinics to provide the PUP program to opioid dependent clients.

Associate Professor Dawe has published extensively in leading international journals including the *British Journal of Psychiatry, Psychopharmacology* and the *Journal of Clinical and Consulting Psychology*. Professor Dawe has received three early career awards including the Early Career Travel Award from the College of Problems of Drug Dependence and the Tracey Goodall Early Career Award from the Australian Association of Cognitive and Behaviour Therapy.

Nat Wright MBChB, FRCGP, DRCOG

Nat is currently the GP advisor to the National Treatment Agency. This entails working with the NTA quality directorate to develop the primary care drugs agenda. He is also the clinical director for the Leeds Integrated Community Drug Treatment Services. This involves providing clinical leadership, direction, training, mentoring, research and development support to over 50 practices in Leeds which are part of the shared care scheme for drug users. From 1996–2003 he was the lead partner at the NFA health centre for homeless people in Leeds, during which time the practice became a first wave beacon practice and an NHS executive approved research practice. He is the chair of the RCGP Health Inequalities Standing Group and has published extensively on the topics of substance use, homelessness, health inequalities and primary care.

Dave Marteau MA, RMN

Dave is a registered psychiatric nurse who has been working in addiction since the mid-80s. He has written a number of articles and one book on the treatment of dependence. He is currently the clinical substance misuse lead for male prisons (England and Wales).

Michael Farrell MBBch, BAO, MRCP, MRCPsych

Dr Michael Farrell is a Senior Lecturer and Consultant Psychiatrist at the Maudsley Hospital and National Addiction Centre, Institute of Psychiatry, Kings College London. He is responsible for a community based drug and alcohol service as well as inpatient services.

His research interests include treatment evaluation, with a particular focus on the treatment of drug dependence, and psychiatric epidemiology with a particular interest in psychiatric co-morbidity. He has a particular interest in aspects of prison-related drug problems and is an policy advisor to the Department of Health Prisons Task Force.

He has been a senior policy advisor to the Department of Health in England and has worked as a consultant with the World Health Organization as well as being a member of the WHO Expert Advisory Committee on Drug Dependence and Alcohol Problems. He is also an Assistant Editor of the journal *Addiction*.

CHAPTER 1

Overview of dependence, treatment, and outcome

Clare Gerada

Introduction

Because drug users are a heterogeneous group of people there is no one-fits-all
method of treatment. Treatment needs to be flexible enough to cater for the differences within this group whilst ensuring that any intervention is evidence based
and effective. The treatment for drug use goes beyond the prescription of medication, although prescribing remains a powerful and effective intervention. The
primary care team is well placed to deal with many of the physical, psychological,
and social needs of the drug user.

Terminology

In the field of addiction there are a number of terms currently in use to describe
the taking of both illicit and licit drugs; the terminology changes over time, often
dictated by the prevailing mood of political correctness. For example, the term
'addict' was a medical term used to distinguish those who used drugs owing to
a medically defined dependence as opposed to the criminal context of drug use.
Since then, the term addict has developed derogatory connotations and has been
replaced by various new terms such as user, misuser, abuser, problem drug user,
dependent user and so on, each meant to distinguish different consequences of
use – from non-problematic 'use' through to problematic 'misuse' or dependence.

Throughout this book the authors have tried to be consistent, using the word 'substance' to describe licit (legal) or illicit (illegal) products, including alcohol and nicotine; using the term 'drug' to describe mainly illicit products such as opioids, cannabis, and stimulants, though also included are benzodiazepines that are not prescribed; and using the term 'medicines' to describe any prescribed products.

Opioid *vs.* opiate

The term opioid indicates not only the naturally occurring opiates, which are derived from the opium poppy, but also their synthetic analogues such as methadone and pethidine.

Patient, client, substance user

As with the terminology describing the behaviour of taking drugs, there has also been confusing and conflicting terminology describing the person entering drug and/or alcohol treatment services.

A recent study undertaken in a large treatment centre asked service users which name they preferred between 'client', 'patient', or 'service user'. The majority preferred the term 'patient'. They were also asked if they considered themselves to have mental health problems. The majority (59%), felt that 'substance misuse' was in the category of mental health problems, though paradoxically most did not consider themselves to have a mental health problem. Broadly similar results were found for those attending alcohol services, but not tobacco cessation services.[1]

Classification of dependence

As there are a variety of terms to describe substance use so there is a spectrum of substance use behaviours, and over time clinicians and researchers have taken different approaches to understanding and describing them. The dependence syndrome was first proposed for alcohol use and is now incorporated in both the UK tenth revision of the *International Classification of Diseases* (ICD)[2] and the American fourth edition of the *Diagnostic Statistical Manual* (DSM)[3] classification systems.

The latest versions of both these systems (ICD-10 and DSM-IV) use the same approach to both alcohol and drugs of use (including nicotine), and both systems make a distinction between the dependence syndrome and other harmful patterns of substance use (see below for definitions and diagnostic criteria). The criteria for the dependence syndrome are similar in the two systems (though this has not always been the case. The criteria for the categories 'harmful use'

(ICD-10) and 'substance abuse' (DSM-IV) differ, with the emphasis on negative social consequences of substance use in the DSM classification, and on the physical and mental health consequences in the ICD-10 classification (see Box 1.1).

Box 1.1 **Drugs recognised by ICD-10**

✓ Alcohol

✓ Opioids (including naturally occurring opiates, synthetic or semisynthetic opiates, and opiate agonist-antagonists)

✓ Cannabinoids

✓ Sedative hypnotics

✓ Cocaine

✓ Other stimulants (including amfetamines, anorectic drugs, khat)

✓ Hallucinogens

✓ Tobacco

✓ Volatile solvents

✓ Multiple drug use and other psychoactive drugs

Dependence, neuroadaptation, tolerance

The terms 'addiction' and 'dependence' are often used interchangeably to describe a constellation of behavioural, physical, and psychological factors associated with drug/alcohol use. Strictly speaking, the term dependence, when used alone, is a state of bodily adaptation to the presence of a particular psychoactive substance (tolerance) and manifests itself in physical disturbances or withdrawal symptoms when the drug is withdrawn. The term 'neuroadaptation' is gaining increasing acceptance to describe this phenomenon. Many, but not all, medicines cause neuroadaptation and, of those that do, not all are subject to misuse. Many people are treated for painful conditions with opioids; often they will exhibit tolerance and even experience withdrawal symptoms when stopping the drug but only a small proportion will become 'addicted' to the drug.

By 'addiction', or 'dependence syndrome', we mean a specific psychological state in which the drug takes up an overriding importance in the person's life. When they do not have the drug, they crave it. They plan their days around ensuring a regular supply, sometimes spending many hours obtaining their drug of desire. Other personal goals and interests no longer seem important when the

3

supply is threatened. If they manage to stop using the drug for any length of time, relapse is followed by a rapid return of the habit at the same intensity as before the period of abstinence (reinstatement).

A dependence syndrome can occur with activities other than drugs, for example gambling, playing computer games, or even shopping. The potential of a drug to create addiction or dependence is determined by a number of factors: its potency (especially the strength of the hedonistic or pleasurable effects), the immediacy of the onset of its effect (not exclusively the property of the drug but also related to its route of use), the predictability of the effects of the drug, and its elimination half-life.

Of the illicit drugs, heroin is deemed to score highest in its addictive potential, with its most potent of opioid effects, its short elimination half-life of only a few hours and its rapid onset of action, especially after smoking or intravenous use. In comparison, methadone has a lower addictive potential, being less potent in its effect and having a slower onset of effect, particularly when taken by mouth. Not only does methadone have a lower addictive potential but it also directly reduces dependence on heroin, insofar as heroin use is often driven by the fear of, or experience of, withdrawal. Methadone reduces this fear and therefore removes the need for drug seeking.

Tolerance

Tolerance is a behavioural state: the way the body usually adapts to the repeated presence of a drug. Higher doses of the psychoactive substance are required to reproduce the original or similar effects. Tolerance may develop rapidly (to LSD, for example) or slowly (to alcohol or cannabis). The drug must be taken on a regular basis and in adequate quantities for tolerance to occur.

Tolerance can occur to different effects of the same drug: for example, a high degree of tolerance develops to the actions of opioids that cause analgesia and respiratory depression so that the effects of opioids are not apparent even when the individual is consuming high daily amounts if that dose level has been reached gradually. Little or no tolerance develops to the action of opioids on the pupil size or bowel activity, however, so that the same individual usually displays a typically constricted pupil and suffers from constipation – the latter a troublesome and common complaint in patients on methadone maintenance programmes.

After a relatively short period of abstinence (for example around two weeks in the case of opioids) tolerance is lost and the dose that was taken before this period of abstinence can now prove to be a fatal overdose. Tolerance is usually a feature of a dependence syndrome.

The clinical diagnostic criteria for dependence syndrome adopted by the World Health Organization (WHO) and contained in the *International Classification of Diseases* (ICD-10) and the American *Diagnostic and Statistical Manual of Mental*

Disorders (DSM-IV) emphasise both the physical factors (such as tolerance) and psychological aspects (subjective awareness of compulsion to use, diminished capacity to control drug use and salience of drug seeking behaviour) as important aspects of a dependence syndrome.

Validity of diagnostic categories

The concept of the dependence syndrome was originally the description given to the pattern of cognitive, behavioural, and physiological symptoms seen in those who consumed alcohol over long periods of time and in large amounts. The applicability of this description when used to describe the effects of other drugs of abuse has been questioned. There is relatively little controversy regarding its use for opioid and benzodiazepine drugs, as both can produce a clear increase in tolerance and characteristic withdrawal syndromes. Its use for drugs such as cannabis, nicotine, cocaine, and amfetamines,* however, has been less certain.

A large study of alcohol, opioid, cocaine, and cannabis users conducted by the World Health Organization in 12 countries found the 'dependence' and 'abuse' constructs to be broadly general across alcohol, opioids, cocaine, and cannabis, but the use of this two-dimensional model was found to fit cocaine use less well than that of the other three substances.[4]

For tobacco addiction, it may be more sensible to use the terms 'dependence' and 'failed cessation' in that there is no equivalent to 'misuse' in nicotine usage (though if nicotine is ever made an illicit substance this of course could result in the user engaging in acquisitive crime to obtain it!). Recent research on cannabis use has supported the validity of the dependence syndrome, though the definition of a withdrawal syndrome remains unclear.

Classification of substance misuse and dependence

ICD-10 (International Classification of Diseases)

Harmful substance use

Actual damage should have been caused to the mental or physical health of the user in the absence of diagnosis of dependence syndrome.

Substance dependence (three or more in the past year)

▶ A strong desire or sense of compulsion to use

---

*In 2004 the British Approved Name (BAN) for amphetamines was modified to accord with the Recommended International Non-proprietary Name (rINN), amfetamines.

▶ difficulties in controlling substance-taking behaviour in terms of its onset, termination, or levels of use

▶ a physiological withdrawal state when use has ceased or been reduced, as evidenced by the characteristic withdrawal syndrome, or use with the intention of relieving or avoiding withdrawal symptoms

▶ evidence of tolerance, such that increased doses are required in order to achieve effects originally produced by lower doses (clear examples of this are found in alcohol-dependent individuals who may take daily doses sufficient to incapacitate or kill non-tolerant users)

▶ progressive neglect of other pleasures or interests because of substance use, increased amount of time necessary to obtain or take substance, or to recover from its effects

▶ persisting with use despite clear evidence of overtly harmful consequences.

DSM-IV (*Diagnostic Statistical Manual*) (*US classification*)

▶ Substance abuse (1 or more criteria for over 1 year) and never met criteria for dependence.

▶ recurrent substance use resulting in a failure to fulfil major role obligations at work, school, or home

▶ recurrent substance use in situations in which it is physically hazardous

▶ recurrent substance-related legal problems

▶ continued substance use despite having persistent or recurrent social or interpersonal problems caused or exacerbated by the effects of the substance.

Substance dependence (3 criteria or more over 1 year)

1. Tolerance: a need for markedly increased amounts of the substance to achieve intoxication or desired effect or markedly diminished effect with continued use of the same amount of the substance.

2. Withdrawal: the characteristic withdrawal syndrome for the substance or the same (or closely related) substance is taken to relieve or avoid withdrawal symptoms.

3. The substance is often taken in larger amounts or over a longer period than was intended.

4. There is a persistent desire or unsuccessful effort to cut down or control substance use.

5. A great deal of time is spent in activities necessary to obtain the substance, use of the substance, or recovering from its effects.

6. Important social, occupational, or recreational activities are given up or reduced because of substance use.

7. The substance use is continued despite knowledge of having a persistent or recurrent physical or psychological problem that is likely to have been caused or exacerbated by the substance.

Reprinted with permission from the Diagnostic and Statistical Manual of Mental Disorders, Fourth Edition, Text Revision, copyright 2000. American Psychiatric Association.

Natural history of drug use

Getting started

The different definitions described in ICD and DSM classifications are designed to distinguish problematic from non-problematic use, as not every one who uses drugs or alcohol goes on to develop problems and even of those who do develop dependent problematic use many may not have lifelong problems. Drug use, especially in adolescence, is in the main experimental and transient, seen by many as a 'rite of passage' between childhood and adulthood.

What factors therefore influence experimental use becoming problematic use? A prospective American study conducted a series of interviews on a sample of young people aged between 15 and 16 years. These adolescents were asked to describe patterns of initiation, persistence, and cessation in drug use and were then followed up over a period of time spanning 19 years, from adolescence to adulthood. A school survey was administered at age 15–16 and further interviews with participants and school absentees were conducted at ages 24–25, 28–29, and 34–35. Retrospective continuous histories of 12 drug classes were obtained at each follow up.

The results showed that there was no initiation into alcohol and cigarettes and hardly any initiation into illicit drugs after the age of 29, the age at which most use ceased. The largest proportion of new users after this age was observed for prescribed psychoactive drugs, such as benzodiazepines. Among daily users, the proportion of heavy users of alcohol and cannabis declined but not of cigarettes. Cigarettes were the most persistent of any drug used.[5]

Factors that predicted cessation of use in adulthood paralleled those that predicted lack of initiation in adolescence: conventionality in social role (e.g. job, family responsibilities), social context unfavourable to the use of drugs (e.g. employment, communities where alcohol use was banned), and good health.

Peer influences were found to be the major predictor of experimental drug use and also likely to influence the evolution into more regular drug use (see Table 1.1). Initiation of use before the age of 15 is associated with more developmental disruption.[6]

Table 1.1   **Predictors of drug initiation in adolescence**

Individual factors	Prior delinquent behaviour
	Peer group influences
	Risk taking behaviours
Parental factors	Poor quality of relationship
	Inconsistent parenting
Lack of participation in conventional activities	Such as employment, education, relationships

Continued use

Since cessation of drug use typically takes place at a different phase in the life cycle from initiation, that is in early adulthood rather than adolescence, factors important for persistence at a later phase of the life cycle may be equivalent to factors important for explaining initiation at a younger age. Whereas conformity to social roles in adolescence involves satisfactory academic performance, in adulthood the new social roles include being married or in a stable relationship and working. It is highly likely that adults' roles such as marriage and stable employment are not compatible with illicit drug use.

The level of drug use is also a predictor of future drug use; the more used, the more likely problematic use is to develop. Once an individual is dependent, drug use is generally a chronic condition, interspersed by periods of relapse and remission; it takes many attempts to achieve permanent abstinence.

Just as there is no one path towards successful abstinence, so there is no single risk factor for problematic drug use. There are a number of complex social factors, including the influence of intimate partners, parents, friends, and work and other activities that can significantly affect the pattern of drug use. The severely dependent long-term heroin or cocaine user is likely after five to ten years of continuous use to be less amenable to change and have less access to social support networks necessary to support changes in use. Repeated involvement with the criminal justice system, long-term unemployment, and increasing social isolation further entrench their drug-using behaviour. Strategies needed for this group are likely to involve significant social, physical, and psychological interventions. If abstinence is going to occur it is more likely to happen earlier than later in a drug user's career.

Principles of treatment

Treatment aims

There are many possible aims of treatment. For those patients who meet criteria for harmful use (ICD-10 criteria) or misuse (DSM-IV criteria) but do not meet criteria for a dependence syndrome, psychosocial approaches are the mainstay of treatment.

Pharmacological interventions currently have limited application, except in treating coexisting conditions such as depression or anxiety, which may be inhibiting progress towards less harmful use. Pharmacological interventions aimed at treating the substance use disorder itself, many of which will be discussed in detail in this book, are of most value in patients who have developed the features of the dependence syndrome, and are targeted at the following areas of patient management:

▶ management of withdrawal symptoms

▶ reduction of physical, social, and psychological harms to the individual and the public associated with illicit drug use by prescribing a substitute drug or drugs (for example, methadone maintenance treatment in which aims may include cessation of injecting, reduction or cessation of illicit heroin use, and reduction or cessation of other high risk behaviours)

▶ relapse prevention and maintenance of abstinence (for example oral naltrexone, cognitive behavioural therapy)

▶ prevention of complications of substance use (for example, hepatitis B immunisation, the use of thiamine to prevent Wernicke's encephalopathy and Korsakoff's syndrome).

General principles of treatment

▶ No single treatment is appropriate for all individuals.

▶ Treatment needs to be readily available, and begin where the user presents.

▶ Treatment should over time address the multiple needs of the individual, physical, psychological, social, and educational.

▶ Treatment modalities used will change over time and at different times during treatment.

▶ Retention in treatment is most predictive of a good outcome.

▶ Substitute medications, such as methadone and buprenorphine, are important elements of treatment for many patients, especially when combined with counselling and behavioural therapies.

▶ Patients with coexisting problems, such as mental health problems, should have these dealt with alongside their drug misuse problems.

▶ Treatment does not need to be voluntary to be successful.

▶ Recovery from drug addiction takes time, and addiction is a chronic relapsing condition often requiring multiple episodes of treatment.

▶ Trained and competent clinicians should provide treatment.

Models of behaviour change

Prochaska and DiClemente developed a model of behavioural change that has become influential in the field of addiction.[7] The model hypothesis is that interventions are most effective when mapped to the state of readiness for change that the user is at. The model also helps to define the clinician's expectations and helps to foster a more realistic relationship between the clinician and the patient, and views change as a process rather than an event – the change process being characterised by a series of stages of change. It may be helpful to explain these stages of change to less informed members of the primary care team, in the hope that they too will see the potentials for intervention even if the patient does not want to stop drug use. By engaging in harm reduction strategies the clinician may be able to nudge the reluctant user gently into abstinence. The Prochaska and DiClemente model divides the individual state of readiness into the following states:

▶ *Precontemplators* do not want to stop and are not concerned enough about the associated risks to change their use. The interventions available are concentrated on harm reduction advice, information about needle exchange schemes, and provision of hepatitis B immunisation.

▶ *Contemplators* are concerned about their drug use and are considering change but have not yet decided to stop. These individuals would benefit from motivational interviewing and other behaviour therapies, nudging them gently into the action stage.

▶ The *action* stage is one in which people decide to stop and put their plan into action; substitution therapies are vital interventions during this phase.

▶ *Maintenance* of the behavioural change: addictive behaviour involves cycles of change with efforts to stop being punctuated by relapse. Maintaining the effects of the treatment needs to involve a range of psychosocial and pharmacological interventions. Marlatt and Gordon described the cognitive behavioural approach called relapse prevention, which aims to develop coping strategies that can help to maintain the phase of change.[8]

Harm reduction

The ultimate aim of treatment is stop or reduce the use of illicit or harmful drugs and to prevent or reduce the harms resulting from drug use. The emphasis on harm reduction is a legacy of the response to the HIV problem: the establishment of needle exchange schemes, outreach clinics, and methadone maintenance programmes. The theme of harm reduction has continued now for over two decades and is the backbone of UK treatment policy.

The Task Force[9] defined the outcomes of treatment into three main domains. These domains act as a guide to the harm minimisation steps that clinicians and commissioners can use when delivering or designing services (see Box 1.2).[9] This will be discussed more fully in Chapter 15.

Box 1.2   **Treatment outcome domains**

Outcome domain	Measure
Drug use	Abstinence from drugs
	Near abstinence from drugs
	Reduction in the quantity of drugs consumed
	Abstinence from street drugs
	Reduced use of street drugs
	Change in drug-taking behaviour from injecting to oral consumption
	Reduction in the frequency of injecting
Physical and psychological health	Improvement in physical health
	No deterioration in physical health
	Improvement in psychological health
	No deterioration in psychological health
	Reduction in sharing injecting equipment
	Reduction in sexual health risk taking

continued over

Outcome domain	Measure
Social functioning and life context	Reduction in criminal activity
	Improvement in employment status
	Fewer working/school days missed
	Improved family relationships
	Improved personal relationships
	Domiciliary stability/improvement

From: Task Force to review services for drug misusers[9]

The 'British System'

The United Kingdom is in the unique position of having minimal restrictions on how doctors manage drug users.[10] Doctors have the freedom to prescribe almost any drug and restrictions apply only to the prescription of heroin, cocaine, and Diconal, which require a Home Office licence when used for the purpose of treating addiction.

This relative freedom is often referred to as the 'British System', the origins of which arose with the Rolleston Report in 1926, which argued that addicts were patients and not criminals and should receive drugs on prescription, contrasting sharply with the situation in the USA.

Today, the British System allows practitioners the freedom to take account of possible social and criminal justice gains as part of their prescribing decisions and hence gives doctors the flexibility to respond to the changing nature of drug problems. This flexibility does not negate the duty of care for the individual or the need to adhere to good practice guidance and safe prescribing.[11]

Practical aspects of prescribing

The *British National Formulary* (BNF), issued free to all general practitioners, contains a wealth of information concerning the overall management of addiction as well as laying out guiding principles when prescribing any medication in the United Kingdom. These principals are:

1. To avoid creating dependence caused by introducing drugs to patients without sufficient reason.

2. To see that the patient does not gradually increase the dose for a drug given for good medical reasons to the point where dependence becomes likely. The prescriber should keep a close eye on the amount prescribed to prevent

patients from accumulating stocks that would enable them to arrange their own dosage or even supply their families and friends.

3. To avoid being used as an unwitting source of supply to addicts. Methods include visiting more than one doctor, fabricating stories, and forging prescriptions.

1999 Clinical Guidelines

The Department of Health's *Drug Misuse and Dependence Guidelines on Clinical Management* (1999)[12] is the authoritative publication for primary care practitioners on the treatment of substance misusers. It is used as a reference source throughout this book. It is likely that the health professional reading this book is already familiar with the 1999 National Clinical Guidelines. These were written nearly a decade after the previous guidelines (1991), which had coincided with both a rapid increase in the number of drug users presenting for care and a predicted HIV crisis amongst injecting drug users.

In 1994, Gerada carried out a small local survey in south London and found that 50% of all drug users in the area were being treated by only 5% of general practitioners, most of whom were largely untrained and unsupported, a trend that was common in other parts of the country (Gerada, unpublished data). The guidelines were written predominantly for a general practitioner audience and aimed to provide a framework from which to work safely, though of course they are relevant to any professional group working in the addiction field. They laid down the minimum responsibilities of the prescriber, which were as follows:

1. Prescribing is the particular responsibility of the doctor signing the prescription. This responsibility cannot be delegated.

2. A doctor prescribing controlled drugs for the management of drug dependence should have an understanding of the basic pharmacology, toxicology and clinical indications for the use of the drug, the drug regime and therapeutic monitoring strategy if they are to prescribe responsibly.

3. The clinician has a responsibility to ensure that the patient receives the correct dose and that appropriate efforts are taken to ensure that the drug is used appropriately and not diverted onto illegal markets. Particular care must be taken with induction onto any substitute medication, especially where self-reporting of dosage is being relied on.

4. Supervised consumption is recommended for new prescriptions for a minimum of three months and should be relaxed only when the patient's compliance is assured.

THE MANAGEMENT OF SUBSTANCE MISUSE IN PRIMARY CARE

5. The prescribing doctor should liaise regularly with the dispensing pharmacist about specific patients and prescribing regimens.

6. No more than one week's drugs should be dispensed at one time, except in exceptional circumstances.

7. Clinical reviews should be undertaken regularly, at least every three months, particularly if the patient appears unstable.

8. Doctors should ensure that measures are taken to improve compliance. This includes supervised consumption for a period of at least three months, urine testing, daily pick-up, instalment prescribing.

In only a matter of a few years the 1999 guidelines already feel dated. General practitioners are much more involved in the care of drug users in 2005 than they were in 1999, when the role of the specialist GP was not given the attention it deserved. The role of the specialist nurse and the extended role of the pharmacist were hardly mentioned.

Buprenorphine is now considered to be a mainstream treatment option that can, and should, be prescribed by generalist practitioners. The evidence for higher doses of methadone was not considered in 1999 and other treatments, such as naltrexone, were not given the prominence that they merited. Polydrug use is now the norm and not the exception and crack cocaine use is much more prevalent.

The guidelines are due for updating and it is hoped that the next version will acknowledge many of the changes that have happened in the intervening years. Of particular interest is how primary care will be represented on any new guidelines committee.

Assessment

The guidelines emphasise that a good assessment is essential to the continuing care of the patient. Assessment skills are vital to all members of the primary care team. The diagnosis of drug use itself is of central importance. Before substitute treatment is initiated doctors should ensure that they have taken a history, carried out an examination, and undertaken relevant investigations. A good assessment should enable the practitioner to confirm the diagnosis of drug dependence through obtaining a history of drug misuse, examination of the signs of misuse, urine analysis, and other investigations where necessary.

All doctors must undertake assessment commensurate with the complexity of prescribing. Prescribing decisions (drug used, amount, and duration of use) should, in most cases and as a tenet of good practice, be dependent on national clinical guidelines, the level of the doctor's training and experience, and discussion with others involved in the care of the patient.

The assessment of a patient is a continuous process carried out at every consultation over many years. The first assessment should not be prolonged and should not delay the initiation of effective treatment. Before prescribing it is important that the clinician remembers three golden rules:

1. Confirm the diagnosis of dependence, through history taking, urine analysis, and where appropriate corroboration with previous health professionals.

2. The responsibility for the prescription is always that of the prescribing doctor (or nurse or pharmacist) and this responsibility cannot be delegated.

3. If using substitute medication, start low and increase the dose slowly.

Essentials of a good assessment

History taking should elicit, as accurately as possible, information about the past and current drug taking behaviour. It should include the reason for presentation, past and current drug use, history of injecting, risk of HIV and other blood-borne diseases, medical history, and psychiatric, forensic and social history. The history should also determine previous contact with treatment services.

Examination should include an assessment of motivation, general and mental health, and family and social situation.

Urine analysis should be regarded as an adjunct to the history taking and examination in confirming drug use and should be obtained before the onset of prescribing and randomly throughout treatment. Hair analysis uses a single strand of hair and can yield information spanning a period of several weeks or months.

The patient should be reviewed in detail at least every three months.

Prescribing issues

Prescribing substitute medication is a useful tool in changing the behaviour of some drug users towards abstinence or towards intermediate goals of reducing the harm to themselves or others. If opioids are prescribed, the 1999 Clinical Guidelines recommend liquid preparations such as methadone 1 mg/ml to avoid the risks associated with injecting crushed tablets or melted suppositories, for example, and to reduce the risk of potential sale on the black market. Drugs that are capable of being injected, such as tablets, carry a greater risk of being dangerously misused by the patient or sold on the black market. The clinical guidelines recommend that tablets should not be prescribed to drug users.

The most common source of problems when prescribing to drug users is the prescription of open-ended prescriptions of drugs without clearly defined and agreed goals. Prescribing too little leads to lies and manipulation and too much can lead to drugs leaking onto the illicit market.

The prescribing doctor should, ideally, see the patient on each occasion that a prescription is issued. Other doctors, such as the patient's general practitioner, should be informed of any prescription. This is important to avoid duplication.

Doctors in the private sector must ensure that their patients have sufficient legitimate sums to pay for the cost of treatment and the cost of the prescriptions. Doctors in this sector must be aware of the potential pitfalls of receiving payments for drug dependency treatment. A private prescription for controlled drugs must not be construed as a supply of drugs in exchange for money. There is a risk that patients may try to finance their consultations and prescriptions by selling higher-value controlled drugs on the black market. It is good practice for doctors in the private sector to communicate with the patient's NHS general practitioner. The more the clinician deviates from established good practice the greater is the onus on the clinician to justify it.

Improving the outcome of treatment

Inherent to successful treatment is its ability to help people overcome drug problems. Despite the growth in treatment services over the past two decades the provision is still patchy across the country and the Audit Commission report, *Changing Habits*,[13] found that a significant number of drug users struggled to get the help they need. It identified that many treatment services had long waiting lists and limited treatment options that drove potential patients away. Care often failed to consider drug users' wider social problems and some treatment was delivered inconsistently and not in line with good practice, for example, some clinicians offered fixed short-term detoxification only.

Factors associated with good outcome are multifactorial, relating to the service itself, such as minimising barriers to entry, having well-trained staff, and having a commitment to providing high quality medical and psychosocial services. Other factors identified as fostering improved outcomes were related to the actual treatment provided, in particular providing optimal daily doses of substitute medication.

Whereas the Audit Commission report looked predominately at secondary care services, it is likely that many of the factors that promote good outcome in specialist settings will be similar for primary care settings. Flexible appointment systems, with a mixture of advanced access (appointments on the day) and booked appointments will attract and maintain users in treatment. Informed staff, systems that allow for sharing of information about patients, the ability to discuss significant events, and reception and administrative staff who understand the ethos of care with drug users all smooth the sometimes turbulent early and relapse stages of the users' treatment. Continuity and consistent care will also retain the user in treatment. It is the author's belief that a well-organised primary care practice should be able to accommodate even the most chaotic patients.

Comparative rates for treatment compliance and relapse

It is perhaps surprising to many clinicians that the overall treatment of opioid addiction, as measured by compliance in treatment and rate of relapse, is as successful as treatment of other chronic diseases such as diabetes, hypertension, and asthma. The outcome, in terms of abstinence at six months is greater for opioid addiction than that for tobacco or alcohol addiction.[14]

Conclusion

Treating drug users is ripe with challenges, but it also provides clinical satisfaction. The very contact between a user and a health professional can bring about enormous changes. Treatment in its broadest sense can (and does) save many lives. There are many interventions available and a competent general practitioner, primary care nurse, or pharmacist can provide most of them. We hope that this book will ensure that the most effective treatment is given.

Further reading

Hamid Ghodse. *Drug and Addictive Behaviour: A guide to treatment.* Second Edition. Oxford: Blackwell Science, 1995.

Lingford-Hughes A R, Welch S, Nutt D J. BAP Guidelines. Evidence-based guidelines for the pharmacological management of substance misuse, addiction and comorbidity: recommendations from the British Association for Psychopharmacology. *J Psychopharmacol* (Oxford) 2004; **18**(3): 293–335.

References

1. Keaney F, Strang J, Martinez-Raga J, Spektor D, *et al.* Does anyone care about names? How attendees at substance misuse services like to be addressed by health professionals. *Eur Addict Res* 2004; **10**(2): 75–9.

2. World Health Organization. The ICD-10 Classification of Mental and Behavioural Disorders: Clinical Descriptions and Diagnostic Guidelines, Tenth Revision. Geneva: WHO, 1992.

3. American Psychiatric Association. *Diagnostic and Statistical Manual of Mental Disorders, Fourth Edition.* Washington, D.C.: APA, 1994.

4. World Health Organization. *WHO Expert Committee on Drug Dependence, thirtieth report.* (WHO Technical Report Series, No. 873). Geneva: WHO, 1998.

5. Chen K, Kandel D B. The natural history of drug use from adolescence to the mid-thirties in a general population sample. *Am J Public Health* 1995; **85**(1): 41–7.

6. Kandel D B, Raveis V H. Cessation of illicit drug use in young adulthood. *Arch Gen Psychiatry* 1989 Feb; **46**(2): 109–16.

7. Prochaska J O, DiClemente C C. Stages of change in the modification of problem behaviors. *Progress in Behavior Modification* 1992; **28**: 183–218.

8. Marlatt G A, Gordon J R. (Eds). *Relapse prevention: Maintenance strategies in the treatment of addictive behaviours.* New York: Guilford, 1985.

9. Department of Health. *The Task Force to Review Services for Drug Users: Report of an independent review of drug treatment services in England.* London: HMSO, 1996.

10. Strang J, Gossop M. The 'British System': visionary anticipation or masterly inactivity? In: Strang J, Gossop M. (Eds). *Heroin Addiction and Drug Policy.* Oxford: OUP, 1994.

11. Zador D. Injectable opiate maintenance in the UK: is it good clinical practice? *Addiction* 2001; **96**: 547–53.

12. Department of Health; The Scottish Office Department of Health; Welsh Office; Department of Health and Social Services, Northern Ireland. Drug Misuse and Dependence – Guidelines on Clinical Management. London: HMSO, 1999.

13. Audit Commission. *Changing Habits: The Commissioning and Management of Community Drug Treatment Services for Adults.* London: Audit Commission, 2002.

14. O'Brien C P, McLellan A T. Myths About the Treatment of Addiction. *Lancet* 1996; **347**: 237–40.

CHAPTER 2 | # Drug Policy in the United Kingdom

Alex Laffan and Clare Gerada

IN THIS CHAPTER

Introduction ‖ *UK drug policy today* ‖ *Law and enforcement policy: reducing supply and prohibiting use* ‖ *Treatment policy* ‖ *Treatment models involving coercion* ‖ *Drug treatment and testing orders* ‖ *Education policy: protecting young people* ‖ *Conclusion*

Introduction

Alcohol and psychoactive substances have been woven into every society since the beginnings of the human race. Alcohol has been made, drunk, and used to excess as far back as records go, and probably since the first fallen apple fermented on the ground. Tobacco (*Nicotiana*), hemp (*Cannabis sativa*), opium poppy (*Papaver somniferum*), and other plants containing drugs have been chewed, smoked, and turned into drinks, almost as long as alcohol has been brewed.

In 5000 BC, Sumerian tablets speak of a herb called the 'joy plant'. Opium was known in Mesopotamia and Assyrian medical texts mention it. In 500 BC, Herodotus, the Greek historian, records that certain Siberian tribes achieved trances induced by inhaling fumes from burning hemp plants. Tobacco was carried from Virginia to England by Sir Walter Raleigh, whose pipe smoking prompted Elizabeth I to remark, 'I don't like this herb.'

Different governments, monarchs and religious leaders have repeatedly had to decide whether to sanction the use of different psychoactive substances or to allow full or limited use. The most recent example close to home is the plan to restrict individuals' right to smoke tobacco in public places.

History is peppered with different attempts at preventing importation of drugs and restricting their use, some placing harsher restrictions than others; tobacco smoking has even had the ultimate sanction of the death penalty attached to it. In 100 BC the Roman senate attempted to suppress alcoholic excesses and orgies, connected with the worship of Bacchus, by law. In 1796 the Chinese government made opium smoking punishable by death responding to decades of excess and problematic smoking of the drug by its population.

Over the centuries, attempts to deal with addiction through prevention and treatment have been tried with varying success. In the 1850s the hypodermic syringe was introduced in the belief that morphine injected by a syringe was non-addictive because it did not 'reach the stomach'. In 1878 cocaine was introduced to the United States, as it was believed to be a treatment for morphine addiction, a belief that persisted for many decades. Cocaine became illegal in the United States in 1914, but not before many became addicted to it.

The past hundred years have seen, perhaps unsurprisingly in a modern world of greater governmental interference, unprecedented levels of both national and international lawmaking regarding psychoactive substances. Since the Hague Convention of 1912, the international supply of drugs has faced continually better resourced monitoring and prevention. In the latter part of the 20th century treatment methods for those addicted to illicit, and licit, drugs have received greater funding and attention, both in the United Kingdom and worldwide.

This chapter explores the United Kingdom's current attitude to drugs regarding tackling supply, providing treatment, and reducing harm to both individuals and communities. It will also analyse how these policies have developed over the 20th century in the United Kingdom and whether, with an increasing emphasis on the criminal justice system as a centre for punishment and rehabilitation, we have finally found a successful drugs policy.

UK drug policy today

The present government's commitment to increasing the number of people in treatment, albeit through the criminal justice system, goes some way to answering those who suggest that today's drugs policy is little more than 'prevention, prohibition and punishment'.[1] There is a worryingly small amount of money spent, however, on researching new and improved treatment methods and on evaluating the effectiveness of current methods. Injectable prescribing in the United Kingdom is a radical, unique policy based on a small amount of research. Until education and prohibition can be better refined the number of young people starting to take drugs shows little sign of receding and treatment services look set to perform a continuous cycle of rehabilitation for new drug users.

In 2002 the government announced an update to its 1998 strategy, *Tackling Drugs to Build a Better Britain*,[2] which retained the original four-point focus: preventing young people from using drugs by prohibition and education; reducing the prevalence of drugs by tackling supply; reducing drug-related crime including advancing treatment within the criminal justice system; and reducing demand for drugs by getting more problematic drug users into treatment. The document also stated that this would be achieved by 'focusing on the drugs that cause the most harm'. It is hardly surprising that the strategy maintains these commitments, as it is difficult to see how a drug policy could operate without a combination of these building blocks. Without prohibition, the UK treatment system would become saturated and education would be undermined; without treatment and harm reduction, drug related illness and deaths would rise; without education, young people might fail to associate drug use with danger.

Law and enforcement policy: reducing supply and prohibiting drug use

The prohibition of drug use and drug dealing remains, financially, the cornerstone of UK policy. Domestic enforcement and international supply reduction together account for 75% of the UK's £1.4 billion budget for tackling drug misuse. While the lengthy sentencing of some drug users has been reduced in deference to treatment, drug trafficking into the United Kingdom and drug dealing once inside the UK remain areas of criminal behaviour that are treated with little tolerance. Reducing the supply of illegal drugs is expensive and often seemingly impossible.

The international element of the problem makes it increasingly difficult for a domestic government to control alone and the UK government is at the forefront of countries in the international community pushing for greater global cooperation. Reducing international trafficking accounts for about 13% of the United Kingdom's spending on drug misuse, while stifling supply within the UK takes up a significant amount of the 62% spent on domestic enforcement.

The government points to a number of apparent successes to justify this spending. In 2000 there was a 53% increase in the number of cocaine seizures and a 30% increase in the number of heroin seizures. Equally the seizure of drug-related assets between April 2001 and March 2002 rose by 20% to £18.9 million.

Specific local interventions, for example in the south London Borough of Lambeth, show some promising results where local action plans have reduced community drug supply. Local politicians and services there met with the home secretary to decide a policy for tackling crack cocaine dealing. In the six months after its implementation robberies were reduced by 33% and over 100 'crack house' raids took place.

Meanwhile the government continues to use the law as a deterrent, with those caught drug trafficking or dealing remaining subject to harsh penalties – life imprisonment for class A drugs and 14 years for class B and C drugs.

Targeting suppliers as distinct from the actual drug users has been cemented in British drug policy since the 1971 Misuse of Drugs Act, which distinguished between the two for the first time.[3] Since then, sentences for dealers have been far more severe than for users, increasingly so following the reclassification of cannabis in early 2004, which allows recreational users to escape an official punishment whereas suppliers may be sentenced for 14 years.

Strategies for reducing production in foreign countries and tackling international supply are usually formed on the basis of international agreements and therefore Britain's ability to enact its own policies are often subject to the cooperation of the international community.

The Hague Convention of 1912 was the starting point for a century of international regulation of drug production and transportation. The Geneva Conference on Opium in 1924/5 further raised the barriers on importing and exporting drugs. In 1946 international drugs policy fell under United Nations jurisdiction and continued apace, with an international opium protocol agreed in 1953, which severely restricted poppy and coca production.

Yet it is the 1961 Single Convention that forms the real basis of international drug policy today, limiting cultivation, manufacture, importation, and possession of drugs as well as introducing strict record keeping and prescriptive measures. While the Single Convention is perhaps not as rigid as it might seem, it has ensured that the United Kingdom has little room for manoeuvre when dealing with drug trafficking. Yet when the United Kingdom is continually at the forefront of the United Nations in pushing for stricter international controls on drug production and supply, this has not been a contentious issue in the United Kingdom. By investing personnel resources into seizing drugs, using the force of the law to deter potential dealers, and targeting specific areas where dealers are known to operate, the UK strategy seems to encompass all the available avenues for reducing drug supply in the United Kingdom. When this is combined with continuing international cooperation and enforcement in reducing the production of illegal drugs at source, and work to block key international trafficking routes, reducing supply is clearly a massive operation. The extent to which the United Kingdom has worked, domestically and internationally, to reduce supply raises questions about its apparent lack of success.

While increases in customs and police seizures, and isolated local examples, look impressive on paper, supply reduction efforts have consistently failed, ever since their inception, to raise the price of drugs, in real terms, or to deter use. Contrary to some popular literature, a rise in price is more likely to result in a fall in use than in the widely expected rise in crime. Increases in the price of alcohol and tobacco have had a significant effect on consumption.

A study conducted before World War II predicted similar results for other drugs. Unfortunately supply reduction policies have failed to achieve reduced misuse. Between 1986 and 1996 the price of heroin in the United Kingdom fell from around £90 per gram to £60 per gram without any reduction in purity. The same pattern is seen in the United States. Thus the rise in seizures in the United Kingdom should not be interpreted as a fall in drug supply.

Without the serious deterrents in place to prohibit the production of drugs in countries such as Burma and Afghanistan (which together account for between 90 and 94% of world heroin production), and barriers to entry into consumer countries, drug supply would only increase. However, prices are still falling with these comprehensive measures in place and it is reasonable to ask whether large sums of money are being well spent, especially as production reducing programmes such as crop substitution and crop destruction are unlikely to have any effect on consumer countries and their retail drug prices.

Interdiction, the report concludes, can be effective only if it covers all smuggling routes. Such measures are surely beyond the United Kingdom's limited budget and will only eat into more cost-effective solutions such as treatment and rehabilitation.

If supply reduction is not working then what about the other side of the prohibition coin, namely reducing recreational drug use? There are several notable aspects of the United Kingdom's changing attitude towards the criminal status of the drug user, but the most important is the focus on class A drugs. In early 2004 the House of Commons voted with the government to reclassify cannabis as a class C drug, effectively permitting the use of the drug without fear of serious legal consequences. To supply cannabis still carries a substantial punishment, of up to a 14-year jail sentence, but the recreational user will normally receive only a caution. The police, meanwhile, will have more time and money to arrest, and refer to treatment, users of class A drugs, which, as the government repeatedly stresses, cause most destruction to communities and individuals. Nevertheless the United Kingdom remains dedicated to the continuing prohibition of all illegal drugs as a deterrent to uptake and continued use.

Another aspect of domestic enforcement is the noticeable shift in drug policy away from health issues and towards criminal justice issues, evident in the growing responsibility of the Home Office, as opposed to the Department of Health.

The United Kingdom has also adopted a prohibition policy on the basis of international agreements, sometimes at the expense of expert advice at home. Drug prohibition reached Britain in the First World War, following the Hague Convention of 1912, and has developed on the back of international agreements ever since.

There have been domestic developments as well, usually in response to popular pressure. The 1964 Drugs Act was the first post-war piece of drug legislation and controlled amfetamine use. Yet it is the 1971 Misuse of Drugs Act that remains the centrepiece of British drug law, albeit somewhat outdated in its strict sentencing of 'recreational' drug users, which has long been ignored by the courts. The 1961 Single Convention that has dictated British policy on trafficking has long been quoted by home secretaries as committing Britain to a policy of prohibition for drug possession as well. In fact, this has been obligatory only since 1988 and even then, as the Dutch have shown, there is plenty of room for manoeuvre.

While the government has made its priority on class A drugs clear, some are not satisfied. On the one hand some see the government's strategy as too focused on the criminal justice system and on the other hand some see the government as being 'soft' on drugs and encouraging cannabis use. At the time of writing it is impossible to judge whether the reclassification of cannabis will cause a marked increase in its use.

Meanwhile, there is little evidence that the government's emphasis on criminal justice has stigmatised the drug user, especially when there is a sustained effort to increase the number of drug users in treatment. While offenders in general have become subject to a greater degree of drug testing and compulsory treatment within the criminal justice system, the current strategy has not vilified drug addicts in the way heroin addicts were in the early 1980s.

The number of drug users, however, is not decreasing. The number of young people trying drugs is a continuing, and growing, problem and suggests that law enforcement alone is not having the desired effect. The government's focus on class A drugs may be a step in the right direction but until the number of users of these drugs falls it cannot be deemed a success.

Treatment policy

On the whole, public opinion across the world favours the prohibition of drugs, seeing this as the only way of limiting the uptake of drug use. Prohibition, however, is far less cost effective than treatment. It would be naive to suggest that the United Kingdom's treatment services would be equipped to cope with the massive increase in drug users that might result from an end to prohibition.

Treatment, however, clearly works, reducing damage to communities and individuals; yet treatment commands only 13% of the United Kingdom's drug misuse budget.[4] Treatment services in the United Kingdom have expanded since their introduction in the 1960s, lagging considerably behind the imposition of prohibition. Nowadays, treatment services and the criminal justice system are designed to work alongside each other, one to deter and one to ensure that those who cannot stop using drugs are at least prevented from causing damage to themselves and communities.

The first specialist clinic was set up in 1964 by John Owens in Birmingham, dispensing heroin to addicts. This sparked off a considerable growth, throughout the 1960s and 1970s, of voluntary services and specialist drug and therapeutic residential communities. From 1968 to 1972 drug dependency units were established in major cities affected by drugs. Alongside the formation of these units was the implementation of the 2nd *Brain Report* recommendation of restricting prescribing rights of heroin to licensed doctors, in effect to doctors who worked within the units and hence only to psychiatrists.

Following the rapid increase of treatment services in the 1960s and 1970s, the 1980s saw the development of a network of services that defined the roles of specialist drug services and gave new responsibilities to general practitioners in treating drug misusers, an area which continues to develop.

In 2004, the government set ambitious targets aimed at drawing drug users into treatment. By 2002 it was on target to double the number of drug users in treatment between 1998 and 2008, while the National Treatment Agency was set up in 2001 to oversee the expansion of drug treatment services in the United Kingdom.

Future goals remain to reduce waiting times (currently 2.8 weeks for priority cases), an expansion of cocaine services, the medical supervision of heroin prescribing, greater involvement of GPs, more referrals from the criminal justice system, and improving prison-based treatment. It is noticeable also that the main goals of treatment are more focused on reducing crime in the community than on the health benefits of abstinence.

HIV and harm reduction

Perhaps the biggest influence on increasing treatment, and in particular treatment provided by general practitioners, was HIV/AIDS, with the Advisory Council on the Misuse of Drugs Part 1 stating in 1988:

> HIV is a greater threat to public and individual health than drug misuse. The first goal of work with drug misusers must therefore be to prevent them acquiring or transmitting the virus. In some cases this will be achieved through abstinence. In others, abstinence will not be achievable for the time being and efforts will have to focus on risk reduction. Abstinence remains the ultimate goal but efforts to bring it about in individual cases must not jeopardise any reduction in HIV risk behaviour which has already been achieved.[5]

This report led to the development of community-based needle and pharmacy syringe exchange schemes all over Britain. The report articulated the policy of directing treatment towards abstinence by achieving intermediate goals such as:

▶ stopping injecting with unsterile equipment

▶ taking drugs by mouth or inhalation

▶ taking prescribed rather than illegal drugs.

The report advocated a comprehensive approach to the prevention of the spread of HIV, and the reversal of the then abstinence orientated (detoxification) prescribing policy as it legitimised longer-term prescribing to enable users to stop injecting.

The arrival of HIV/AIDS meant that this harm reduction approach to treatment had taken on a new, arguably more important role. The essence of harm reduction has always been to protect the non-drug-taking community from the crimes committed by drug misusers, but for the first time, in the 1980s, the general public's health was seen to be at risk from drug users' injecting behaviour. The spread of HIV from shared injecting equipment was increasing rapidly across the world and British drug policy was suddenly demanded to coax drug users out of hiding and into needle exchange schemes where sterile equipment was available to be used only once and then discarded. The creation of needle exchange schemes has been remarkably successful in containing HIV and reducing unsafe injecting, and as a public health intervention can be seen alongside the action of John Snow removing the Broad Street pump handle in the 19th century. For drug users who cannot stop injecting, the government is prepared to endorse more controversial treatments such as injectable methadone and heroin.

Harm reduction is popular and successful, reducing both crime and drug-related deaths, which include HIV and hepatitis contracted from sharing needles. The enormous success in stemming the spread of HIV among injecting drug users has surely cemented harm reduction as a central part of British drug policy and perhaps will see the development of safe injecting rooms and supervised injection services as the obvious next steps, as discussed in Chapter 15. The essence of harm reduction can even be seen in the government's policy on alcohol, which, instead of attempting to cut down alcohol consumption, has catered for more flexible licensing hours in the hope that it will reduce the number of drunken people simultaneously emptying onto the streets and causing disturbance.

Evidence for treatment

'Treatment works!' may seem to be a platitude but it is a vital message to give to government bodies responsible for funding drug treatment services. Without evidence for it, monies would continue to be diverted into reducing supply rather than reducing demand and providing treatment.

To 'prove' treatment works requires investment in long-term studies, such as the National Treatment Outcome study, which has its origins in a request from the minister of health in 1994 for a reappraisal of the effectiveness of the national (UK) drug misuse treatment services. The study was a prospective, longitudinal, cohort study and monitored the progress of individuals recruited in one of four treatment settings. Outcomes were based on self-report use of drugs and alcohol and across a number of outcomes presented in terms of change in injecting risk behaviour, psychological health, and criminal behaviour. At five-year follow up the study was able to conclude that drug treatment reduced drug use by 40–60% and arrests for violent and non-violent criminal behaviour as much as 50%, and that for every £1 spent on treatment £3 was saved in criminal justice costs.[6,7] Improvements in drug misuse were largely maintained at four and five years after treatment, with 47% of those who had attended drug residential rehabilitation services and 35% of those who attended community drug treatment reporting abstinence from illicit opiate use. The study also found that less than half (44%) of those who attended drug treatment for problems with crack cocaine were still misusing crack at four to five years follow up.

Treatment therefore does work, though to work effectively it needs to be delivered by well trained staff, delivering effective evidence-based interventions. The latest data to come out of the study show further clear economic benefits of treating drug users in England. While addiction treatment cost £2.9 million in the two years prior to index treatment and a further £4.4 million in the subsequent two years, crime costs fell by £16.1 million during the first year, and by £11.3 million during the second year. In other words, for every £1 spent on treatment, society saves anything from £9.50 to £18 on crime costs. This is a vast improvement on previous estimations.[8]

Whereas there is evidence of the effectiveness of treatment and adequate budgets devoted to treating patients, there is a lack of detailed clinical research into different treatment methods. The Home Affairs Select Committee's report on the government's drug policy in 2002 called for evaluations into the prescription of heroin prescribing, treating cocaine use, and new treatments for opioid users, and for a pilot scheme of safe injecting houses for heroin users. Although the government has promised to focus research on these issues a lack of funding will impede effectiveness.

High quality research in the United Kingdom is lacking, and research using primary care patients or clinicians virtually non-existent. Much of the evidence cited in this book is from the United States and Australia, which, although useful, can sometimes not be easily transferable to a UK setting. Following foreign trends does not necessarily tackle problems. The establishment of a national task force on crack cocaine in the United Kingdom in 1989 in response to USA problems was unnecessary; it was disbanded after a year and left the real amfetamine problem unchecked, with the crack cocaine problem arriving into the United Kingdom only a decade later.

Box 2.1   **National Treatment Outcome Research study hierarchy
of treatment goals**[9]

✓ Reduction of psychological, social and other problems related to drug use

✓ Reduction of psychological, social or other problems not directly attributable to drug use

✓ Reduction of harmful or risky behaviour associated with the use of drugs, including sharing equipment

✓ Attainment of controlled, non-dependent, or non-problematic use

✓ Abstinence from main problem drug(s)

✓ Abstinence from all drugs

Figures show that research funding made up just 0.02% of the United Kingdom's drug misuse budget although some extra funding has since been found. This low sum compares dramatically with that of the United States which funds 85% of the world's research on drug use and drug addiction.

Treatment models involving coercion[10]

Programmes involving coercion have been used in the United States for many years. US 'drug courts' initiatives were developed out of local courts' recognition that, on the one hand, problem drug use created significant criminal and social problems and that, on the other, users had increasingly tough and inflexible penal responses to their drug dependency. Repeated imprisonment and recourse to punishment was clearly failing to tackle the causes of these problems effectively.

In response a scheme was developed that involved treatment instead of punishment, although non-compliance with treatment would result in the user being redirected through the criminal justice system, usually to a custodial sentence. Within this US system, drug users dealt with by drug courts were typically required to participate in treatment for a year or more, have at least three contacts per week with the treatment provider, and submit one or more urine test per week (at least in the early stages of treatment). Treatment providers and case managers were then required to provide monitoring reports to the judge by whom decisions about whether to proceed with a custodial sentence were made.

The weight of the US research supported the drug courts initiative as an effective crime prevention option and found that patients involved with drug courts had higher retention rates than criminal justice patients in general, and that criminal behaviour was substantially reduced during participation in drug courts programmes. Rates on recidivism for those undertaking a courts programme was also reported as lower than for others not involved in such programmes.

Many of the studies, however, took account of only those who had completed the programme and excluded programme drop-outs from the analysis, thus introducing significant positive bias.

In England, drug treatment and testing orders have been loosely modelled on the US drug courts system and aim to divert drug users from prison into community based treatment services. The prevention of reoffending is the main goal of these orders alongside the usual treatment goals concerning personal and public health. As with the US drug courts, the orders aim to break the cycle of 'use-dealing-imprisonment-use-dealing-imprisonment' found amongst many drug users.

Even with only three pilot sites, funded to develop the orders, there was limited evidence of success. There was a great deal of inconsistency in service provision, namely in patient inclusion/exclusion criteria, intensity, nature, and flexibility of the interventions delivered, expectation of drug use for patients/clients on orders, consistency and effectiveness of urine testing, and response to breaching the order's conditions.

At present, the conclusion reached on drug treatment and testing orders must be that whereas drug dependent offenders can be coerced into treatment, the overall outcome of success is hugely variable and inevitably will depend on the skills of the practitioners involved in care provision and the capacity for multi-agency working, factors that are not unique to these orders. A general practitioner caring for a patient on a drug treatment and testing order should clarify the following issues with the user and their key worker:

1. Who supervises the urine test (ideally this should be the key worker)?

2. What level of supervision for urine testing is acceptable? (It may be against many GPs' principles to witness a patient urinate.)

3. If patients disclose that they are using additional illicit heroin or other drugs what course of action should the GP take? (There may be issues about doctor–patient confidentiality unless clearly stated from the outset.)

4. Should the GP report other behaviour (e.g. continued prostitution, shoplifting, domestic violence) to the key worker?

Criminal Justice Interventions programme

The programme, which began in April 2003, focuses on those parts of the country with high levels of acquisitive crime. These include offences such as theft, burglary, car crime, shoplifting, deception, and begging. The programme aims to take advantage of opportunities within the criminal justice system for accessing drug-misusing offenders – many of whom are difficult to access by other approaches – and moving them into treatment, away from drug use and crime.

The programme ensures that expansion of individual interventions is accompanied by continuing support systems for dealing with drug-misusing offenders.

The programme involves:

▸ arrest referral schemes – partnerships between the police, local agencies, and drug action teams that encourage problem drug users to take up appropriate treatment after arrest

▸ drug testing schemes, which test for heroin and crack cocaine use among those who have committed 'trigger offences', thus identifying problem drug users early in their involvement with the criminal justice system

▸ drug testing and treatment orders – community sentences (not prison sentences) that divert offenders out of crime by requiring drug treatment, compulsory drug testing, and court reviews of progress.

THE MANAGEMENT OF SUBSTANCE MISUSE IN PRIMARY CARE

Education policy: protecting young people

The final major aspect of drug policy in the United Kingdom is education and young people. Treatment services for young people are now available in 80% of drug action teams, while sport and arts programmes are being used in 57 disadvantaged communities to provide an alternative to drugs.

The government is committed to continuing education with a major new communications campaign launched in the spring of 2003 driving home the risks of using class A drugs and encouraging young people and their parents to seek advice and help. By March 2004 all primary and secondary schools in England should have developed a drug education policy, while dealers supplying class C drugs to children will be dealt with as severely as those dealing in class A and class B substances. Meanwhile, the compulsory testing and treatment of those in the adult criminal justice system will increasingly be matched for those in the youth justice system.

In the 1960s school-based drug prevention programmes were focused on the provision of factual information to scare young people away from drugs and their risks. By the 1970s, with information dissemination arousing as much curiosity as fear, there was a shift towards personal development. This included a focus on decision making and values clarification and instead of being drug-specific, was intended to be applied by the students themselves to decisions such as whether to take drugs.

Since then more drug-specific policies have been reintroduced, complemented by disturbing images and high-profile case studies, such as that of Leah Betts whose death in 1995 from ecstasy received a great deal of publicity in the hope of warning other young people of the dangers of this drug.

Evidence that education works does exist, but is very limited. It constitutes around 13% of the drug misuse budget but has shown unrewarding results. A £7.5m investment by the government over five years from 2002 to determine the most effective approach to delivering drug education will be welcomed if it can produce a reformed strategy with results to match.

At the moment, education is failing in its main goal of reducing teenage drug uptake. The details of drug use among 11–15-year-olds is given in Chapter 3, but in summary the number of children smoking, drinking alcohol, and taking illegal drugs is increasing. The biggest reason for drug taking among this age group is 'to see what they were like', which suggests education is not succeeding. The government has agreed with the Home Affairs Select Committee that shocking images of the harm caused by drugs should continue to be used, although they need to reflect reality. It is impossible to say whether extensive use of these images will have a better effect. Education methods are discussed in greater detail in Chapter 17, which focuses on all aspects of young people and drugs.

Educational programmes have been evaluated far less fully and rigorously than treatment programmes, in part because of the complexities of carrying out longitudinal studies in this area and disentangling all the potential variables.

Where there has been evaluation, effects have been short-lived and unsatisfactory – as the drug uptake figures for teenagers suggest. In the United States there has been some measured success where school-based interventions have been combined with attempts to change attitudes within the local community as a whole. Again, as with supply reduction measures, such lack of success raises doubts about whether large amounts of funding are being well spent. For now, it seems reasonable to allow the government to complete its review into the most effective methods of education before passing further judgement.

Conclusion

Many experts have been disappointed with the use of criminal justice as a way of preventing and treating drug users as opposed to using more inclusive methods. This policy, however, has made good use of the wide scope to rehabilitate drug users within the criminal justice system, and the number of patients in treatment is increasing at an encouraging rate. This has, in turn, been overshadowed by a recent Audit Commission report suggesting that up to 80% of offenders on drug testing and treatment orders are reconvicted in the first two years after release, though in a relatively new system a tightening and tidying of guidelines may make for more promising results.

More research is needed into new methods of treatment to refine the services available, but the general efficacy of treatment is proven. Realistically, the prohibition of currently illicit drugs remains an obligation for any government when popular opinion and international agreements are taken into account. The effects of reclassifying cannabis cannot yet be judged, but a focus on class A drugs has long been called for and police should be able to arrest and refer more serious users. Enforcement and reducing supply is, however, expensive. Although enforcement can funnel users into treatment, tackling international production and supply has been singularly ineffective. Even with the large budget available the problem cannot be solved without even greater international funding. A re-evaluation of policy and financial distribution is needed.

Education, too, must be subject to serious scrutiny. The £7.5 million government allocation should be enough to succeed, but if this still fails to achieve reductions in teenage uptake of drug use a more radical reconsideration of the education policy will be needed.

Drug use is not spiralling out of control in the United Kingdom, but neither is it falling and the number of young people taking drugs is rising. Treating older drug users effectively can only be of limited overall benefit when more and more young people will be in the treatment services of tomorrow.

Further reading

Carnwath T, Smith I. *Heroin Century.* London: Routledge, 2002.

Working party of the Royal College of Psychiatrists and the Royal College of Physicians. *Drugs, Dilemmas and Choices.* London: Gaskell, 2000.

Strang J, Gossop M (Eds). Heroin Addiction and the British System: Volume 2 Treatment and Other Responses. Oxford: Routledge, 2004.

References

1. Buchanan J, Young L. The war on drugs – a war on drug users? *Drugs Education, Prevention and Policy* 2000; **7(4)**: 2000.

2. Home Office. *Tackling Drugs to Build a Better Britain, Updated Strategy.* London: HMSO, 2002 (available at: www.drugs.gov.uk).

3. Davenport-Hines R. *The Pursuit of Oblivion. A Global History of Narcotics 1500–2000.* London: Weidenfield & Nicolson, 2001.

4. Working party of the Royal College of Psychiatrists and the Royal College of Physicians. *Drugs, Dilemmas and Choices.* London: Gaskell, 2000.

5. Healey A, Knapp M, Austin J, *et al.* Economic Burden of drug dependency. Social costs incurred by drug users at intake to the National Treatment Outcome Research Study. *Br J Psych* 1998; **173**: 160–5.

6. Gossop M, Marsden J, Stewart D, Treacy S. Outcomes after methadone maintenance and methadone reduction treatments: two years follow-up results from the NTORS. *Drug and Alcohol Dependence* 2001; **62**: 255–64.

7. Bell J, Hall W, Byth K. Changes in criminal activity after entering methadone maintenance. *Br J Addict* 1992; **87**: 251–8.

8. Godfrey C, Stewart D, Gossop M. Economic analysis of costs and consequences of the treatment of drug misuse: 2 year outcome data from National Treatment Outcome Research Study (NTORs) *Addiction* 2004; **99(6)**: 697.

9. Department of Health. *Task Force to review services for drug misusers: report of an Independent Review of Drug Treatment Services in England.* London: Department of Health, 1996

10. Turnbull P J, McSweeney T, Webster R, *et al. Drug Treatment and Testing Orders: Final evaluation report.* Home Office research Study 212. London: HMSO, 2000.

CHAPTER 3

Prevalence and patterns of drug use in Britain and Europe

Clare Gerada

Introduction

How many people in Britain use illicit drugs? This question is deceptively easy to ask but difficult to answer. Reliable information on the extent and patterns of drug use and age of first use in the general population and specific populations is difficult to obtain, especially as people differ in their willingness to disclose personal use of illegal substances, even when anonymity is promised. To provide numbers, epidemiologists use a range of techniques and combine information drawn from different sources.

National Drug Treatment Monitoring System

In the United Kingdom, figures for drug users presenting for treatment are drawn directly from the National Drug Treatment Monitoring System, a development of the regional drug misuse databases, which have been in place since the late 1980s. National figures for England[1] report the number of users in treatment with drug agencies and GPs as around 140,900 for the year 2001/2.

The monitoring system collects data on drug users presenting for treatment and those in treatment, though not on how many people are addicted to or having problems with drugs – the hidden population of users. To find this hidden population it is important to devise measures that find out firstly, how many people are in treatment as a whole and secondly, how many people have drug-related problems but are not seeking help.

Estimating the number not in treatment

There are statistical tools that can be used to make intelligent estimates of hidden populations of drug users.

Capture–recapture

A statistical technique known as the capture–recapture method can be used to estimate hidden populations. The method was originally used to estimate population sizes, such as the number of salmon in a pool.

The method involves 'tagging' a captured population and then in given settings calculating the overlap between tagged and untagged populations. Used with drug users these settings would include various treatment settings, including non-statutory sectors. The size of the overlap between samples allows a statistical model to be created, which can then be used to estimate the size of the wider drug-using population.

Using this method, several studies have estimated the number of problematic drug users in their area. For example, in 1984 Hartnoll[2] collected data on the number of opiate users in north London who had attended a drug clinic and those admitted to hospital for infectious diseases. Comparing the sources, they found that a fifth of the hospital sample had also attended the drug clinic. The researchers used this ratio to estimate that the total number of opioid users was five times the number who attended the drug clinic.

Social survey data

Important data on the prevalence of drug use has been provided by a wide range of local and national surveys, which measure different aspects of a person's drug use, such as:

▸ any use during a person's lifetime (lifetime prevalence), often called 'lifetime experience'

▸ any use during the previous year (past 12 months prevalence), often called 'recent use'

▸ any use during the previous month (past 30 days prevalence), often called 'current use'.

The figures for lifetime use are always higher than for the other two groups, as this group includes everyone who has ever tried drugs, no matter when. Recent use figures are generally lower but reflect more accurately the current situation. A combination of lifetime experience and recent or current use can provide insight into drug-use patterns.

National surveys used in the United Kingdom are the British Crime Survey (covering England and Wales), the Scottish Crime Survey, and the Northern Ireland Crime Survey. All of these are based on representative samples of the households in the countries they represent.

There are a number of surveys that focus on vulnerable groups, for example care leavers,[3] youth homelessness and substance use,[4] substance use by young offenders,[5] and school surveys.[6]

Drug use in the United Kingdom

General population

The lifetime prevalence of the use of most drugs has remained relatively stable, though amfetamine and LSD use appears to be declining steadily, whereas cocaine and ecstasy appear to be increasing slightly.

Levels of drug use are not static and change according to vogue, price, availability, and demographics of the local population.

Figure 3.1 **Lifetime prevalence of use of different drugs among users of any drug by year[7]**

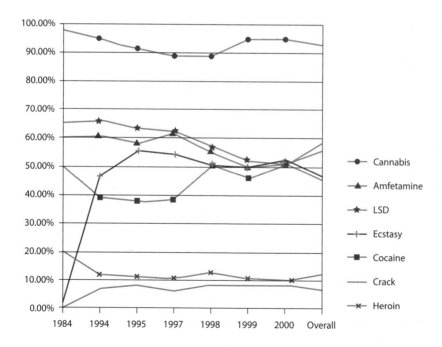

Children

For all children aged between 11 and 15 years in England the latest figures available (2003) show that the prevalence of taking drugs in that year increased slightly from the previous year from 20 to 21% though the prevalence of taking drugs in the past month, surveyed in 2003 (12%), was about the same as in 2002. The prevalence of drug use increased sharply with age; only 8% of 11-year-olds had used drugs in the past year compared with 38% of 15-year-olds, with cannabis by far the most commonly used illicit drug. One per cent had used heroin in the past year and 1% had used cocaine. In total 4% had used a Class A drug.

Table 3.1 **Prevalence of drug use in children in England, 2003**

Age of children surveyed	Percentage of children reported to have used a drug in the past year/England
11-year-old	8
13-year-old	15
15-year-old	38

Young people

Levels of drug use by young people have been fairly static over the past few years, with only cocaine use in the past year (2003) showing an increase in use. The overall prevalence of taking drugs amongst 16–24-year-olds in the past year (2003) actually decreased slightly between 2001/2 and 2002/3 (from 30% to 28%).

Among young people cannabis is the most commonly used drug in the United Kingdom with figures at around 26% of 16–24-year-olds having used cannabis in the past year. In England and Wales, ecstasy is the next most popular drug with 6% having used it, followed by cocaine at 5%, and amfetamines at 4%. Scottish figures show that LSD is the most popular drug after cannabis, with 3% having used it. In Northern Ireland, 7% of 16–29-year-olds had used ecstasy in the past year and 5% had used amfetamines and hallucinogens.

Vulnerable groups

Drug use by care leavers is much higher than drug use by the general population. Ward et al., in 2003,[3] surveyed care leavers aged between 14 and 24 years old and found that three-quarters of the sample had ever used a drug and over half had used a drug in the past month. Not surprisingly, levels of drug use by the young homeless are much higher than by young people in general. Wincup et al., in 2003,[4] sampled 160 homeless 16–25-year-olds and almost all (95%) had ever used drugs and equally almost all (89%) had used drugs in the past year and past month (76%), many of them using cocaine, heroin, and/or amfetamine together with cannabis. This means that when a young homeless person presents to primary care, drug misuse should be considered even if the patient does not volunteer this information.

The Youth Lifestyle Survey[8] found that about a fifth of young people admitted to some form of offending and that self-reported drug use was the strongest predictor of serious or persisting offending.

Drug use in the offending population

Drug use by the offending population is common. Drug misuse is both a cause and a consequence of contact with the criminal justice system. The largest relevant survey is the NEW-ADAM survey,[9] which carries out voluntary drug testing and interviews on samples of arrestees. The 2001 survey found that 65% of all arrestees tested (1,435) were positive for some form of drug, 34% positive for opiates, and 15% for cocaine.

Other studies from surveys of prison populations indicate similarly high rates of drug use prior to imprisonment, the rate being highest for young offenders, where six out of ten had used some drug before entering prison. Among women drug offences were more common, at one in five.[10]

Drug use in UK compared with other European countries

Figure 3.2   **Cannabis, ecstacy and amfetamine use in Germany, UK and France**

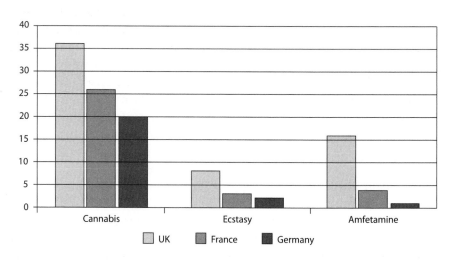

Source: European Monitoring Centre for Drugs and Drug Addiction, 2003

Britain has often been portrayed as the drug capital of Europe, with repeated claims from the media and others that it has higher cannabis use, higher cocaine use, and higher alcohol use than its European neighbours. Indeed at first reading it does appear that Britain has a high level of cannabis, ecstasy, and amfetamine use compared with most other members of the European Union (EU).

It is notoriously difficult, however, to make comparisons in use of illicit drugs across different nations. There are many factors that can interfere with establishing accurate comparisons. For example, sources of variation may reflect the differences in the urban and rural populations (where drug use is more prevalent in urban populations), age patterns/birth cohorts (these will affect measures of different drugs used as well as actual numbers using across the total population), the extent of the converging of lifestyles of young men and women (the more convergent the higher the levels of use by women), and sociocultural factors, including income. As well as natural variation, the tools used to measure prevalence will vary across each country and hence comparative analysis across different countries using different survey tools need to be made with caution, in particular where differences are small. Despite methodological limitations, however, some common patterns of drug use throughout the EU can be identified.[11]

The European Monitoring Centre for Drugs and Drug Addiction produces an annual report on the state of drugs in Europe (it does not currently include new member states), attempting to bring coherence to the methods of collecting the data. Trends identified by the 2003 report[11] are illustrated below.

Cannabis

In all countries in the EU, cannabis is the most commonly used drug, with many countries reporting lifetime prevalence rates in more than 20% of the general population. A conservative estimate would suggest that at least one in every five adults in the EU has tried the drug. Cannabis use has increased year on year across most of the EU, though it does appear that rates are now levelling off and stabilising, albeit at historically high levels. In young people cannabis taking may be the norm rather than the exception.

Some evidence of a convergence in patterns of use is also found, although rates still vary considerably, with France, Spain, and the United Kingdom, in particular, reporting relatively high levels of use, and Finland, Sweden, and Portugal reporting comparatively low figures. In all countries, estimates of the prevalence of recent use (within the past year) among the adult population remain below 10%.

When young adults are considered, rates of use rise considerably. In all countries, recent use prevalence peaks in the 15–25-year age group, with France, Germany, Ireland, Spain, and the United Kingdom all reporting that over 20% of this age group have used cannabis in the past 12 months. Lifetime use estimates are higher, with most countries reporting lifetime prevalence estimates of between 20 and

35% in young people. The number of people using cannabis on a regular basis is small in overall population terms (generally less than 1%), although higher rates of regular use may be found in young people, and in particular in young men.

Amfetamines and ecstasy (MDMA)

Europe remains an important area for the production and use of amfetamines and ecstasy but not methamfetamine, the use of which is largely restricted to Australasia, South-east Asia, and America. After cannabis, the most commonly used drug in EU countries is either ecstasy or amfetamine, with rates of lifetime experience among the adult population ranging between 0.5 and 5%. In the past, prevalence of amfetamine use was generally higher than prevalence of ecstasy use, but this difference is now less apparent. In school populations, lifetime experience of inhalants (e.g. volatile gas use, glue sniffing) is second only to that of cannabis and in general is considerably higher than experience of either ecstasy or amfetamines.

As with cannabis, the highest rates of lifetime and recent use are found in young adults. A number of indicators suggest that ecstasy use has continued to spread in some sections of urban youth in Europe. Some studies have found extremely high prevalence rates among such groups, although a pronounced increase in use of the drug is not generally observable in the wider population.

The numbers of people treated for an amfetamine problem in Europe varies widely: just under a third of drug users in treatment in Sweden and Finland are amfetamine users, compared with around 9% in Germany and 3% or less in all other countries. In almost all countries rates of demand for treatment related to ecstasy and to a certain extent amfetamine use are very low. A small number of deaths in Europe can be directly attributed to the use of ecstasy, but overall the numbers remain low in comparison with deaths related to opioid. Although there have been some fluctuations in recent years, and possibly signs of stabilisation in some areas, both amfetamine and ecstasy seizures (numbers and quantities) have increased substantially in the EU over the past decade. In Finland, Sweden, and Norway, amfetamines are the second most commonly seizied drug (after cannabis).

Cocaine and crack cocaine

Survey data suggest an increase in cocaine use, especially in the smokable 'crack' form, in the United Kingdom and, to a lesser extent, in Denmark, Germany, Spain, and the Netherlands. Cocaine use, and increases in use, appear to be more common among young people living in urban areas. National figures may therefore reflect local trends in some major European cities to only a limited extent. Seizures have increased steadily since 1985. Similarly, the quantity of cocaine seized has generally exhibited an upward trend over the same period, although figures tend to fluctuate from year to year.

The prevalence of use of crack cocaine in Europe appears to be relatively low, although sporadic local reports suggest a problem among marginal groups in some cities, for example within the sex industry. We know, however, that the health impact of crack cocaine use is disproportionately greater than that caused by cocaine powder use so the impact on health and social care services even with low prevalence use is likely to be significant. The increasing number of cocaine users is already placing demands on treatment services, which are not well equipped to manage stimulant users.

Heroin and injecting drug use

Afghanistan accounts for around 70% of global opium production. Opium grown in South America is destined for the North American market. Afghan production has been disrupted for one reason or another in recent years, with significant reductions during the Taliban-imposed prohibition on poppy production in 2000.

Although few in terms of overall numbers, heroin users are responsible for a disproportionate share of the health and social problems resulting from drug consumption; regular injecting of heroin has a far greater health and social care cost than any other drug. In most countries in the EU, with the exception of Sweden and Finland where amfetamine use is more prevalent, problem drug use remains characterised by the use of heroin, often in combination with other drugs, so called 'polydrug use'. As estimation in this area is difficult, and the precision and reliability of estimates vary considerably, caution is required both in interpreting trends and in making comparisons between countries.

National estimates of problem drug use vary between two and ten cases per thousand of the adult population (that is between 0.2 and 1%). No common trend in the number of problematic drug users in the EU can be observed, although studies suggest that in at least half of EU countries some increase has occurred since the mid-1990s.

Probably around half of problem drug users in the EU are drug injectors, i.e. around 600,000–900,000 of the EU's estimated 1–1.5 million problem drug users. The proportion of injectors varies considerably between countries and has changed over time, with levels of injection falling in almost all countries during the 1990s, although there is some evidence of more recent increases. The figures for the United Kingdom give estimates of injecting drug use varying between two and five cases per thousand of the adult population (or 0.2–0.5%).

Drug related deaths

It is well documented that heroin users are at a substantially greater risk of premature death than their non-heroin using peers. The number of drug related deaths in the United Kingdom rose throughout the 1990s and early 2000s as it has in many other countries.[12, 13]

Longitudinal studies suggest annual mortality rates of about 1.2% of heroin users. The excess mortality among heroin users varies between 6 and 20 times that expected in the population for an age–sex matched group.

The longest cohort study in the literature[14] has followed up a group of 128 heroin addicts attending London clinics for 22 years, of whom 43 have died, with 18 deaths attributed to overdose. The average death rate was just under 2%.

Darke and Zador reviewed the literature on deaths attributed to heroin overdose. These typically occurred in older, heroin dependent males not in drug treatment at the time of death. Most fatal cases were in those who had been using heroin for a considerable number of years – and not, as one might expect, in the young novice or inexperienced user. Fatalities involving heroin alone were in the minority and typically there were other drugs found at post-mortem – principally alcohol and benzodiazepines.[15]

A number of studies touching on drug related deaths in the UK have been published in recent years.[12] Key findings emerging from these studies are that:

▶ Illicit methadone accounts for more than half of all methadone related deaths, with most occurring at weekends.

▶ Polydrug use is not only a feature of opioid related death but also of fatalities involving ecstasy. Most ecstasy deaths occur at a time of celebration.

▶ The risk of death is considerably higher in the first week following release from prison and there is a risk of overdose the week after successful completion of inpatient detoxification.

In more recent years the death rate in drug users has fallen, no doubt in part owing to the implementation of many of the recommendations from the Advisory Council on the Misuse of Drugs (ACMD)[14] report on reducing drug related deaths. The ACMD examined many potential causes of drug related deaths, including the inadequacy of general practitioners in the use of methadone. They made far-reaching recommendations including a need to clarify the definition of a drug related death, modernisation of data collection and analysis, issues relating to methadone treatment, prevention of viral diseases and road accidents, and improvement of services in prison and on release. Some of the recommendations have been implemented by the Department of Health – in particular the improvement in reporting drug related deaths and the production of guidance to drug action teams on developing local confidential inquires into drug related deaths in order that better information and improvements in services for drug users would reduce the number of deaths.[16]

Conclusion

For decades drug policy in the United Kingdom has concentrated on improving access to treatment and the prevention of drug related harms. In recent years the emphasis has begun to shift towards preventing crime and hence criminal justice initiatives, including drug treatment and testing orders, have been introduced. The success or otherwise of UK drug policy is discussed in greater detail in Chapter 2.

It is clear from the figures, however, that while drug use may not be increasing at a record-breaking rate, overall drug use in the United Kingdom is disturbingly high, especially when one includes cannabis use. The problem is shared across the EU, albeit in most countries at a slightly lower level than the United Kingdom, and is an issue that will undoubtedly receive more debate and more international cooperation in the future. Meanwhile, the role of the primary care practitioner in the United Kingdom remains to increase the capacity for treatment, picking up the inevitable pieces that no drug policy will ever be able to wipe out completely.

Further reading

Office for National Statistics. *Drug Use, smoking and drinking amongst young teenagers in 1999.* London: ONS, 2000 (available at: www.statistics.gov.uk).

Gabbay, M. (Ed). *The Evidence-Based Primary Care Handbook.* London: Royal Society of Medicine, 1999.

European Monitoring Centre for Drugs and Drug Addiction. INSIGHTS. *Reviewing current practice in drug-substitution treatment in the European Union.* EMCDDA, November 2000 (available at: www.emcdda.org).

References

1. Department of Health. Provisional Statistics from the National Drug Treatment Monitoring System in England, 2001/02 and 2002/03 UK. London: DOH, 2003.

2. Hartnoll R, Daviaud E, Lewis R G, Mitcheson M C. *Drug Problems: Assessing local needs. A practical manual for assessing the nature and extent of problematic drug use in a community.* London: Drug Indicators Project, 1985.

3. Ward J, Henderson Z, Pearson G. *One problem among many; drug use among care leavers in transition to independent living.* Home Office Research Study; **260**. London: Home Office, 2003.

4. Wincup E, Buckland G, Bayliss R. *Youth homelessness and substance use: report to the drugs and alcohol research unit.* Home Office Research Study; **258**. London: Home Office, 2003.

5. Hammersley R, Marsland L, Reid M. *Substance use by young offenders the impact of normalisation of drug use in the early years of the 21st century.* Home Office Research Study; **261**. London: Home Office, 2003.

6. Balding J. *Young people in 1995.* School Health Education Unit: University of Exeter, 1996.

7. Department of Health. *Statistics on young people and drug misuse: England.* London: HMSO, 2003.

8. Flood-Page C, Campbell S, Harrington V. Miller J. *Youth Crime: findings from the 1998/99 Youth Lifestyles Survey.* Home Office Research Study; **209**. London: Home Office, 2000.

9. Bennett T, Holloway K, Williams T. *Drug use and offending: summary results from the first year of the NEW-ADAM research programme.* Home Office Research Findings; **148**. London: Home Office, 2001.

10. Lader D, Singleton N, Meltzer H. *Psychiatric morbidity among young offenders in England and Wales.* London: ONS, 2000.

11. Annual Report 2003: *The state of the drugs problem in the European Union and Norway.* European Monitoring Centre for Drugs and Drug Addiction (available at: www.emcdda.eu.int).

12. Griffiths C. *Deaths related to drug poisoning: results for England and Wales, 1997 to 2001.* Health Statistics Quarterly (Spring 2003): **17**; 65–71.

13. The Advisory Council on the Misuse of Drugs. *Reducing drug related deaths, 2000.* London: HMSO, 2000.

14. Oppenheimer E, Tobbutt C, Taylor C, Andrew T. Death and survival in a cohort of heroin addicts from London Clinics. *Addiction* 1994; **89**: 1299–1308.

15. Darke S, Zador D. Fatal heroin 'overdose': A review. *Addiction* 1996; **91(12)**: 1765–72.

16. Department of Health. *Guidance for Drug Action Teams on developing local confidential inquires into drug- related deaths.* London: HMSO, 2003 (available at: www.doh.gov.uk).

CHAPTER 4

Controlled drug prescribing by general practitioners in England

David Roberts and Clare Gerada

IN THIS CHAPTER

Introduction

Controlled drugs are an important part of the prescribing armoury for general practitioners and, as well as for the treatment of addiction, they are used for analgesia, epilepsy, symptomatic treatment in palliative care, and attention deficit/hyperactivity disorder (ADHD) in children. Although the actions of the convicted former GP Harold Shipman, who used fraudulently obtained diamorphine to murder patients over a 23-year period, were unique, his use of controlled drugs did expose the apparently unrestricted freedom that doctors in the United Kingdom have when using the so-called 'The British System'. Dame Janet Smith, chairwoman of the Shipman Inquiry,[1] has, in her fourth report of the Shipman Inquiry recommended practices and procedures to tighten the mechanisms for audit and monitoring and the implementation of measures to identify potentially fraudulent or inappropriate prescribing at an early stage. Shipman and his actions will be discussed in Chapter 24. This chapter will concentrate on examining the patterns of prescribing of controlled drugs using the results of prescribing data from English general practitioners.

General trends in controlled drug prescribing 2002/3

Using data from the Prescribing Pricing Authority 2002/3 it has been possible to examine in greater detail the prescribing patterns by general practitioners of controlled drugs.[2] The data are only for prescriptions issued by English GPs on NHS (FP10) prescriptions and hence do not include any hospital generated items or prescribing from private practice. The prescription indicates nothing about the condition that the drug was used for and therefore this can be deduced only from the usual indication for the drug in question. Over 2.7 million prescriptions for controlled drugs were issued by English GPs in the year 2002/3, representing 0.44% of all prescriptions of all categories of prescribed (controlled and non-controlled) medicines issued for that year. The increase in the quantities of controlled drugs prescribed by general practitioners was 8% on the previous year.

Analgesics account for 60% of controlled drug prescriptions. Nearly a third of all controlled drug items prescribed were for methadone solution for the treatment of addiction (Figure 4.1).

Figure 4.1   **Summary of controlled drug prescriptions issued on NHS prescriptions by English GPs 2002/3**

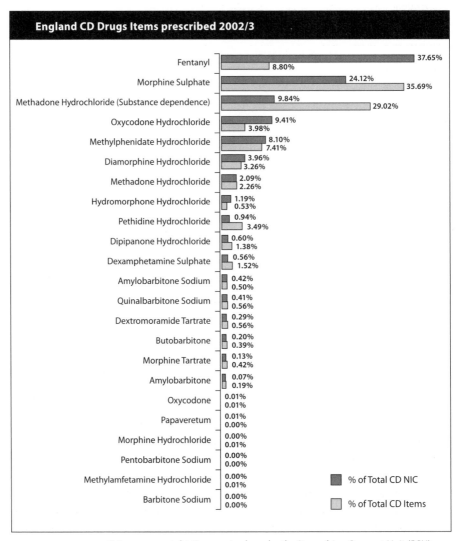

Source: Analyses by the Prescribing Support Unit (PSU) based on information systems at the Prescription Pricing Authority (PPA)

Though general practitioners prescribed over 300 different controlled drug preparations, only 40 drugs accounted for 80% of all preparations and of these morphine sulphate was the most frequently prescribed drug (970,000 items), accounting for over 35% of all controlled drug items. Fentanyl, morphine sulphate, oxycodone hydrochloride, and diamorphine hydrochloride all show prescribing growth for items, with significant increases in fentanyl and oxycodone hydrochloride (see Table 4.1).

Table 4.1 **Analgesic drugs prescribed in England 2002/3**

Drug	Items	Items' growth from previous year (%)
Oxycodone hydrochloride	108,420	60.15
Fentanyl	239,612	26.61
Morphine sulphate	971,447	4.97
Diamorphine hydrochloride	88,854	2.13
Dipipanone hydrochloride	37,518	-5.74
Methadone hydrochloride	61,621	-6.40
Pethidine hydrochloride	94,983	-7.38
Dextromoramide tartrate	15,171	-8.74
Hydromorphone hydrochloride	14,458	-13.82
Morphine tartrate	11,413	-16.94
Morphine hydrochloride	246	-32.23
Oxycodone	211	-37.94
Papaveretum	125	-42.40
Total	**1,644,079**	

Analgesics

Over 1.6 million items prescribed were for 13 different analgesic drugs. Five drugs (fentanyl, morphine sulphate, methadone hydrochloride (substance dependence), oxycodone hydrochloride, and methylphenidate hydrochloride) dominate controlled drug prescribing, and account for over 90% of total controlled items. All bar methylphenidate hydrochloride are analgesics. Methadone preparations are classified by the Prescription Prescribing Authority as drugs used in substance misuse treatment; all other formulations are classified as analgesics (Table 4.2).

Table 4.2 **Analgesics prescribed 2002/3**

Drug	% of controlled drug analgesic items
Fentanyl	14.57
Morphine sulphate	59.09
Oxycodone hydrochloride	6.59
Diamorphine hydrochloride	5.40
Methadone hydrochloride	3.75
Hydromorphone hydrochloride	0.88
Pethidine hydrochloride	5.78
Dipipanone hydrochloride	2.28
Dextromoramide tartrate	0.92
Morphine tartrate	0.69
Papaveretum	0.01
Oxycodone	0.01
Morphine hydrochloride	0.01

© Crown copyright

Specific analgesic drugs

Diamorphine

It may surprise practitioners that the United Kingdom is one of the few countries in the world that recommends the use of diamorphine as a medicine. This decision was the subject of considerable debate and discussion during the 1950s but, on the advice of the UK medical profession, its continued availability as a medicine was retained. This decision was reaffirmed by the Advisory Council in the Misuse of Drugs in 1973.[3]

Diamorphine has many advantages over other analgesics and has an important place in palliative care. It is highly effective when rapid analgesia is required, as it is highly water-soluble and hence very large doses can be given in little volume and can be given via subcutaneous infusion pumps. Outside the United Kingdom other treatments are used, such as hydromorphone or fentanyl. It is likely that the high volume of diamorphine items prescribed can be accounted for by prescriptions from doctors involved in hospice care. For example, the number of prescriptions issued for diamorphine 500 mg (prescribed in high doses by Shipman) is relatively small compared with the 130,000 cancer deaths per year in England and Wales.

Oxycodone

Oxycodone is a central nervous system depressant and appears to work through stimulating the opioid receptors in the central nervous system that activate responses ranging from analgesia to respiratory depression to euphoria. It is derived directly from thebaine, an opium constituent. Like many opiates, oxycodone can give a pleasurable 'high', with inherent dangers such as dependence and overdose. In its pill form, sold as OxyContin, the drug is released slowly, giving a sustained 'high' typically over 12 hours. This effect has made it a drug of choice among some opiate users, something the media in the United States has reported following a number of overdoses and cases of reported dependency.

The drug is usually swallowed. Injection can cause tissue and vein damage (as well as the risks normally associated with injecting). Prescribing for oxycodone in England increased dramatically from 2001/2 to 2002/3, with percentage increases varying across the country between 23 to 105%.

Oxycodone acquired its nickname 'Hillbilly heroin' because of disproportionately high addiction rates among rural communities, becoming endemic in poor, sparsely populated areas such as the Appalachian valley (the poorest region of the United States). The drug, meant for oral use, is frequently ground up and then injected or snorted. It has been associated with many hundreds of deaths in North America. The drug is increasingly popular as a drug of misuse in Canada and there are fears that increased prescribing of this drug in the UK may lead to diversion and abuse. In March 2002 the first British death attributed to oxycodone abuse was reported by Tony Thompson [*The Observer*, Sunday March 24th 2002] 'a pretty 18 year old from Hull who dreamt of becoming a model ... joined friends for a night out on the town ... they began drinking wine and beer and smoking cannabis ... a variety of pills were doing the rounds and at some point Samantha swallowed up to seven oxycodone'. She died some time later having been laid on a mattress by her friends 'to sleep it off'. General practitioners in the United Kingdom need to exercise caution when prescribing this drug so that it does not inadvertently become diverted or abused.

Drugs used in the treatment of addiction

Methadone

Although overall methadone prescribing decreased, prescribing for methadone solution, classified by the *British National Formulary* as a drug for the treatment of substance dependence, increased by 8%, with over 370,000 litres prescribed in 2002/3.

The rise in methadone prescribing represents a triumph for general practitioners and a real achievement in their response to treating drug users. The National Drug Strategy target of 30% of general practitioners involved by 2004 has been achieved. Support, through effective shared schemes, training (predominantly through the Royal College of General Practitioners), and the publication of national good practice guidelines have all undoubtedly contributed to the rise in GPs providing evidence based treatment to this patient group.

The audit has shown that although most methadone prescribed by general practitioners is in the form recommended by the clinical guidelines, methadone solution 1 mg/ml (Table 4.3), other preparations, including methadone ampoules, tablets, and higher strength preparations of methadone (e.g. 10, 20, 50 mg/ml), were also prescribed in significant amounts (Table 4.4). These drugs are not recommended in the treatment of addiction as they have a high divertible value and the tablet and higher strength methadone are known to be injected. It is likely that the very high strength preparations are used for pain control: because methadone is a long-acting analgesic it would be a particularly effective analgesic for background symptom control.

Dextromoramide

Dextromoramide tartrate (Palfium™) is a synthetic opiate* developed in 1956. The pharmacological action of the drug is similar to that of other opiates such as morphine and diamorphine in that it has strong analgesic properties although there are differences in its duration of action, effects, and analgesic properties compared with other drugs in the same class. Historically, in the United Kingdom and elsewhere, dextromoramide was popular with opioid dependent people. Doctors often prescribed it to patients who were unable to obtain heroin, either on the illicit market or by prescription. Its increasing use was reflected in an increasing number of primary dextromoramide addictions.

At present dextromoramide is rarely used and comprises less than 1% of all opiate prescriptions dispensed in the treatment of opiate addiction in England and Wales and has now been discontinued owing to shortages of ingredients for manufacture.[4]

---

*Dextromoramide is strictly speaking an opioid. An opioid is any drug that has agonist effects at the opioid receptor whilst opiates are those opioids found in opium (e.g. morphine, codeine) or semi-synthetic derivatives such as diamorphine.

Table 4.3   **Oral methadone prescriptions 2002/3**

Preparation	Items	Total quantity of oral methadone prescriptions
Methadone HCl_oral sol 1 mg/ml	673,175	319,103,909
Methadone HCl_oral sol 1 mg/ml S/F	113,199	56,587,316
Methadone HCl_oral conc 10 mg/ml S/F	1,180	209,029
Other preparations	2,422	92,8675
Total	**789,976**	**376,928,929**

© Crown copyright

Table 4.4   **Non-oral methadone prescriptions 2003/4**

Preparation	Items	Total quantity of non oral methadone preparations
Methadone HCl_tab 5 mg	28,860	3,457,970
Methadone HCl_inj 50 mg/ml 1 ml amp	9,897	196,877
Physeptone_tab 5 mg	7,606	781,806
Methadone HCl_inj 10 mg/ml 1 ml amp	6,393	253,665
Methadone HCl_inj 10 mg/ml 2 ml amp	2,222	41,444
Methadone HCl_inj 10 mg/ml 5 ml amp	1,967	35,829
Methadone HCl_inj 10 mg/ml 3.5 ml amp	1,504	25,221
Other preparations	3,172	
Total	**61,621**	

© Crown copyright

Stimulants

The increase by 20% of stimulant prescribing reflects general practitioners' adherence to the recent National Institute for Clinical Excellence (NICE) guidance on the use of methlyphenidate for the treatment of childhood attention deficit/hyperactivity disorder (ADHD) (Table 4.5).

Table 4.5 **Stimulant prescriptions 2002/3**

Drug	Items	Items' growth compared with previous year (%)
Methylphenidate hydrochloride	201,674	19.95
Dexamfetamine sulphate	41,262	−2.75
Methyl amfetamine hydrochloride	153	8.93

© Crown copyright

NICE recommends that treatment should be initiated only by child and adolescent psychiatrists or paediatricians with an expertise in ADHD, but continued prescribing and monitoring may be performed by general practitioners under shared care arrangements with specialists.

Private prescribing

There is currently no equivalent to the Prescribing Pricing Authority for private prescriptions and hence no easy way of calculating the type or volume of controlled drugs issued on private prescriptions. This is likely to change if the recommendations made by Dame Janet Smith in the fourth report of the Shipman Inquiry are implemented when all controlled drugs, whether generated through NHS or private prescribers, will be subject to audit.

At present the only way of examining private prescribing data is by manually collecting data of drugs dispensed through community pharmacists. An analysis of this nature was undertaken by Strang and Sheridan[4] and data derived from community pharmacies in 1995 showed that private prescriptions were significantly more likely than NHS prescriptions to be for methadone tablets or ampoules (33% of all prescriptions in both cases), to be for substantially higher daily doses, and to be collected on a weekly or fortnightly basis. The differences in prescribing between NHS and private practitioners were most apparent for methadone ampoules. So, whilst the mean daily doses for NHS and private prescriptions for oral methadone mixture were 44.3 mg and 55.2 mg, respectively, and for NHS and private tablet prescriptions were 51.9 mg and 82.5 mg these different amounts did not reach statistical significance at the 0.05 level. However, for NHS and private methadone ampoules prescriptions, the mean daily doses were 62.4 mg and 117.8 mg and this did reach significant levels. The volume of private prescriptions for dextroamfetamine sulphate and other controlled drugs is not known.

Conclusion

Overall the prescribing of controlled drugs across England conforms to good practice guidance and to known changes in treatments for a number of conditions. Most of the prescribing observed is unremarkable, and demonstrates on a national level adherence to good practice.

References

1. *The Shipman Inquiry, Fourth Report: The Regulation of Controlled Drugs in the Community.* Cm 6249. London: HMSO, 2004.

2. Prescribing Support Unit. *Audit of Controlled Drugs Prescribing in England for Financial Year 2002–2003.* Prescribing Support Unit, 2004. Data presented to the Shipman Inquiry.

3. Ghodse H. Pain, anxiety and insomnia – a global perspective on the relief of suffering. *Br J Psychiatry* 2003; **183**: 15–21.

4. Sheridan J, Strang J, Barber N, Glanz A. Role of community pharmacies in relation to HIV prevention and drug misuse: findings from the 1995 national survey in England and Wales. *BMJ* 1996; **312**: 272–4.

CHAPTER 5

General practitioners and the care of drug users: past, present, and future

Clare Gerada and Linda Harris

IN THIS CHAPTER

Introduction || Changing climate || Drug policy and primary care || Measures to increase the response of GPs in the care of drug users || Does treatment in primary care work? || Have things got better? || Results from 2001 survey of random sample of English GPs and their involvement or otherwise in the care of drug users || Are there problems with GP involvement? || Specialist primary care practitioners || Conclusion

Introduction

Primary care has been described as the 'front-door' to the NHS through which most of the population access health and, increasingly, social care. Ninety-eight per cent of the population is registered with a GP and 60–70% of this registered population will see their GP each year. Collectively 1–1.5 million patient contacts are made by about 30,000 GPs and around 20,000 primary care nurses every day, each contact lasting an average of 13.3 minutes. Each person sees their GP on average five times a year, with women more likely than men to consult (six and four respectively). On average, GPs see around 117 patients a week and practice nurses, 105.[1] This makes the GP and the primary care nurse vital components of any mental health and drug strategy and a useful early warning sign of developing health problems.

One of the most distinctive characteristics of primary care in the United Kingdom is that it is a readily accessible service (97% of patients are able to see a GP within two working days), accessed by self-referral, provided to a registered population usually involving all members of a family, and provided in a community setting by general practitioners and primary care nurses working with a wider health care team.

Many countries have developed primary care services with variations in the structure and organisation, mode of payment of GPs, gatekeeper function, and relationship to secondary specialist services. Where primary care is most developed, such as the Netherlands, Denmark, the United Kingdom, and Canada, the GP forms the core and focal point of the primary health care team.[2] He or she is the first point of contact for most patients, including drug users, and provides generalist and increasingly specialist care to these patients. In these countries the GP provides personal care for individuals in the context of their families, community, and culture and exercise their professional role by promoting health, preventing disease, and providing cure, care, and palliation.

Changing climate

Since the 1990s, primary care in the United Kingdom has undergone considerable change in organisation, services, and payment structure. A plethora of new organisations and strategies has been launched in recent years. Change continues with the introduction of a new General Medical Service (nGMS) contract for GPs in April 2004.

Beginning with the introduction of fund-holding and the purchaser–provider split of the early 1990s, these major changes continued with the 1997 NHS Primary Care Act and the changes in the organisation of primary care laid out in *The New NHS, Modern, Dependable*.[3] The Primary Care Act heralded the ability of other professional groups, such as nurses, to provide primary care services, not necessarily through the traditional surgery environment. For example, through nurse-led walk-in clinics offering care to any patient, and NHS Direct, a nurse-led telephone advice and information service.

The most recent government plan – the NHS Plan – heralds new roles for nurses and GPs, in particular through the development of intermediate (general practitioners with special clinical interest) practitioners, able to offer new ways of providing services to their colleagues.[4]

By February 2004 over 1400 nurses and nearly 100 pharmacists had been trained as supplementary prescribers and can prescribe any medication in the *British National Formulary* (except controlled drugs or unlicensed medicines) in partnership with a doctor and within the limits of a clinical management plan for the patients. Changes in regulations will give much greater prescribing rights to nurses and pharmacists; these rights include controlled drugs.

At the time of writing GP commissioning, or strictly speaking *practice based commissioning* is about to be reintroduced, giving practices and doctors the ability, again, to control budgets and commission services to meet their population needs.

Drug policy and primary care

For drug users, primary care is seen as being readily accessible and less stigmatising than traditional specialist addiction services and research shows that patients prefer care from a competent GP than from other professionals.[5,6] Government policy has promoted GPs as an important part of modern health care for drug users and the past two decades have seen numerous policy documents, health service circulars, and government strategies laying the foundations for effective primary care involvement.[7]

The World Health Organization (WHO),[8] as long ago as 1973, listed some of the crucial reasons why GPs are well placed to deliver primary care to those with mental illness, including drug and alcohol misuse. Policy makers have consistently prioritised the care of drug misusers by GPs and a number of policy documents, statements, and key publications have been produced to this effect over the past decade.

The 1984 National Clinical Guidelines predicted, 'GPs are increasingly likely to see patients presenting with drug related problems in view of the increasing incidence of opioid addiction,' and, 'we wish to encourage as many GPs as possible to treat these patients and to help them in every possible way'.[9] These first guidelines stated their concern that some doctors, both in general practice and in the hospital services, 'are unwilling or reluctant to see drug misusers or advise on drug related problems'. The prediction of increasing numbers of patients presenting with drug related problems was not surprisingly correct, with the 1980s seeing a substantial increase in the incidence of drug use. The view from policy makers now being that all staff within health and social services, the criminal justice system, and education will encounter drug users in the course of their work and that *all* drug users have the same entitlement to services as any other patient.[10]

The view discussed above must be contrasted with previous decades when, far from wanting more GPs involved, the profession was in part blamed for the increase of drug misuse. GPs were seen as part of the problem, not as part of the solution,[11] and specialist clinics for the treatment of opiate dependence were set up as a response to the 'over zealous' prescribing by GPs.[12] To illustrate this point, the ACMD report in 1982 'Treatment and Rehabilitation' (the precursor of the 1984 Clinical Guidelines) hardly makes mention of general practitioners other than to admonish them for overriding the 'strict non-prescribing policy of *hospital based clinics* and [doctors in general practice] seeing it as their duty to consider giving opioid prescriptions to drug users on their lists'. The report goes on to state that these general practitioners do so in the 'knowledge that they are acting in conflict with the clinical policy of their local hospital-based service but also in the belief that they are using a method of treatment approved by experts elsewhere'. By implication therefore the Advisory Council of the Misuse of Drugs (ACMD) were discouraging general practitioners to work with drug users other than 'in a structured system under the direction and supervision of the consultant in charge who takes ultimate responsibility for patient care'.[13] This recommendation has of course changed, not just with the rise in numbers of drug users needing care, but also with the advent of the threat of HIV infection. The rise of HIV and AIDS amongst injecting drug users provided an urgency to deliver services and a realisation that the treatment of drug users could no longer be seen as predominantly the domain of specialist addiction psychiatrists.[14, 15]

As in the 1980s, leaders in the field were advocating general practice involvement. The ACMD in 1993 identified that GPs were the key to early and easy access to care for drug users, and that they were central to the overall strategy of reducing drug related harm. This report identified negative attitudes held by GPs and lack of training as the major barriers to effective GP involvement,[16] and went on to remind GPs of their contractual responsibilities to 'provide general medical services to all patients on their list, including drug users' and that 'they [GPs] should be encouraged to respond to the specific needs of this particular group'.

The Department of Health published the new *Guidelines on the Management of Drug Misuse and Dependence* (often referred to as the 'Orange Guidelines') in 1999 after a gap of nearly ten years adding its collective voice to the rights of drug users to receive appropriate care and stressing the responsibilities of all doctors to provide effective safe care.[17] The document offered a template for safe practice, in particular promoting shared care or collaborative working between different professional groups and between different levels of expertise.

The UK government's 1998 White Paper, *Tackling Drugs to Build a Better Britain*,[18] set out the government's ten-year strategy for tackling drug misuse. It had four key themes: prevention, treatment, reducing availability, and fighting drug-related crime. It emphasised the rights of drug misusers to receive treatment, including from primary care, and identified treatment in primary care as an important facet in delivery of this strategy. A key target was set: to increase participation of drug misusers in treatment by 66% by 2005 and by 100% by 2008. In recent years the Task Force, the Audit Commission and the Home Affairs Committee have all recommended an increase in the involvement of GPs to meet current treatment challenges.[19-21]

With a few notable exceptions[22, 23] it seemed, certainly in the 1990s, that GPs were slow in responding to these recommendations, although it is hardly surprising that faced with little or no training, no investment in primary care services, negative attitudes,[24] and fears of violence and of being overwhelmed,[25] that GPs were apparently largely disengaged with this patient group.

Measures to increase the response of GPs in the care of drug users

To engage GPs, policy makers have had to address a number of fundamental principles, these are:

▶ to provide role legitimacy

▶ to provide support

▶ to ensure that practitioners are trained and resourced.

Role legitimacy

This is perhaps the most important of these three principles. Without practitioners feeling they have a role to play in the care of drug users, no amount of additional resources, structures, or training will produce change. There is little doubt that GPs have a legitimate role, though for many this meant the provision of general medical services only (for example treatment of acute episodes of illness).

Throughout the 1980s and 1990s, a small cadre of GPs worked hard to reverse the lack-lustre response by GPs in providing anything other than general medical services only. These doctors, under the auspices of the Royal College of General Practitioners (RCGP), set up a national annual conference for primary care practitioners working with drug users, which will in 2005 celebrate its tenth anniversary. The conferences have always been oversubscribed and even with delegate capacity increased year on year capacity cannot match demand.

Through the conferences and other mechanisms, an informal network of support among primary care practitioners, in particular among GPs, has developed that provides information and shares good practice across the country. This informal network sowed the seeds for the current structure of RCGP regional leads, a national training programme, and a web-based resource and help line (www. smmgp.demon.co.uk).

Perhaps the turning point in the profession's acknowledging that it had a legitimate role to play in the care of drug users was the publication of a joint statement, in April 2000, from the two major organisations that represent the voice of general practice, the RCGP and the General Practitioners Committee (GPC) (a subcommittee of the British Medical Association). This statement reflects this shift in attitude (at least on paper) in primary care's involvement in the care of drug users.

The RCGP and GPC believe that GPs should offer appropriate care to all patients on their lists. Where patients have problems with substance abuse, appropriate care will include aspects of primary care normally provided by the practice health care team, shared care with other services and referral to other appropriate services. Certain GPs may develop particular expertise in the care of substance abusers, and the number and location of these doctors should, ideally, be sufficient to avoid substantial workload falling onto only a few GPs. In supporting the development of this expertise, the Health Departments must ensure the provision of appropriate training in this field; facilitate professional support; resource the adequate provision for support services, including specialist service; and offer appropriate financial additional remuneration for such work. (RCGP/GPC Policy Statement on care of substance abusers, 2000.)

Role support (shared care, GPs with special clinical interest, clinical guidelines)

Government policy, in relation to primary care/drug misuse treatment has concentrated on the provision of shared care to support GPs in their care of drug users. The Department of Health defined shared care as 'the joint participation of GPs and specialists (and other agencies as appropriate) in the planned delivery of care for patients with a substance misuse problem, informed by an enhanced information exchange beyond routine discharge and referral letters'.[26] It may involve the day-to-day management by the GP of a patient's medical needs in relation to his or her drug misuse. Such arrangements would make explicit which clinician was responsible for different aspects of a patient's treatment and care; they may include prescribing substitute drugs in appropriate circumstances. This can be considered as joint participation in the care of drug users that goes beyond the simple exchange of letters.

There are many models of shared care: most centre on liaison nurses providing GPs with a range of support depending on the needs of the GP, the complexity of the patient, and access to other services etc.[27] A joint working group of the Royal College of Psychiatrists and GPs concluded that effective shared care could be achieved if some or all of the following measures are in place: close contact between GP and specialist, integrated training, audit, locally agreed management protocols, and well defined responsibility for control and monitoring of prescribing.

In the shared treatment of drug users the following are practical examples currently in operation:

▸ Consultant-led specialist service with full-time medical facilitator and nursing support. Patients assessed and stabilised at a clinic and then referred to participating GPs for opiate and benzodiazepine prescribing with a treatment plan that involves regular contact with a named key worker. Random urine testing and sanctions for continued illicit drug use. Changes in medication negotiated with community drug worker and case conferences called to address complications that arise. The specialist service manages only a small number of patients with complex needs.

▶ Staged care with drug team led by consultant (psychiatrist, specialist GP, or professional allied to medicine) assessing and commencing treatment with central prescribing for an agreed limited period followed by GP taking over prescribing with support of a key worker attached to the practice or from specialist service. In some instances GP clinical assistants are involved in the assessments.

▶ Liaison team (led by consultant psychiatrist or GP with special clinical interest) with a team of suitably qualified staff (alcohol and drug specialists) employed by specialist provider. The team is based in primary care and facilitates and supports GPs to manage the treatment of drug users. The team is peripatetic and aims to enable the GPs to treat the users rather than members of the team taking over care themselves.[21]

▶ A 'one-stop' clinic led by specialist general practitioner and employing a range of additional services, such as psychologists social workers, drug and alcohol workers.[28] In some locations the GP sees referrals and carries out assessments on behalf of other GPs within a locality.[23] In this latter example, methadone maintenance clinics are run jointly by GPs and drug counsellors in two Glasgow practices. The patients are seen in separate clinics within general practice rather than during normal surgeries – which might otherwise inadvertently cause problems of stigmatisation and congregation of drug users. The GP is mainly involved in initial assessment of patients, stabilisation on methadone, and then with inter-current illness and serological testing.

The 1999 *Clinical Guidelines* defined three categories of doctor: the 'generalist', the 'specialised generalist' (defined as a practitioner whose work is not primarily concerned with drug misuse treatment, but who has developed a special interest in treating drug misusers), and the 'specialist' (defined as a practitioner who provides expertise, training and competence in drug misuse treatment as their main activity).

The Royal College of General Practitioners has recently recognised the role of general practitioner with special clinical interest in substance misuse. The growth of general practitioners with special clinical interest has added another layer to those able to support generalist practitioners in the shared care of drug users.[29] There are examples of GPs who are informally regarded as 'expert' within their own practice or immediate locality.[15, 30] What is new, and both exciting and potentially threatening, is that primary care organisations can now commission these doctors to provide care outside the confines of the practice. Trusts will be able to, according to local need and expertise, define the number of practitioners, specialty areas, terms and conditions, pay, and service level agreements of these doctors.

How these new roles develop and how they achieve the aims of reducing waiting times and provide fulfilling roles for GPs needs to be evaluated. Primary care organisations will need to understand and use the new expertise wisely to ensure that they are not merely replacing consultant specialist opinion with a cheaper, less experienced one, though mindful that GPs are able to provide specialist services themselves.[31]

Role adequacy

Few of those working with drug users have received any training in relevant areas. Lack of training inevitably leads to fear and prejudices, which in turn fosters negative responses towards this patient group. Lack of training also means that GPs are ill-prepared to understand the place of drugs in our society, particularly amongst young people. The amount of training medical students receive in substance misuse declined by half between 1987 and 1996 and has fallen again by 2004.[32] The most recent survey (2004) has shown that medical students were receiving on average six hours of formal training in substance misuse over their entire training.[33]

The Royal College of General Practitioners has developed a national training programme to meet the requirements of both the generalist and the special interest GP and in time it is hoped that every medical school will place drug misuse on its curriculum (Box 5.1).[34]

Box 5.1   **Royal College of General Practitioners National Drug Misuse Training Programme**

Training aimed at general practitioners, nurses, prison doctors, pharmacists, expert patients	
The training programme is in two parts, Certificate 1 and Certificate 2.	
Part 1	Certificate 1 is aimed at the generalist practitioner wishing to obtain training such that they will be able to identify, assess, refer, and provide harm reduction treatment. Certificate 1 is in two sections: section 1 e-learning (multiple choice questions based on case scenarios) and section 2 face-to-face day-long training delivering a common curriculum. Only by achieving a 70% score in section 1 and completing section 2 will the candidate be awarded Certificate Part 1
Part 2	Certificate 2 is designed for those having completed Part 1 or equivalent level and wishing to extend their training to that required to deliver care at practitioner with special interest level. The course is based on small, mentor-led master classes based on critical reading together with course work, ending in a viva

Special interest master classes	The RCGP provides a programme of special interest master classes, aimed at providing continued professional development for practitioners with special clinical interest

Does treatment in primary care work?

Research into the role played by GPs within this field is limited mainly to local rather than national (with virtually no international) study. The research available is now almost two decades old.[35-39] Most studies are reports of service development with little in respect of outcome. Paradoxically there are many studies looking at attitudes of GPs treating drug users and opinions on drug users being treated by their GP.

The only study comparing outcomes in general practice with those provided by specialist services was drawn from a sample of the National Treatment Outcome Research Study.[40] At six-month follow up similar improvements were observed in patients receiving methadone treatment within general practice and those treated at specialist services. Frequency of heroin use fell to less than half that at intake with significant reductions in the use of other drugs. The authors concluded, however, that these results could not be generalised as the general practices involved were atypical, in that five coordinated shared care for 35 other practices and two provided treatment to a large number of drug users.

Keen[41] reports that after one year of care provided by a primary care service, significant improvements in outcome were observed when measured in terms of reduction in risk-taking behaviour, consumption of illicit drugs (from urine analysis), criminal activity (from criminal records), and drug related deaths. When prescribing, GPs are less likely than specialist services to adhere to national guidelines and less likely to prescribe methadone solution and prescribe for daily dispensing.[42]

The cost of treating drug use in general practice is often assumed to be cheaper than in specialist services. This is an incorrect assumption. Providing methadone maintenance in Glasgow was costed at £2,030 per patient per year in the early 1990s. This was based on an average 20 minutes weekly of counsellor time and three minutes of GP time and included the cost of methadone and dispensing fees.[43]

Hutchinson and colleagues assessed the changes in drug related behaviour of a group of opioid dependent intravenous users who were being treated with oral methadone under supervised consumption as part of a shared care scheme. This one-year cohort study based in Glasgow recruited 204 patients and re-interviewed 73% at six months and 58% at six and twelve months. Twenty-nine per cent of the cohort was continuously on methadone for twelve months and this group showed the most significant improvements in drug related behaviour. The results from the total cohort showed substantial reductions in injecting behaviours and other drug use – crime, injecting related morbidity, and psychological dependence on drugs – with moderate improvement in social functioning. The results were comparable with those from specialist treatment settings and demonstrated the benefits of primary care treatment.[6]

The new general practice contract will drive costs up as payment will now be made to GPs for providing services to drug users on a patient-by-patient basis and to general practitioners with special interest to support these GPs through shared care. How these costs will compare with specialist services, however, are difficult to evaluate as primary care services tend to provide care to larger numbers of patients spread over a number of sites but to a less complex group with no significant co-morbidity.

Have things got better?

Since the first call to arms for GPs in the early 1980s, there has been a rapid expansion in the quality and quantity of care provided by GPs. Certainly in terms of numbers of drug users receiving treatment from general practitioners things have undoubtedly got better. The first national survey of GPs in 1985 found that only 19% of GPs had been consulted by an opioid user in the previous four weeks.[44]

A Scottish survey found that, although 60% of GPs sampled had seen and treated drug users, only three-fifths prescribe methadone within the UK recommended range.[45]

A more recent survey in 2001,[48] and using similar methods, found that half of respondents had seen an opiate user in the previous four weeks and half of these (25% of total) had prescribed some form of opioid substitution therapy, such as methadone or buprenorphine, to at least four patients, a doubling of the mean number from the 1985 survey.[44] Using national prescribing data, nearly three-quarters of a million items for methadone were prescribed by English GPs in 2002/3, representing nearly 30% of all controlled drug prescriptions for that year.

The 2001 survey found that doctors who work in urban or suburban areas are more likely to see opiate misusers, as are male doctors. Doctors seeing opioid users are more likely to describe themselves as more 'specialised', in receipt of local additional remuneration, and to have in place certain policies designed to limit some of the often cited problems such as being overwhelmed with opiate-using patients. Once seen, patients are more likely to be prescribed substitution therapies by 'specialised generalists', male GPs, GPs in receipt of local remuneration, and GPs who work in practices with specialised support. The importance of this kind of support has previously been identified as essential for engaging health professionals in work of this kind.[46, 47] See Tables 5.1 and 5.2.

Results from a 2001 survey of a random sample of English GPs and their involvement or otherwise in the care of drug users[48]

Table 5.1 **Survey question: which of the following applies to your practice?**

Practice policy	Yes		No		Don't Know	
	N	(%)	N	(%)	N	(%)
There is a policy for the management of opiate misusers in a formal shared care arrangement with specialist service (N=1500)	887	(59.1)	571	(38.1)	42	(2.8)
Care of opiate misusers is not part of the work of our practice (N=1316)	479	(36.4)	807	(61.3)	30	(2.3)
There is a limit on the number of opiate misusers who are patients at the practice (N=1178)	223	(18.9)	916	(77.8)	39	(3.3)
There is a limit on the hours during which opiate misusers can be seen by a doctor (N=1151)	114	(9.9)	1013	(88.0)	24	(2.1)

Table 5.2 **Comparison in policy between 1985 and 2001**

Variable	1985	2001
Proportion of GPs who saw at least 1 patient in the previous 4 weeks	19%	50.6% (1011/1997)
Mean number of patients per "active" (ie had seen at least one opiate misuser) GP in previous 4 weeks	2.0	4.08
Proportion of female patients	32% (107/329)	27% (924/3641)
Proportion of patients under 25 years of age	52%	47.2% (1577/3341)
Proportion of new attendees in previous 4 weeks	35% (114/329)	14.9% (519/3477)

Analysis from GP-prescribing data through the e-pact system indicates that an estimated 29,932 drug users were in treatment with GPs for the year 2001. Projected increases for 2004 are that 30,832 users will be in treatment. The percentage of GPs involved in shared care has risen from a mean of 20% across England in 2001/02 to over 35% in 2004/05 (see chapter 4).

Are there problems with GP involvement?

In response to a series of papers in a journal issue dedicated to primary care/drug misuse, Merrill and Ruben wrote a paper entitled 'Treating drug dependence in primary care: worthy ambition but flawed policy?'[49] It is clear therefore that not all would agree with the current drive towards increasing GPs' involvement and that primary care practitioners in the field of addiction need to take note of some of the anxieties raised by fellow GPs and by specialists. The evidence for or against GP involvement is deficient. Treatments given by GPs vary considerably and outcomes are inconsistent and ill defined. Large numbers of drug users are still unregistered and many GPs still do not wish to get involved in this field.

Specialist primary care practitioners

At the time of writing there is much debate amongst a senior cadre of GPs as to what constitutes a primary care addiction specialist. The term 'community consultant' was used in the 1993 Advisory Council of the Misuse of Drugs *AIDS and Drug Misuse Update* in an attempt to encourage GP involvement with drug users within a certain geographical area.[14]

If defined by GPs leading services – providing strategic direction, teaching, training, and supervising others – then there are certainly a small number of GPs around the country who provide this level of input. There are examples of GPs also providing care to patients with complex needs and providing specialist level prescribing interventions, such as injectable methadone and amfetamine substitution treatment.

There are other GPs who, in the absence of any psychiatrist addiction specialist, lead multidisciplinary teams and provide shared care to local GPs. These practitioners, as they exist today, are largely self-taught, developing their skills through clinical experience and developing their knowledge through self-directed learning and/or attendance at conferences. As their roles and responsibilities become better defined they can be used to lead shared care drug and alcohol services, providing support to practitioners with special interest and helping to provide effective evidence based care in primary and community settings.

To date there are around 35 clinicians – mostly GPs but with a smaller number of pharmacists and nurses who could be considered to be providing specialist addiction services. Taking just the GPs, these services vary from providing clinical and managerial leadership to what can only be described as a drug dependence service – with responsibility for providing drug misuse services to a primary care organisation geographical area.

Others limit their services only to drug users in contact with primary care services – so-called liaison or shared care services.

Yet others combine a mix of the two, offering services to primary care as well as providing specific care to, for example, pregnant women through liaison with obstetric services, or homeless patients through liaison with the voluntary sector. What distinguishes these doctors from GPs with special interest is their leadership and development roles and that they, on the whole, provide drug misuse services as a significant part of their working life – with only a few sessions being still in mainstream generalist general practice.

It is important that the definition of a specialist is not solely based on tautological criteria, for example, a specialist being one who provides specialist input or who sees large number of patients. Rather it is important that those who call themselves specialists base this definition on acquired skills, knowledge, and demonstrable competence in the field, albeit that these may be based around the provision of primary care specialist services rather than hospital based.

Conclusion

So what does the future hold for primary care drug misuse treatment? On the positive side, many GPs are willing to be involved in providing general medical care to drug misusers, with evidence of a considerable degree of untapped willingness to be involved. With appropriate support and funding, some of the remaining 'dormant' GPs might be stimulated into more action. Despite more than a decade of actively promoting the vital contribution of the primary care practitioner, however, there remains a substantial minority who remain opposed to such involvement. The new general practice contract, although being a vehicle for driving up standards, may not actually increase the numbers of GPs willing to participate, and the funding of services must remain a serious threat to any expansion.

Perhaps it is time to reverse decades of trying to increase numbers and concentrate on consolidating quality. A recent Audit Commission study into community-based drug treatment services noted, 'GPs will continue to be a key resource in the treatment of drug misuse. The current shift towards primary care means that new partnerships with specialist services make good sense.'[1]

There is a need to provide better coordinated services for drug users, which match their needs. To a large degree GPs have responded to the challenge of the management of drug users and collectively are undoubtedly the backbone of drug misuse treatment services, including the provision of substitute medication. The new Modernising Medical Careers agenda now gives GPs in training many opportunities to extend their training into the substance misuse field, though only time will tell how many of tomorrow's doctors will take up the challenge.

References

1. Audit Commission. *Focus on General Practice in England*. London: Audit Commission, 2002.

2. Gerada C. *Primary Care Service for Mental Health*. In: Ramsay R, Gerada C, Mars S, Szmukler G. (Eds). Mental Illness. A Handbook for Carers. London: Jessica Kingsley, 2001.

3. Department of Health. *The New NHS: Modern, Dependable*. London: HMSO, 1997.

4. Department of Health. *The NHS Plan*. London: HMSO, 2000.

5. Bennett T, Wright R. Opioid users: attitudes towards the use of NHS Clinics, general practitioners and private doctors. *Br J Addiction* 1986; **81**: 757–63.

6. Hutchinson S, Taylor A, Gruer L, *et al*. One year follow up of opiate injectors treated with oral methadone in a GP-centred programme. *Addiction* 2000; **95**(7): 1055–68.

7. Gerada C. Drug Misuse and Primary care in the New NHS. *Drugs: Education, Prevention and Policy* 2000; **7**(3): 213–23.

8. World Health Organization. Primary care of mental illness. Geneva: WHO, 1973.

9. Medical working group in drug dependence. *Guidelines of good clinical practice in the treatment of drug misuse*. London: DHSS, 1984.

10. Department of Health, Scottish Office and Welsh Office. *Drug Misuse and Dependence*. London: HMSO, 1991.

11. Stimson G V, Oppenheimer E. *Heroin Addiction: Treatment Controls in Britain*. London: Tavistock, 1982.

12. Interdepartmental Committee. *Drug Addiction*. Second Report. London: HMSO, 1965.

13. Advisory Council on the Misuse of Drugs. *Treatment and Rehabilitation*. London: HMSO, 1982.

14. Advisory Council on the Misuse of Drugs. *Aids and Drug Misuse Part 1*. London: DHSS, 1988.

15. Advisory Council on the Misuse of Drugs. *Aids and Drug Misuse Part 2*. London: DoH, 1989.

16. Advisory Council on the Misuse of Drugs. *Aids and Drug Misuse Update*. London: DoH, 1993.

17. Department of Health, The Scottish Office Department of Health, Welsh Office, Department of Health and Social Services, Northern Ireland. *Drug Misuse and Dependence – Guidelines on Clinical Management*. London: DoH, 1999.

18. Department of Health. *Tackling Drugs to Build a Better Britain: The Government's 10-Year Strategy for Tackling Drug Misuse*. London: HMSO, 1998.

19. Home Affairs Committee. *The Government's Drugs Policy: Is It Working?* Vol 3. London: HMSO, 2002.

20. Audit Commission. *Changing Habits. the Commissioning and Management of Community Drug Treatment Services for Adults*. London: Audit Commission, 2002 (available at: www.audit-commission.gov.uk).

21. Department of Health. *The Task Force to Review Services for Drug Misuses*. Report of an Independent Survey of Drug Treatment Services in England. London: DoH, 1996.

22. Robertson J. The practical business of treatment 2. Treatment of drug misuse in general practice setting. *Br J Addiction* 1989; **84**: 377–80.

23. Gerada C, Barrett C, Betterton J, Tighe J. The Consultancy Liaison Addiction Service: the first five years of an integrated, primary care based community drug and alcohol team. *Drugs: Education, Prevention and Policy* 2000; **7**: 251–6.

24. McKeganey N. Shadowland: General practitioners and the treatment of opiate abusing patients. *Br J Addiction* 1988; **83**, 373–86.

25. Wilson P, Watson R, Ralston G E. Methadone maintenance in general practice patients, workload and outcomes. *BMJ* 1994: **309**: 641–4.

26. Department of Health Circular EL (95) 114 Reviewing Shared Care Arrangements for Drug Misusers. London: DoH, 1996.

27. Gerada C, Farrell, M. Shared care. In: Robertson R. (Ed). *Management of Drug Users in the Community: a Practical Handbook*. London: Arnold, 1998; 328–52.

28. Cohen J, Schamroth A. General practice management of drug misusers. *The Practitioner* 1989; 1471–4.

29. Royal College of General Practitioners. *General Practitioners with Special Interests*. London: RCGP, 2001 (available at: www.rcgp.org.uk/recgp/corporate/responde/nhsplan/Gpspecialinterests).

30. Carnwarth T, Gabbay M, Barnard J. A share of the action. General practitioner involvement in drug misuse treatment in Greater Manchester. *Drugs; Education, Prevention and Policy* 2000; **7**: 235–50.

31. Lawrence S. Models of primary care for substance misusers: St Martins Practice, Chapletown Leeds – secondary provision in a primary care setting. *Drugs, Education, Prevention and Policy* 2000; **7**: 279–91.

32. Crome I B. The trouble with training; substance misuse education in British medical schools revisited, what are the issues? *Drugs: Education, Prevention and Policy* 1999; **6**: 111–23.

33. Crome I B, Shaikh M (in press). Undergraduate medical school education in Britain III: Can medical students drive change? *Drugs: Education, Prevention and Policy*.

34. Gerada C, Murnane M, The Royal College of General Practitioners Certificate in Drug Misuse. *Drugs: Education, Prevention and Policy* 2003; **10(4)**: 369–79.

35. Bury J K, Ross A, van Teijlingen E, *et al*. Lothian general practitioners, HIV infection and drug misuse: epidemiology, experience and confidence 1988–1993. *Health Bull (Edinb)* 1996; **54**: 258–69.

36. Deehan A, Taylor C, Strang J. The general practitioner, the drug misuser, and the alcohol misuser: major differences in general practitioner activity, therapeutic commitment, and 'shared care' proposals. *Br J Gen Pract* 1997; **47**: 705–09.

37. Davies A, Huxley P. Survey of general practitioners' opinions on treatment of opiate users. *BMJ* 1997; **314**: 1173–4.

38. Martin E, Canavan A, Butler R. A decade for caring for drug users entirely within general practice. *Br J Gen Pract* 1998; **48**: 1679–82.

39. Hutchinson S, Taylor A, Gruer L, *et al*. One year follow up of opiate injectors treated with oral methadone in a GP centred programme. *Addiction* 2000; **95(7)**: 1055–68.

40. Gossop M, Marsden J, Stewart D, *et al*. Methadone treatment practices and outcomes for opiate addicts treated in drug clinics and in general practice: results from the National Treatment Outcome Study. *Br J Gen Pract* 1999; **49**: 31–4.

41. Keen J. Primary care treatment of drug users: the Sheffield experience. *The Journal of Primary Care Mental Health* 2001; **5 (1)**: 4–7.

42. Strang J, Sheridan J. Effect of government recommendations on methadone prescribing in southeast England: a comparison of 1995 and 1997 surveys. *BMJ* 1998; **317**: 1489–90.

43. Wilson P, Watson R, Ralston G E. Methadone maintenance in general practice: patients, workload, and outcomes. *BMJ* 1994; **309**: 641–4.

44. Glanz A, Taylor C. Findings of a national survey of the role of general practitioners in the treatment of opiate misuse: extent of contact with opiate misusers. *BMJ* 1986; **293**: 427–30.

45. Matheson C, Pitcairn J, Bond C M, *et al*. General practice management of illicit drug users in Scotland: a national survey. *Addiction* 2003; **98**: 119–26.

46. Weinrich M, Stuart M. Provision of methadone treatment in primary care medical practices: review of the Scottish experience and implications for US policy. *JAMA* 2000; **283**: 1343–8.

47. Matheson C, Bond C M, Hickey F. Prescribing and dispensing for drug misusers in primary care: current practice in Scotland. *Family Practice* 1999; **16**: 375–9.

48. Sheridan J, Hunt C, Kerr B, *et al.* Caring for opiate misusers: results from the 2001 national survey of general practitioners in England and Wales. Submitted for publication 2004.

49. Merrill J, Ruben S. Treating drug dependence in primary care: worthy ambition but flawed policy? *Drugs, Education, Prevention and Policy* 2000; **7**: 203–1.

CHAPTER 6

The role of the nurse

Jane Haywood and David Harding-Price

Introduction

The role of nursing within modern health care is expanding all the time. The aim of this chapter is to offer the reader an overview of the clinical areas most likely to involve substance users, some information about the National Treatment Agency's 'models of care', and an outline of the role of the nurse in caring for substance misusers in primary care. The complicated issue of nurse prescribing will also be discussed.

It is recognised that there are a wide range of nurses working in primary care from the practice nurse based in the surgery, to the district nurse, health visitor, and community psychiatric nurse working in patient's homes, to the school nurse and the occupational health nurse based in places of work. All of these nurses can have an input into the clinical life of a substance user.

For years now nurses have played a pivotal role in the care of drug and alcohol users supporting medical practitioners in the management of these patients. As health care enters the 21st century nurses and nursing have a range of opportunities, extending from the new General Medical Services contract and the NHS Plan, to develop skills in specialist areas, be that substance misuse, diabetes, or care of the elderly.

Consequently it is an exciting time of opportunity for nurses working in this field, with nursing roles expanding and changing. There are accredited training programmes and modular packages to suit nurses, wherever they may be working.

Managing drug and alcohol users brings into play many of the core components of the role of the nurse, as defined by the International Council of Nurses (1992):

▶ provider of care

▶ counsellor/therapist

▶ educator/resource

▶ advocate

▶ promoter of health

▶ researcher

▶ supervisor/leader

▶ consultant.

Models of care and the role of the nurse

The National Treatment Agency's overall remit is to: 'increase the availability, capacity and effectiveness of treatment for drug misuse in England … and to double the number of people in effective, well-managed treatment from 100,000 in 1998 to 200,000 in 2008'.[1]

From a commissioning and service delivery perspective, services are divided into tiers, 1–4. Depending on their level of expertise, nurses have a role to play in service provision at all of these levels (see Table 6.1).

Tier 1: personal and general medical support
vaccination/communicable diseases
sexual health/health promotion
screening for blood-borne viruses

Tier 2: drug-related advice and information
open access or drop-in services
motivational interviewing/brief interventions
liaison with drug misuse services for acute medical
    and psychiatric sectors
specific assessment and care management

Tier 3: drug specialist care planning and coordination
structured care, planned counselling, and therapy options
community-based detoxification services
community-based prescribing
stabilisation and maintenance prescribing
liaison with drug treatment services

In addition to these roles, for those practices that are providing either a local or a nationally enhanced service for substance misusers this provides the opportunity for primary care practitioners to develop a variety of models to provide seamless care to patients within their surgeries.

The generalist nurse

The 1999 Clinical Guidelines discuss the role of the generalist:

Their skills and techniques range from assessment of drug misusers, counselling, and carrying out other treatment procedures, to health education and teaching. Their clinical and treatment role in drug misuse services is as varied as it is essential.

They also discuss the role of the GP:

... utilizing shared care, places an emphasis on developing close links between the primary health care team and specialist staff in order to:

▸ enhance GP skills in the detection and management of patients with drug misuse problems

▸ reduce referrals to the specialist services for patients with less complex medical needs and hence enable the patient to be treated in primary care for as long as possible

▸ encourage selective referrals to specialist services for patients with more complex needs and problems.

All nurses working in primary care should have a foundation level of knowledge regarding substance misuse. The Royal College of General Practitioners' National Drug Misuse Training Programme Certificate Part 1 can provide any nurse working in primary care with the necessary general knowledge and skills to work with this patient population.

The practice nurse may be the first point of contact users have when they register with the practice. Drug (and alcohol) use in the young homeless is so prevalent that it should be considered to be present until proven otherwise; the nurse can play a vital role in encouraging the young person to seek help.

The new patient screening session is a good place to ask about drug use – obviously only after rapport has been established. We generally ask the question after asking about smoking and drinking behaviour, as for example, 'Do you smoke, how much do you drink in an average week, what about other drugs?' It is useful to remember that before screening for any lifestyle issue it is important to offer the patient a choice before answering. This may seem a paradox, on the one hand trying to offer help and on the other giving permission for non-disclosure. The implications of a record (even in one's youth) of illicit drug use, however, can be significant for future mortgage, life insurance, and employment opportunities and these should be considered and shared with the patient.

Nevertheless, nurses have an important role in prevention. Simple advice from nurses during routine care has been shown to be effective in smoking cessation.[2]

The nurse with special interest

Nurses who develop a special interest in drug or alcohol misuse often start the process of developing a local service within a surgery. Nurses who take on this role should first ensure that they have gained more than basic knowledge about drug or alcohol misuse.

Such nurses can develop early practice interventions, for example, health promotion for safer injecting or completing more complex assessments using recognised assessment tools.[3-5] Nurses working at this level can also be instrumental in developing in-house support for users, for example immunisation of users' children or production of a leaflet providing information about local services. The nurse will also probably have a working relationship with the local secondary drugs/alcohol teams. They are in the best position to refer patients to the most appropriate local service.

Nurses with special interest can also provide other functions including:

▸ improving the skills of GPs and primary care nurses in identifying and managing patients with drug and alcohol related problems, by training and the development of written material

▸ enabling drug and alcohol misusers to access primary health care services

▸ improving the quality of care these patients receive by supporting the implementation of the clinical guidelines

▸ redistributing the care of drug users more equitably across primary care group patches.

Table 6.1 **The different roles that nurses can play within a primary care setting**

Nursing process	Assessing	Planning	Implementing	Evaluation
Generalist nurses	Providing new patient health screen and identifying problems, brief intervention, health promotion	Referring to GP and local drug treatment services	Following up with viral screening and vaccinations, wound care management, family planning	Monitoring audit trail of vaccinations and viral screening
Nurse with special interest	In addition, providing harm reduction information, assessing suitability for primary care treatment, obtaining urine for drug screen	Liaison with specialist agencies and community pharmacist, referring to GP and local drug treatment services	Working with the GP. Goal-setting, support stabilisation, referral to tertiary services, relapse prevention, supporting drug and alcohol detox	Regular monitoring of treatment and achievement of goal with patient and GP
Specialist nurse	In-depth assessment, formulating treatment plan, working with complex needs	Patient contracts and medication concordance, developing a clinical management plan, potential to prescribe independently and supplementarily	Taking the lead in regular patient contact, assessing and changing treatment where necessary and in liaison, patient involvement in service, crisis intervention	Auditing treatment, patient satisfaction surveys, implementing changes to practice protocols, attending Share Care Monitoring Groups (SCMG)

The addiction specialist nurse and clinical nurse specialist

These nurses have developed their interest in substance misuse beyond the provision of localised care in their surgery and most are able to develop their service to a whole locality. Nurses have been a major component of the alcohol and drug addiction workforce for at least two decades. Rassool defined addiction nursing as 'a clinical specialty concerned with the care and treatment interventions aimed at those individuals whose health problems are directly related to the use and misuse of psychoactive substances and to other addictive behaviour such as eating disorders and gambling'.[6]

Specialist addiction nurses working in primary care are ideally placed to respond quickly and meet the needs of general practitioners and other primary care staff. Drawing on previous experience from specialist services, relevant post-registration training, and continuous clinical supervision, such nurses are essential practitioners in supporting and developing shared care often across a wide geographical area.

There are a number of models in which specialist nurses can support the shared care of drug and/or alcohol misusers in primary care settings. Many addiction nurses work within a liaison and consultancy model where the nurse meets the GP to discuss and agree the management plan of patients under shared care. This aims to support the GPs in the management of their patients rather than the nurses taking over the care themselves. The nurse can also facilitate linking the patient and GP with an appropriate agency for continuing non-medical support, being flexible to meet the requirements of the GP.

Jacksley et al.[7] described a clinical nurse specialist service in one London borough, consisting of a five-point model for the role of the specialist nurse in primary care:

▸ one-off expert substance misuse/health assessment with recommendations for treatment

▸ shared care: formal therapeutic package, leading to stabilisation or abstinence, with referral to specialist services (detoxification or rehabilitation if necessary)

▸ continuous support: reviews monthly, two-monthly, and stabilised at three-monthly intervals; rapid response if GP feels client needs to be seen in the interval between review meetings

▸ on-site and immediate information exchange and advice while in treatment at the practice

▸ fast tracking into specialist treatment services for clients who have encountered a crisis.

Nurse prescribing

This is a complex area and one that is still being reviewed and revised, especially in the light of the Shipman Inquiry. Expanding prescribing rights to nurses seems to be a move in a sensible direction. Experienced and trained nurses should be able to provide the whole range of interventions available to doctors, which therefore should include prescribing controlled drugs. To this effect the present UK government is proposing to amend the Misuse of Drugs Regulations 2001 to allow nurses (and pharmacists) to prescribe controlled drugs under a mechanism called Supplementary Prescribing: this allows health professionals other than doctors and dentists to prescribe medicines for individual patients under a clinical management plan, which in essence means that nurses can continue, and make amendments to, prescribing regimens previously agreed by a doctor (independent prescriber). The aim of nurse, extended nurse, and supplementary prescribing is to benefit patients and make better use of the professional health-care workforce. They should offer patients improved access to healthcare staff, with greater convenience as well as increased choice.

Although the legislative changes to enable nurses to prescribe first came into force in 1992, national implementation did not occur until 1998. Nurses were allowed to prescribe only from a limited formulary after completing an appropriate course. Since 1999, preparation for this training has been included in all training for district nurses and health visitors. Prescribing is now an integral role of all district nurses, health visitors, and some practice nurses, and their prescribing status is noted on the professional register held by the Nursing and Midwifery Council. See Table 6.2.

Extended formulary nurse prescribing

Since April 2002, nurses who have successfully completed a specific and longer programme of preparation and training – and have been assessed as having reached the required standard – have been able to prescribe a range of medicines. This includes all general sales list and pharmacy medicines that GPs can currently prescribe, plus a specific list of about 180 prescription only medicines, without obtaining permission from a doctor, to treat around 80 medical conditions. This list is known as the Nurse Prescribers' Extended Formulary. The formulary was expanded in January 2004, following amendment to the Misuse of Drugs Regulations by the Misuse of Drugs (Amendment) (No.3) Regulations 2003 in October 2003, to include six controlled drugs. These were midazolam, diazepam, and lorazepam (schedule 4 controlled drugs to be used for palliative care only), and codeine, co-phenotrope, and dihydrocodeine (schedule 5 controlled drugs). The range of medical conditions that nurses are currently able to prescribe for are set out in the *British National Formulary* (BNF) and *Drug Tariff*. District nurse and health visitor prescribers are not permitted to prescribe controlled drugs unless they have also qualified as nurse prescribers.

When the Advisory Council on the Misuse of Drugs (ACMD) approved the inclusion of the six controlled drugs in November 2001, It recommended the following two provisos:

▶ that all prospective nurse prescribers should receive adequate and appropriate training in the use of the medicines, their potential for misuse, and on how to avoid being manipulated by patients who are addicts

▶ introduction of appropriate legislative provisions to deal with inappropriate prescribing by nurses similar to those that apply to doctors and dentists.

In September 2003 the Committee on Safety of Medicines proposed that the Nurse Prescribers' Extended Formulary should be extended further to allow nurses to prescribe the following additional controlled drugs:

for palliative care:

▶ morphine sulphate

▶ buprenorphine hydrochloride

▶ dextropropoxyphene hydrochloride

▶ diamorphine hydrochloride

▶ dihydrocodeine tartrate

▶ fentanyl

▶ meptazinol

▶ methadone hydrochloride

▶ nalbuphine hydrochloride

▶ oxycodone hydrochloride

▶ pethidine hydrochloride

▶ tramadol

for suspected myocardial infarction:

▶ diamorphine and morphine.

Patient Group Direction (PGD)

The Patient Group Direction scheme has been operating in the NHS since August 2000, and in the private health sector and the prison service since April 2003. Initially it related to all medicines other than controlled drugs.

The Misuse of Drugs (Amendment) (No.3) Regulations 2003 in October 2003 allowed for the scheme to be extended to including the following controlled drugs:

▶ diamorphine for the treatment of cardiac pain by nurses in accident and emergency departments and coronary care units in hospital only

▸ all controlled drugs listed in schedule 4 (except anabolic steroids) and schedule 5 of the 2001 Regulations by the following registered healthcare professionals: nurses, paramedics, health visitors, midwives, ophthalmic opticians, chiropodists, orthoptists, physiotherapists, and radiographers (as set out in schedule 8 of the Regulations).

The recommendation was made with the following caveat: that the use of patient group direction for controlled drugs should be carefully monitored and those authorised to supply by means of patient group direction should receive adequate training on how to avoid being manipulated by addict patients. Injectable forms of controlled drugs for treatment of addiction are excluded.

Supplementary prescribing

The Department of Health implemented legislation on 4 April 2003 to enable nurses and pharmacists who had completed an approved programme of training and preparation to prescribe prescription only medicines, pharmacy medicines, and general sale list medicines.

Independent nurse prescribers under the auspices of the Extended Nurse Prescribing Formulary (ENPF) scheme do not have the status of independent prescribers for the purposes of supplementary prescribing. Supplementary prescribing is not restricted to specific medical conditions but to an agreed treatment plan for an individual patient. Legislation details the particulars to be contained in the clinical management plan (e.g. patient's details, conditions to be treated, medicinal products which can be prescribed, and when the patient should be referred back to the independent prescriber) and requires supplementary prescribers to have access to the patient's medical records. The clinical management plan must be devised in agreement with the patient.

Education and training and registration for supplementary prescribers

Nurses and pharmacists who wish to become supplementary prescribers must complete an accredited education and training programme. The programme comprises a least 28 days' educational training provided by an accredited university, with an additional 12 days' learning in practice supervised by a medical practitioner.

Nurses and pharmacists who wish to train as prescribers need to:

▸ establish a prescribing partnership with a medical practitioner

▸ obtain the agreement of the local hospital trust or primary care trust that a supplementary prescribing partnership will meet a local service need

- ▸ apply to the local Workforce Development Confederation for funding
- ▸ on completion of training, register with the Nursing and Midwifery Council or Royal Pharmaceutical Society as a supplementary prescriber.

Private prescriptions

Nurses who are trained to prescribe from the Nurse Prescribers' Extended Formulary are able to issue private prescriptions for any of the medicines in the BNF. As with prescriptions issued on the NHS, nurses must restrict their prescribing to the medical conditions listed in the BNF and *Drug Tariff*.

Supplementary prescribers may also issue private prescriptions for any medicines covered by the clinical management plan.

Accountability and professional responsibility

Independent nurse prescribers, whether operating within or outside the NHS, are clinically responsible and professionally accountable for the care of their patients and their own actions. Where a nurse is appropriately trained and qualified as an independent prescriber, and prescribes as part of his or her nursing duties with the consent of the employer, the employer may also be held vicariously responsible for the nurse's actions. The Department of Health's *Guide to Implementation of Independent Nurse Prescribing*[8] advises all nurse prescribers to ensure that they have professional indemnity insurance for their prescribing activities, for example through membership of a professional organisation or trade union.

A nurse prescriber who prescribes outside the medical conditions that are covered in the BNF, *Drug Tariff*, and Department of Health guide, or who as a supplementary nurse prescriber works outside the patient's clinical management plan, could be subject to both disciplinary proceedings by the employer and action by the Nursing and Midwifery Council should a charge of professional misconduct follow. If a prescription only medicine is involved, the nurse could also be subject to legal sanction under the Medicines Act.

Support for nurses

The Association of Nurses in Substance Abuse was founded in 1983 by a group of addictions nurses to bring together nurses working in isolation in the drugs and alcohol field. It is a membership organisation, which encourages networking and sharing of ideas and holds an annual residential conference. In addition, local regional meetings take place throughout the year. The association is open to any nurse whose work brings them into contact with patients who use any substance.

The Royal College of Nursing's Mental Health Practice Forum provides all forum members with a quarterly newsletter that contains issues relating to mental health. Following the amalgamation of a number of forums some years ago substance misuse became part of this forum. Members of the Royal College of Nursing can also gain access to a wider professional knowledge base to enable them to develop their own personal practice.

Table 6.2 **Nurse prescribing**

Role	Definition
Independent prescriber	A clinician responsible for the assessment of patients with a diagnosed condition and for decisions about clinical management required, including prescribing
Supplementary prescriber	This was initially defined as a clinician who takes over the continuing care of a patient, which may include prescribing, after initial assessment of an independent prescriber. The final definition has been changed from that used in the consultation document to make it clear that supplementary prescribers (and independent prescribers) have responsibility for their prescribing
Supplementary prescribing	A voluntary partnership between an independent prescriber (a doctor or dentist) and a supplementary prescriber (a nurse, midwife, or pharmacist) to implement an agreed patient-specific clinical management plan, with the patient's agreement. The plan is to be drawn up, following diagnosis of the patient, by the independent prescriber following consultation and agreement between the independent and supplementary prescribers. The scheme applies to both the NHS and private healthcare sector. The supplementary prescriber can, in accordance with the clinical plan, prescribe any prescription only medicines, or, if the product is for parenteral administration, either administer it or give directions for its administration. The exceptions are controlled drugs and unlicensed medicines, although supplementary prescribers could prescribe licensed medicines 'off-label', i.e. for an unlicensed condition or where the unlicensed medicines are part of a clinical trial, which has a clinical trial certificate. A supplementary prescriber's status can be checked against the register held by the supplementary prescriber's professional registration
Nurse prescriber	A person who: (a) is registered in Part 1 or 2 of the professional register and (b) against whose name is recorded in the professional register an annotation signifying that s/he is qualified to prescribe drugs, medicines, and appliances to patients

continued over

Role	Definition
Extended formulary nurse prescriber	A person who: (a) is a first level nurse, (b) against whose name is recorded in the professional register an annotation signifying that s/he is qualified to prescribe drugs, medicines, and appliances from the ENPF
Patient group direction (PGD)	A written direction relating to supply and administration, or administration only, of a prescription only medicine to persons generally (subject to specified exclusions), signed by a doctor or dentist and a pharmacist. There are three main types of PGD: (a) that allows authorised healthcare professionals to supply medicines on behalf of an NHS body, (b) to assist a doctor or dentist providing primary NHS services, and (c) where an NHS body authorises the use of a PGD for the supply of a prescription only medicine by a named person lawfully conducting a retail pharmacy business. In addition, supply of prescription only medicines under a PGD can be made on behalf of an independent clinic / hospital or medical agency, a prison service or a police force

Additional reading

Rassool G H. (Ed). *Substance Use and Misuse: Nature, Context and Clinical Interventions.* Oxford: Blackwell Science, 1998.

References

1. National Treatment Agency. *Models of Care for Treatment of Adult Drug Misusers.* London: NTA, 2002.

2. Lancaster T, Stead L, Silagy C, Sowden A. Effectiveness of interventions to help people stop smoking: findings from the Cochrane Library. *BMJ* 2000; **321**:355–8.

3. Peterson T, McBride A. *Working with substance misusers.* London: Routledge, 2002; 84–91.

4. Rassool G H. *Substance Use and Misuse.* Oxford: Blackwell Science, 1998; 100–4.

5. Department of Health. *Drug Misuse and Dependence: Guidelines on Clinical Management.* London: DoH, 1999; 19–21.

6. Rassool G H. Addiction nursing – towards a new paradigm: the United Kingdom experience. In: Rassool G H, Gafoor M. (Eds). *Addiction Nursing: Perspectives on Professional and Clinical Practices.* Cheltenham: Stanley Thornes, 1997.

7. Jacksley H, Dicker A, Coyne P. GP contract killing you? Time to call a nurse. *Drugs and Alcohol Today* 2004; **4(2)**: 15–18.

8. Department of Health. *Extending independent nurse prescribing within the NHS in England: a guide for implementation.* 2nd Edition. London: DoH, 2004.

CHAPTER 7

The management of drug misuse in primary care: exploring wider opportunities in community pharmacy

Diana Kay Roberts and Janie Sheridan

IN THIS CHAPTER

Introduction ‖ Pharmacists and the management of drug users ‖ Areas of health care where pharmacists can have an impact ‖ Delivering services to drug users ‖ Prescribing services ‖ Supplementary prescribing ‖ Pharmacist prescribing ‖ Information and advice to drugs services ‖ How can pharmacists take on additional roles?

Introduction

This chapter aims to explore the roles community pharmacists can have when treating drug users that go beyond those such as dispensing substitution therapies and the provision of needle exchange.

Pharmacists do not need reminding of their skills and the potential for interventions that they have in addition to their traditional role of dispensing medicines. Pharmacists, possibly even more so than general practitioners, are able to provide multiple brief interventions to patients and often, especially where patients find it hard to access primary care services, are able to provide a first point of contact with the rest of the health services. The new pharmacy contracts will help to consolidate the pharmacist's role as a diagnostician, prescriber, and manager of long-term chronic conditions. Under the new arrangements, pharmacists, like general practitioners, will be paid according to the type and quality of care they provide and will be able to develop special interest areas using their new flexibilities to provide local pharmaceutical services to specific populations of patients. The challenge for community pharmacists is the re-engineering of everyday practice to incorporate the many elements of the extended role against a background of increasing prescription volumes and patient expectation.[1]

Pharmacists and the management of drug users

Traditionally the dispensing of medicines has dominated the role of community pharmacists. With regard to the management of drug misuse this has included dispensing prescriptions for methadone mixture to drug users and, since the mid-1990s, has involved supplying clean injecting equipment and health promotion literature by means of pharmacy based needle exchange schemes.

Since the publication in 1999 of the clinical guidelines,[2] increasing emphasis has been placed on the roles that both community and hospital pharmacists can play in the care and treatment of people in the community who have problems with their drug use. As noted in the guidelines, community pharmacists provide a significant point of contact as part of primary health care services and have regular (often daily) contact with the patient. Hence their role in the care of drug users is crucial, and communication in both directions between pharmacists and other health professionals should be encouraged. Research confirms that at least 50% of community pharmacists are involved in the provision of pharmacotherapies such as methadone for opiate dependent patients,[3,4] and in England and Wales that almost one in five provide needle exchange services.[4]

While pharmacists have embraced these roles, they also have an opportunity to expand them to the management of a wider range of health issues relating to problem drug use. It is timely for pharmacists to consider providing care beyond dispensing and needle exchange, given the contact that they have with patients or potential patients. For example, a drug user not in treatment may attend a pharmacist for clean injecting equipment maybe weekly, sometimes more often, offering numerous opportunities for the provision of health promotion advice and information. A patient in receipt of a methadone prescription may attend the pharmacist, albeit briefly, every weekday for many weeks or months. For this patient, the pharmacist represents the main health professional contact, and for the pharmacist even this brief daily contact can provide ample opportunities for the delivery of extended health care.

The success of extending the role of pharmacists in this area of practice will depend on their becoming more proactive and innovative. In particular they will need to work in collaboration with other key professionals (health, social work, drug services). Pharmacists are so used to working in isolation that they often overlook the potential benefits to themselves and their patients that working in an integrated way with the patient and all those involved in their care and treatment can provide. Again, the opportunities envisaged in the nGMS and new pharmacy contracts may facilitate better collaborative working between health professionals.

Community pharmacists are trained to take a holistic approach when dealing with patients, are in a position to respond to requests from patients for medications to relieve symptoms of self-limiting conditions that are presented to them in the pharmacy, and are able to prescribe both general sales list and pharmacy medicines, where appropriate, as well as providing any necessary advice. They are in a prime position to refer patients as necessary to a GP, dentist, accident and emergency department, or drug service. Finally, because they are situated in the community and have contact with their patients/customers when they are well, as well as when they are ill, they have the opportunity to follow up patients and may therefore be a valuable initial contact point when a relapse occurs.

In practice, patients with chronic long-term disorders probably have as a good a relationship with their local pharmacist as they do with their general practitioner. The extent to which pharmacists can effectively intervene in patient care, however, even to alter or suggest alterations to treatment regimens, is limited by lack of access to patients' medical records, and access to the details of their involvement with other relevant agencies. They may therefore be limited in their ability to recognise events and conditions that require referral to or from other agencies or treatment providers.

The rest of this chapter will consider a number of innovative ways in which management of drug misuse in the community can be expanded to benefit patients and to optimise their care. Two approaches will be taken: the first will explore areas of health care that are of particular relevance to those with problem drug use, and the second will look at other processes and activities that may facilitate the provision of a more comprehensive system of care for patients.

Areas of health care where pharmacists can have an impact

Management of minor ailments schemes

It is important for the pharmacist to recognise that patients on a substitute medication programme for the treatment of substance misuse, and those utilising needle exchange services, may also experience concurrent self-limiting diseases or minor ailments. Requests for the supply of over-the-counter products to treat such conditions may be genuine rather than a ploy to obtain medicines that can enhance illicitly obtained psychoactive substances.

Community pharmacists are ideally placed to develop guidelines and protocols for the supply and/or sale of any necessary treatments and to ensure that the medications proposed do not interact with prescribed methadone, buprenorphine, or other treatment medicines. With the development of minor ailment schemes, which will allow pharmacists to supply such remedies as part of the NHS in specified circumstances, it is essential that patients on drug treatment programmes are not inappropriately excluded from such developments.

The treatment of minor ailments by pharmacists has been a feature of the daily routine of community pharmacy for many generations. Clinical governance issues and the need for pharmacists to use evidence-based practice when responding to requests from the public mean that such requests are now handled in a professional and considered manner. Medicines counter staff are required to undertake specific training and to refer requests to the pharmacists as appropriate.

Pilot schemes undertaken in several primary care trust areas have demonstrated that community pharmacists can help to shift the management of minor ailments from the care of the GP to the community pharmacy and hence reduce the GP's workload.[5] Research indicates, however, that patients on a methadone programme may be refused access to self-medication and treatment for self-limiting conditions such as coughs, colds, headaches, or sleep-disturbances because it is assumed that their requests for antihistamines, decongestants, or analgesics are not genuine.[6,7] It is important to recognise that methadone and buprenorphine patients are not immune to coughs, colds, and headaches. It would be beneficial for such conditions to be treated appropriately by the pharmacist supplying the substitute medication rather than that the patient seeks such medication elsewhere, where the counter staff and/or pharmacists are not aware of the patient's medication history.

Dental health

Research has shown that drug users suffer numerous problems with their teeth yet they often have trouble accessing dental care owing to fear of pain, fear of stigmatisation, previous bad experiences, and cost of treatment.[8-10] Dental problems may result as a consequence of drug use, for example, bruxism caused by stimulant use, or as a result of the lifestyle that is often associated with problematic drug use, or from eating high calorific sugary foods, or having poor general diet, bad dental hygiene, and poor access to health care when problems arise, such as dental abscesses or cavities. Furthermore, opiates may mask dental pain, something that becomes apparent only when the patient stops using opioids for whatever reason. Community pharmacists are in a position to identify dental problems when the user enquires for over-the-counter remedies, and can encourage the person to seek dental treatment.

In a study in London, pharmacists were able to link with local dentists and make direct referrals for drug users to NHS dental care.[11,12] Methadone is often cited as a 'cause' of dental problems and many patients will request sugar-free methadone solution. It is true that methadone solution has the potential to provide an environment in which tooth decay occurs, as the solution is acidic and has high sugar content, and because opiates reduce saliva flow, a risk factor for dental decay. Both sugar-free and sugar-based solutions of methadone are acidic and can cause erosion of dentine.

It is important that patients are aware that they need to practise good dental hygiene whichever formulation they are taking. Giving the advice to suck the methadone solution through a straw and to rinse the mouth with plenty of water after the dose is swallowed, or to chew sugar-free gum, can all minimise the risks of tooth decay.[13] Other problems may be associated with the use of sugar-free formulations, not the least being the ease with which it can be injected, and that some of the sweetening agents used in sugar-free preparations have laxative effects which can be severe where large doses result in a considerable volume of mixture being consumed on a daily basis.

Prevention of overdose

Accidental overdose is a risk for drug users and a common occurrence. Most drug users have witnessed overdose in a friend or drug-using peer. The National Treatment Agency and the Department of Health have responded to the ACMD report on drug related deaths to help minimise the number of accidental deaths. One measure has been the introduction of simple, unambiguous advice on what to do if a user is present when a fellow user overdoses.[13] Pharmacists can reinforce these endeavours by the provision of oral and written advice to those receiving medication and to needle exchange clients on how to avoid overdose and what to do if they are present when someone else experiences one. Materials that are suitable for use include those published by DrugScope, Exchange, HIT (a Liverpool based organisation that delivers effective interventions on drugs, alcohol, sexual health, community safety and other public health concerns), and the Department of Health-funded 'Talk to FRANK' 24-hour drugs information and telephone helpline, frank@talktofrank.com, and the Scottish equivalent, 'Know the Score'. It has been argued that naloxone should be made more generally available, for example to those who are likely to witness opioid overdoses. The ACMD drug-related deaths report was of the view that, as a matter of principle, naloxone should be made more widely available, but that careful consideration should be given to prevention, first aid, and resuscitation (placing person in recovery position, keeping airways open etc).[14] Whether or not pharmacists are willing to be trained to supply and administer naloxone under patient group directions is open to debate.[15] Pharmacists could certainly be involved, however, in drawing up patient group directions for the supply and administration of naloxone by nurses in the NHS, prisons, or some other settings where overdoses may occur.

Pharmacists should ensure that all medicines are stored safely so that accidental poisoning of of children is prevented. Again, the provision of both oral and written advice/information can be helpful in reinforcing safety messages, as can the addition of warning labels on dispensed methadone or buprenorphine containers.

Nutrition

Drug users may not eat a balanced diet, and may often miss out on meals and consume high levels of sugary foods.[16,17] Concurrent alcohol dependency can increase their risks of developing nutritional deficiencies including anaemia. Pharmacists can provide advice on healthy eating, and may refer patients to a doctor or a dietician for the provision of prescribed vitamin supplementation or advice on over-the-counter products.

Drug users often ask for dietary supplements, such as high calorie drinks. There is no empirical evidence to guide the clinician in either prescribing or selling these products, and they are probably best avoided except in the most nutritionally deprived individuals. In otherwise healthy, non-debilitated individuals, dietary supplements are no substitute for a balanced diet. When discussing the use of supplements in the homeless population, Wright suggests that they should be considered only when the body mass index falls below 19.[18] Community pharmacists should consider contacting their local dietician for specific information to supply to drug users. It may even be possible to develop such information as a joint project between the local pharmacy, drug, and dietetic services.

Constipation

One of the most common and uncomfortable adverse effects of opioids (prescribed or otherwise) is constipation. Unlike some of the opioid effects, tolerance to this does not always occur. Patients on opioid substitution therapy report constipation as a common adverse effect. Asking patients who are on a methadone prescriptions about their bowel habits could be something routinely undertaken by the pharmacist. Patients should be told early on in treatment that constipation is likely to be a problem. Dietary advice and laxative treatment where appropriate can be provided by their pharmacist. Patients should be advised to increase the amount of fruit and vegetables that they eat and reduce the amounts of alcohol. Laxatives that work by softening stools will be more helpful than those that act on muscle tone.

Sleep problems

Psychoactive drugs often interfere with sleep patterns. The most obvious culprits are caffeine, cocaine/crack, and amfetamines, though any drug can cause this problem, even benzodiazepines when they are taken in high doses. Many drugs interfere with normal sleep, especially following a reduction of dose, such as during detoxification. Sleep disturbance after an opioid detoxification is often cited as one of the major causes of relapse.[19]

Although the prescribing of drugs to aid sleep may be inappropriate for many drug users, advice on sleep hygiene, the use of sleep diaries and herbal remedies, plus a listening ear are all useful interventions that can be provided by pharmacists. An informative leaflet on sleep is available from HIT on 0870 990 9702. Or: www.exchangesupplies.org/publications/sleep/sleepintro.html.

Sweating

Sweating is a common long-term problem in methadone patients; histamine release may be a partial cause of this phenomenon. The sweating can be severe and is often present in the absence of other histamine-related effects, which suggests that other mechanisms may be involved. Whereas sedating antihistamines may be helpful in both inducing sleep and in countering the sweating caused by histamine release, they are also known to potentiate the effects of methadone and have been specifically sought by drug users for this purpose and therefore should be avoided.[20]

Excessive sweating can be a cause of severe distress to patients on high doses of methadone. Wearing loose cotton clothing, avoiding coffee and strong tea or soft drinks that contain high amounts of caffeine, and cold baths can sometimes be helpful. Taking methadone early in the day rather than later may also be helpful in reducing night sweats.

Smoking cessation

A high proportion of drug users smoke. In one American study of methadone maintenance patients, more than 90% of the patients smoked cigarettes and many others also smoked cannabis.[21,22] Research has indicated that many patients in methadone treatment are interested in quitting smoking and are interested in smoking cessation services being offered in treatment programmes.

Community pharmacists have been shown to be effective in enhancing smoking cessation and are knowledgeable about smoking cessation products. There may be a useful role for pharmacists working in collaboration with drug treatment services that wish to instigate smoking cessation services for their patients to develop enhanced services that involve smoking cessation.[23]

The pharmacist should bear in mind that it may be inappropriate to promote smoking cessation as a high priority goal at a time when the patient has many other more pressing problems to deal with. It may be more appropriate to discuss smoking cessation options once a successful detoxification has been completed rather than before. Nicotine is notoriously difficult to give up and is, based on the number of cigarettes smoked before lifelong addiction, arguably the most addictive drug used. Additional advice on how and when to offer information about the various treatments that are available to assist smoking cessation should be explored.

Hepatitis

The incidence of hepatitis B and C among injecting drug users is of concern, as they can be transmitted by the sharing of contaminated injecting equipment. Co-infection with hepatitis A may lead to serious consequences for those who already have liver damage. Whereas no vaccination is available against hepatitis C, both hepatitis A and B are preventable conditions.

Giving advice on hygiene to needle exchange clients can help to reduce infection. Vaccination against hepatitis A and B is possible for those not already infected. Many injecting drug users have not been vaccinated and many are not aware of their hepatitis B status. Pharmacists should be encouraged to ask whether the user has ever been tested and/or vaccinated, and make the appropriate referral for testing and immunisation. Where a pharmacy needle exchange has a private consulting room on site it may be possible to allow the room to be used for a nurse- or pharmacist-based vaccination facility using patient group directions to administer hepatitis B and the combined A&B vaccine using accelerated regimens. Such an innovative arrangement has been running in Lanarkshire since November 2002.[24] The vaccination programme was carried out in stages: such that the vaccination regimens in one pharmacy were completed before the two nurses involved moved on to start the programme in the other pharmacies.[24]

Children of problem drug users

It is important that pharmacists, like all professionals who work with the drug-using population, recognise that the wellbeing of children is of paramount importance and overrides the duty of confidentiality to their parents or other patients. The Advisory Council on the Misuse of Drugs in their major report, *Hidden Harm*,[25] considered the particular problems faced by the children of drug users. Although the role of pharmacists was not specifically mentioned in the report, there are nevertheless a number of ways in which pharmacists could assist both the parents and their children. These include:

▶ contributing positively to the stabilisation of the parent's drug use through the provision of methadone and/or needle exchange services

▶ alerting the GP when the patient is not well or is behaving abnormally

▶ asking about the home situation

▶ observing the condition of any children brought into the pharmacy

▶ advising that children are registered with a GP

▶ advising on safe storage of medicines and injecting equipment in the home

▶ providing contraception advice

▶ providing advice on immunisation for both parent and children

▶ referring pregnant drug users to antenatal services if necessary

▶ monitoring of pregnant drug users

As mentioned earlier in this chapter, pharmacists should also encourage safe storage of medicines and injecting equipment in order to prevent accidental harm to children in the home environment. Pharmacists should consider reporting childcare concerns to GPs, social workers or key drug workers, or in exceptional cases, directly to the police.

Saliva testing for drugs

Patients who have been on a substitute prescription for some time may be ready to progress from daily-supervised supply and administration of their medication to a structured take-home regimen. Prescribers, drug workers, and even pharmacists, however, may have reservations as to the suitability of such a relaxation. Urine testing to ensure compliance with the medication regimen and assurance that illegal drugs are not being consumed is inappropriate in the community pharmacy setting.

A pilot study in Glasgow has demonstrated that it is possible to use saliva tests to monitor such patients.[26,27] At the end of the trial 13 of the 22 (60%) patients were either still on twice weekly dispensing or had reduced to weekly dispensing – with supervision once a week. The majority of these patients had kept their jobs, found jobs during the period, or commenced vocational training. In addition, over the study period, the pharmacy concerned experienced a reduction in workload due to the reduction in daily-supervised doses.[26]

Delivering services to drug users

There are many ways for pharmacists to become involved in delivering services to drug users. One such example is the Four Way Berkshire Agreement service.[28] This scheme, developed by a pharmacist, provides a mechanism for helping professionals comply with good prescribing practice and improve multiprofessional collaboration. The scheme provides remuneration for GPs and pharmacists and also establishes well-defined channels of communication. In addition, the community pharmacist has a prime role in providing supervised consumption of methadone and shared care, and also in helping track patients and monitor outcomes. The new community pharmacy and GP contracts, and the introduction of extended, enhanced and additional services, should increase the potential for pharmacy involvement.

Prescribing services

Patient group directions

A patient group direction (PGD) is a written direction relating to the supply and administration, or administration only, of a prescription only medicine to persons generally (subject to specified exclusions) and is signed by a doctor or a dentist, and a pharmacist.[29] Over recent years pharmacists have demonstrated their ability to supply prescription only medicines under the auspices of such directions, notably for the supply of emergency hormonal contraception, nicotine replacement therapy, and flu vaccination.[30-32] Consideration could be given to developing PGDs for the following situations:

▶ provision of antibiotics to treat injection related injuries

▶ supply and administration of naloxone for opioid induced overdose

▶ administration of hepatitis B or the combined hepatitis A and B vaccination to pharmacy needle exchange (PNEX) clients/patients.

Although it is recognised that not all pharmacies have an appropriate private area to undertake all three of the above activities, it is apparent that an increasing number of pharmacies are making such facilities available. In the case of the vaccination it may be more acceptable to facilitate a nurse to use a private area to administer the vaccinations under a PGD drawn up locally. This arrangement has already been shown to work effectively in the Lanarkshire Health Board area in Scotland.

Medication reviews

Although most reviews have targeted the elderly or patients on long-term medication for cardiovascular or respiratory conditions, there is no reason why consideration should not be given to pharmacists undertaking medication reviews for patients on methadone or buprenorphine programmes. Some of these patients may be receiving concurrent medications that interact with methadone or buprenorphine or they may develop problems that necessitate the administration of additional medications. In such cases, for instance, women taking oral contraceptives or patients receiving medication to treat HIV/AIDS, tuberculosis, epilepsy, hepatitis C, or alcoholic liver disease, it is important to monitor the patient to reduce the possibility of adverse drug reactions.

The future?

The proposed introduction of computer generated prescriptions and record keeping for controlled drugs and the electronic transfer of prescriptions should release time to allow pharmacists to take an even more proactive clinical role in the care of all patients, including those with drug or alcohol use problems. Dame Janet Smith, however, in the fourth report of the Shipman Inquiry has expressed some reservations that the systems currently available are sufficiently robust to be used for controlled drugs.[33,34] We hope that Dame Janet's concerns will be resolved so that pharmacists can spend less time on administrative matters and can devote more time to patient care. One welcome recommendation from this report is that in the future pharmacists should be able to endorse corrections to technical errors on prescriptions for controlled drugs without the patient's having to return to the prescriber.

Supplementary prescribing [35, 36]

The Department of Health has defined supplementary prescribing as a voluntary partnership between an independent prescriber (e.g. a GP) and a supplementary prescriber (e.g. a pharmacist) to implement an agreed patient-specific clinical management plan with the patient's agreement.[37,38] Whilst the controlled drugs other than those in schedule 5 are not covered by supplementary prescribing arrangements at present, nevertheless, there is a range of other medications that could be prescribed as part of an agreed management plan for named individual patients with drug misuse problems. Models that have already been developed for supplementary prescribing include structured medication reviews for older people. There is no reason why similar protocols could not be developed for patients on methadone or buprenorphine maintenance programmes.

Pharmacist prescribing

In addition to the introduction of schemes that allow pharmacists to supply and administer medicines using PGDs and the introduction of supplementary prescribing by pharmacists in accordance with an agreed care plan, the Department of Health has confirmed that it is moving forward with the development of independent pharmacist prescribing.[39,40] Whilst the indications are that such prescribing will exclude medications that are controlled drugs, there remains a range of chronic conditions that drug misusers suffer from for whom it may be appropriate for pharmacist prescribers to order medications other than controlled drugs.

Information and advice to drugs services

Although pharmacist-led medicines information centres are well established in hospitals throughout the United Kingdom and elsewhere, the expertise of such centres is, with some notable exceptions, in the field of medicines rather than substances liable to misuse. Those pharmacists who have acquired relevant knowledge and expertise in the field of substance misuse have already demonstrated their potential to provide valuable support and information to local drugs agencies and their clients.[41–43]

How can pharmacists take on additional roles?

What is needed to facilitate these developments? In the first place, a willingness and acceptance of these roles among pharmacists is essential. Appropriate levels of competence need to be described, and training put in place to enable pharmacists to achieve and maintain them.

Pharmacists should be proactive in forming partnerships with local drugs service providers, including GPs, specialist drugs services and nurse-led needle exchanges. The expansion of shared care arrangements to encompass these additional interventions would ensure that all partners in the care of a client are aware of what has taken place.

In its report on the commissioning and management of community drug treatment services for adults, the Audit Commission reported that pharmacists can play an important role in the management of drug misusers, but noted that research has shown that many (pharmacists) are an underused point of contact to the drug misusing population and would benefit from a closer working relationship with prescribing services.[44] The only way those services can become more aware of the important role that pharmacists have in the treatment and care of drug misusers is if the pharmacists themselves take the initiative and contact services with a description of what they can offer.

The provision of acceptable levels of privacy to encourage and enable appropriate discussion to take place is essential. Such facilities enhance the level of services that can be offered to all pharmacy clientele and not just drug users. When taking on additional roles in the field of substance misuse it is essential that pharmacists ensure that they have optimum levels of security to protect themselves, their staff, and the premises. Useful advice on how to optimise security and deal with difficult situations can be obtained from local police community safety officers.

Additional reading

Department of Health (2004)
www.dh.gov.uk/PolicyAndGuidance/MedcinesPharmacyAndIndustry/Prescriptions/
SupplementaryPrescribing/fs/en

NatPACT (2004) Chronic disease management compendium of information
http://.natpact.nhs.uk/news

Sheridan J, Strang J. (Eds). *Drug Misuse and Community Pharmacy*. London: Taylor and Francis, 2003.

References

1. Ghalamkari H. Pharmacists are willing to extend their roles and change their practice. *Pharm J* 2004; **273**: 82.

2. Department of Health. *Drug Misuse and Dependence: Guidelines on Clinical Management.* London: HMSO, 1999.

3. Matheson C, Bond C. Motivations and barriers to community pharmacy services for drug misusers. *Int J Pharm Pract* 1999; **7**: 256–63.

4. Sheridan J, Barber N, Glanz A. Role of community pharmacies in relation to HIV prevention and drug misuse: findings from the 1995 national survey in England and Wales. *BMJ* 1996; **313(7052)**: 272–4.

5. South East Regional Forum of Local Pharmaceutical Committees. *Improvement, Expansion and Reform: Modernising Primary Care.* 2nd ed. Wadhurst: JMH Publishing, 2004; 12.

6. Roberts K, Coggans N, King J. Do problem drug users only purchase 'over-the-counter' (OTC) medications for the purpose of misuse? In Proceedings of 11th International Conference on the Reduction of Drug Related Harm. Jersey: 9–13 April 2000. Poster 133.

7. Akram G, Roberts K. Pharmacists' management of over-the-counter medication requests in methadone patients. *Journal of Substance Use* 2003; **8(4)**: 215–22.

8. Metsch L R, Crandall L, Wohler-Torres B, *et al.* Met and unmet need for dental services among active drug users in Miami, Florida. *J Behav Health Serv Res* 2002; **29(2)**: 176–88.

9. Molendijk B, Ter Horst G, Kasbergen M, *et al.* Dental health in Dutch drug addicts. *Community Dent Oral Epidemiol* 1996; **24(2)**: 117–19.

10. Sheridan J, Aggleton M, Carson T. Dental health and access to dental treatment: a comparison of drug users and non drug users attending community pharmacies. *Br Dent J* 2001; **191(8)**: 453–7.

11. Sheridan J, Carson T, Aggleton M. Providing dental health services to drug users: testing a model for a community pharmacy advice and referral scheme. *Pharmaceutical Journal* 2003; **271(7621)**: 180–2.

12. Greater Glasgow NHS Board. Methadone and teeth. Health promotion leaflet. Glasgow: Greater Glasgow NHS Board.

13. Derricot J, Preston A, Hunt N. Overdose exchange campaign. London: DoH, 2002.

14. Advisory Council on the Misuse of Drugs. *Reducing Drug Related Deaths.* London: HMSO, 2000; 80–1.

15. Mackie C M, Healy A-M, Roberts K. A comparison of community pharmacy methadone services between Dublin and Glasgow: extent of service provisions in 1997/98 and views of pharmacists on existing provision and future service developments. *Journal of Substance Use* 2004; **9(5)**: 235–51.

16. Best D, Gossop M, Lehmann P, *et al.* Eating too little and smoking and drinking too much. Wider lifestyle problems among methadone maintenance patients. *Addiction Research* 1998; **6**: 489–8.

17. Zador D, Lyons Wall P M, Webster I. High sugar intake in a group of women on methadone maintenance in south western Sydney, Australia. *Addiction* 1996; **91(7)**: 1053–61.

18. Wright N. *Homelessness: A Primary Care Response.* London: Royal College of General Practitioners, 2002.

19. Staedt J, Wasmuth F, Stoppe G, *et al.* Effects of chronic treatment with methadone and naltrexone on sleep in addicts. *European Archives of Psychiatry and Clinical Neuroscience* 1996; **246(6)**: 305–9.

20. Roberts K, Gruer L, Gilhooly T. Misuse of diphenhydramine soft gel capsules (Sleepia®): a cautionary tale from Glasgow. *Addiction* 1997; **94**: 1575–7.

21. Clemmey P, Brooner R, Chutuape MA, *et al*. Smoking habits and attitudes in a methadone maintenance population. *Drug and Alcohol Dependence* 1997; **44**: 123–32.

22. Calsyn D A, Saxon A J. An innovative approach to reducing cannabis use in a subset of methadone maintenance clients. *Drug and Alcohol Dependence* 1999; **53(2)**: 167–9.

23. Maguire T A, McElnay J C, Drummond A. A randomised control trial of a smoking cessation intervention based in community pharmacies. *Addiction* 2001; **96(2)**: 325–31.

24. Lanarkshire Health. Annual report of the Hepatitis B Vaccination Programme 2003–2004. Lanarkshire Health, 2004.

25. Advisory Council on the Misuse of Drugs. *Hidden Harm. Responding to the Needs of Children of Problem Drug Users.* The report of an inquiry by the Home Office. London: ACMD, 2003.

26. Dickson S. (2003) The suitability of buccal fluid oral testing in a community pharmacy drug misuse setting. Personal Communication.

27. Buxton A. The National Health Service Pharmacy Contract in England. *Pharm J* 2003; **271**: 406–8.

28. Walker M. Shared care of opiate substance misusers in Berkshire. *Pharm J* 2001; **266**: 545–52.

29. Royal Pharmaceutical Society of Great Britain. *Medicines, Ethics and Practice: A Guide for Pharmacists.* 28th ed. London: RPSGB, 2004; 11.

30. Emergency hormonal contraception: users welcome pharmacy supply. UKCPA conference report (editorial). *Pharm J* 2003; **271**: 751.

31. Kempner N. Pharmacists' role in smoking cessation. *Pharm J* 2003; **260**: 273.

32. Hind C, Peterkin G, Downie G, *et al*. Successful provision of influenza vaccine from a community pharmacy in Aberdeen. *Pharm J* 2004; **273**: 194–6.

33. Smith J. The Shipman Inquiry. Fourth report: the regulation of controlled drugs in the community. Command Paper Cm 6249. London: Stationery Office, 2004.

34. Bellingham C. How supplementary prescribing helps both in acute and chronic hospital care. *Pharm J* 2004; **272**: 640–1.

35. Bellingham C. New pharmacy contract must let pharmacists develop over time. *Pharm J* 2004; **272**: 514.

36. National Pharmaceutical Association. Supplementary prescribing: progress to date. *Professional Practice Matters* Summer 2004: 4–6.

37. Department of Health (2004). Useful information available at: www.dh.gov.uk/Policyand Guidance/MedicinesPharmacyandIndustry/Prescriptions/SupplementaryPrescribing/fs/en

38. ETP still on target for 2007 (editorial). *Pharm J* 2004; **272**: 664.

39. Independent prescribing for pharmacists to start in 2005 (editorial). *Pharm J* 2004; **273**: 571.

40. Scott J, Kennedy E J, Winfield A J, Bond C. Role of the pharmacists at a drug counselling and needle exchange service. Presentation at 9th International Conference on the Reduction of Drug Related Harm. Sao Paolo, Brazil, 1998.

41. Scottish Drugs Forum. The benefits of having a pharmacist on the team. *SDF Bulletin* September 1998; 6.

42. Wills S. *Drugs of Abuse.* London: Pharmaceutical Press, 1997.

43. Gerrett D, Anderson D, Cullen A M S. The pharmacists' role in drug abuse. *Br J Pharm Pract* 1987; **9**: 422–31.

44. Audit Commission. *Changing Habits: the Commissioning and Management of Community Drug Treatment Services for Adults.* London: Audit Commission, 2002.

CHAPTER 8

Management of opioid addiction: evidence-based treatment

Clare Gerada and Jenny Keen

IN THIS CHAPTER

Introduction || *Prevalence of opioid users in general practice* || *Opioid treatment options* || *Opioid withdrawal/detoxification* || *What to choose for detoxification* || *Maintenance treatment for opioid dependence* || *Relapse prevention* || *Conclusion*

Introduction

Chapter 9 describes practical treatment issues in the management of opioid addiction. This chapter deals with the generalities of opioid treatment, including the evidence base for various treatment options. To be effective the practitioner must be aware of the reasoning behind treatment choices. There is, however, a serious lack of sound evidence on which to base many of our prescribing decisions and even where evidence does exist it seldom includes primary care patients or practitioners as part of the research methodology.

Prevalence of opioid users in general practice

The number of opioid users on a typical general practice list is generally estimated at around 1–5/1000, with at least 50% of all general practitioners having seen a heroin user in the previous month. The number of drug users registered with a practice varies according to the geographic location, the special interest of the practitioner/s and the ability of the clinician and the practice to extend care to this patient group. Even where the general practitioner has a significant interest in the care of drug users, the number of heroin users will still only be in the region of 0.5–1% of the registered list.

Opioid treatment options

There are, and should be, various options available to the clinician when treating opioid dependency (Table 8.1). Over the years the vogue for different options has varied, though as time progresses it has become clear that substitute treatment based on high dose maintenance therapy should be the treatment of choice in the majority of individuals. Nevertheless, it is important for the clinician to have a clear understanding of other treatment options and where they may be used.

Methadone is perhaps the best-known treatment for opioid substitution. It was synthesised in Germany during World War II as a substitute for morphine when supplies of opium from Turkey were cut off by the United States and their allies. Since then methadone has been thoroughly researched and carefully evaluated. It has received more scientific scrutiny and evaluation than any other medical treatment or human service programme in the addiction field. Most evaluations have shown that, when correctly implemented, the treatment is capable of producing remarkable improvements in patients who were previously dysfunctional heroin addicts. Methadone maintenance patients throughout the world have been restored to productive lives, relationships with families and children have been re-established, many have furthered their educations, obtained employment and improved their physical and mental health.

Until the development and use of methadone as a maintenance medication in the mid-1960s, the primary use of methadone in the treatment of addiction was to withdraw addicts from heroin, a procedure that differs from maintenance and exploits only a few of the potentially useful properties of the medication. In the United Kingdom, the Advisory Council on the Misuse of Drugs report in 1982, *Treatment and Rehabilitation*, acknowledged rather reluctantly that 'whilst recognising abstinence as an ideal, some clinicians are prepared to continue maintenance prescribing over an indefinite period of time to enable stabilisation of behaviour'.

Buprenorphine, a partial opioid agonist/antagonist, is gaining popularity as an option to methadone for both detoxification and maintenance and the evidence base for its effectiveness is growing.

Opioid withdrawal/detoxification

The symptoms of heroin withdrawal, if untreated, reach a peak within 36–72 hours after the last dose and subside over about five days. In contrast, the symptoms of methadone withdrawal peak at around 4–6 days and do not substantially subside for 10–12 days. There is evidence of a protracted withdrawal opioid syndrome with milder symptoms persisting for many months.

Table 8.1 **Summary of treatment options for opioid dependence**

Stage of treatment	Options
Withdrawal/ detoxification	The opioid dependent individual is taken off the drug, either abruptly, or gradually so as to eliminate physical dependence with the minimum of discomfort from withdrawal. Detoxification alone cannot be expected to achieve long-term abstinence and is best considered as a precursor to, or first stage of, treatment
	Options available include tapered doses of methadone or buprenorphine or an alpha-2-adrenergic agonist, such as lofexidine. Other medications: antiemetics for nausea and vomiting, antidiarrhoeals, and analgesics for muscle cramps. Some clinicians use dihydrocodeine for short-term detoxification, though evidence for effectiveness of this is limited
Maintenance	Wealth of evidence for the effectiveness of high dose methadone in combination with psychosocial support in number of outcomes. Also evidence growing for effectiveness of maintenance on buprenorphine for opioid substitution treatment
Relapse prevention	Naltrexone treatment is a useful adjunct to other psychosocial interventions to prevent relapse

Methadone at gradually tapering doses

Methadone detoxification as opposed to maintenance was at one time the favoured treatment for opioid dependent drug users. The 1991 Clinical Guidelines hardly mentioned maintenance as a treatment option, stating instead, 'There is at least a small proportion of patients for whom this [maintenance] is a helpful approach ... it is a specialised form of treatment best provided by, or in consultation with, a specialist drug misuse drug service.' Unfortunately, in some areas detoxification is still the only pharmacological intervention sanctioned by specialist addiction services and a number of general practitioners insist that their patients undertake detoxification rather than maintenance substitution treatment.

In prisons detoxification (though not always with methadone), often carried out over a few days, is the most common treatment intervention provided. There is, however, some evidence that with well-motivated patients and where the rate of methadone reduction is not too rapid, gradual tapering of methadone can be effective in reducing withdrawal symptoms and can lead to heroin abstinence.

The conclusions of studies comparing different methadone withdrawal reduction schedules showed that different types of methadone withdrawal schedule produced different responses in terms of time course of withdrawal, the severity of withdrawal response, and possibly in terms of subsequent engagement in treatment. Severity of withdrawal was lower if a linear rather than exponential reduction was followed. Lower rates of treatment dropout were found if patients were well-informed, if the regime was doctor-regulated rather than self-regulated, if the regime included contingency management, and if counselling was provided.[1]

When to use methadone detoxification

Detoxification should be seen as a brief (although an important) bridge between maintenance and relapse prevention in the treatment of opiate addiction and not as a treatment for dependence by itself. Mattick and Hall suggest that the criteria for assessing the effectiveness of detoxification should be based upon:

1. rates of completion of the process

2. severity of withdrawal symptoms (both psychological and physical distress)

3. medical complications, rather than for example, relapse rates.[2]

This means that outcome is not based on long-term abstinence, implying that detoxification alone is not an effective treatment if abstinence is the final outcome measure.

Buprenorphine for treatment of withdrawal

A systematic review of studies comparing buprenorphine with other withdrawal regimens was carried out in 2004 by Gowing *et al.*[3] The overall conclusion was that buprenorphine regimens resulted in lower withdrawal severity than benzo-diazepines or alpha-2-adrenergic agonists and with less adverse side effects.

Alpha-2-adrenergic agonists

A systematic review of the use of alpha-2-adrenergic agonists in patients with opioid dependence found that methadone dose reduction was more effective than alpha-2-adrenergic agonists in improving treatment retention and amelioration of withdrawal symptoms. Methadone detoxification took longer than with alpha-2-adrenergic agonists. Clonidine and lofexidine were equally effective but hypotension was less likely to occur with lofexidine. There were more adverse effects for clonidine than for methadone and clonidine does not currently have a licence for use in opiate detoxification.[4]

What to choose for detoxification

Given the evidence of effectiveness of different treatments used in detoxification the following criteria can be used by the clinician when choosing the drug for detoxification treatment:

Desired duration of treatment

▶ If short duration of treatment is the aim, alpha-2-adrenergic agonists are preferable to methadone.

▶ Methadone treatment is more successful if carried out slowly with gradual stepwise reduction rather than rapid reductions in dose.

Adverse effects

▶ Buprenorphine is preferable to alpha-2-adrenergic agonists if there are concerns of bradycardia or hypotension.

Withdrawal severity

▶ Buprenorphine results in lower severity of withdrawal symptoms than alpha-2-adrenergic agonists.

Specific patient groups

▶ Methadone can be used during pregnancy and there is emerging evidence that buprenorphine is safe and effective though it does not have a Medicines and Healthcare Products Regulatory Agency (MHRA) licence (formally medicines control licence) for use during pregnancy. Alpha-2-adrenergic agonists should not be prescribed during pregnancy.

In situations where a quick detoxification is planned, and methadone contraindicated, experienced practitioners would suggest buprenorphine as the first line treatment.

Maintenance treatment for opioid dependence

The objectives of maintenance treatment are to:

▶ suppress signs and symptoms of opioid withdrawal

▶ extinguish opioid drug craving

▶ block the reinforcing effects of illicit opioid 'blockade'.

Methadone maintenance

There are a number of treatment options available for maintenance treatment. The use of methadone is the most researched treatment for heroin dependence, was the first widely used opioid replacement therapy designed to treat heroin dependence, and is used in many countries (see Figure 8.1). There are Cochrane reviews comparing the effectiveness of methadone maintenance therapy with no opioid replacement therapy, the most recent published in 2003.[5] Other reviews include those by Farrell.[6]

Numerous studies, several with double-blind placebo controlled design, clearly demonstrate that long-term treatment with methadone and buprenorphine are effective treatments for opioid dependence, reducing illicit drug use, risk of HIV, death, crime, and unemployment, and improving social stabilisation, retention rate in treatment, and patients' contribution to society.

Studies of the effectiveness of methadone maintenance programmes, however, vary widely in terms of the nature and quantity of psychosocial support delivered in addition to the medication, and in terms of the degree of supervision of methadone consumption. It is also important to note that the research evidence has been based on programmes with supervised consumption of methadone, while in practice many treatment programmes, especially those in primary care and private practice settings, have no supervised consumption or indeed additional psychosocial support systems. See Box 8.1.

Box 8.1   **Benefits of methadone maintenance treatment for the management of opioid dependence[5]**

✓ Reduced levels of opioid use

✓ Reduced levels of crime

✓ Reduced levels of injecting and other risk behaviour

✓ Improved quality of life

✓ Increased sense of wellbeing

✓ Better physical health

✓ Reduced drug-related death rate

✓ Reduced non-opioid misuse

High dose methadone

The advantages of high dose methadone maintenance treatment have been recognised internationally for many years though it is only recently that this has been on the agenda in UK treatment settings. Unfortunately a large number of patients in the United Kingdom have to tolerate inadequate doses of methadone, placing them at higher risk of death and other complications, not least relapse into injecting drug use.

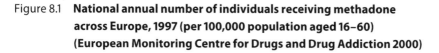

Figure 8.1 **National annual number of individuals receiving methadone across Europe, 1997 (per 100,000 population aged 16–60) (European Monitoring Centre for Drugs and Drug Addiction 2000)**

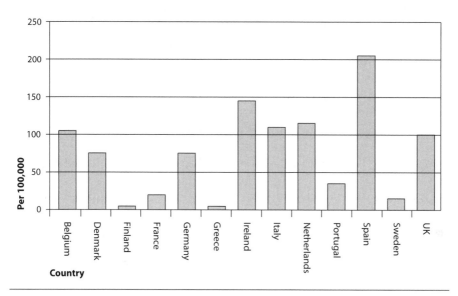

Over the years there have been clinical trials comparing various doses of methadone for maintenance treatment and it is consistently reported that patients receiving a higher methadone dose compared with those at lower doses exhibit better outcomes. Studies have shown that an adequate dose of methadone is typically 80–100 mg/ml. Many methadone maintenance treatment programmes, however, prescribe low dosages of methadone for political, psychological, philosophical, or moral reasons.

Another point of disagreement amongst prescribers is the use of dosages of over 100 mg/day. A review of methadone dosages strongly suggests that methadone dosages higher than, and sometimes greatly higher than, 100 mg/day may be beneficial in some patients. Current guidance to treatment providers such as the Department of Health 1999 Clinical Guidelines, models of care and the recent National Treatment Agency *Research into Practice* briefings on methadone maintenance treatment all emphasis the greater benefits associated with daily methadone doses of 60–120 mg (and higher doses in exceptional cases).[7]

For general practitioners there has always been an anxiety about increasing doses of methadone and many GPs have placed an arbitrary ceiling of 40–60 mg/ day. Methadone maintenance treatment is a worthless exercise if individuals who need high doses of methadone to keep away from crime and illicit drugs are denied this because of a general unwillingness to prescribe over a certain amount. This does not mean indiscriminately placing a patient on high starting doses of methadone. The dose increase should be incremental and safeguards such as supervised ingestion and daily dispensing should reduce the fear of diversion.

Although the evidence supports higher doses there is no consensus on ceiling dose. Individuals vary in their metabolism and so-called 'fast metabolisers' may require higher doses. Some commonly prescribed medications enhance methadone metabolism.

At very high doses it is advisable that the primary care practitioner works closely with the specialist service that may have the facilities to admit patients for dose titration. Therapeutic plasma level monitoring may provide additional guidance, though this form of monitoring is rarely used and impractical in those patients with poor venous access.

Methadone tablets

The 1991 and 1999 Clinical Guidelines, the Department of Health Task Force, and the Advisory Council on the Misuse of Drugs (2000) have all advised that tablets should not be prescribed, as they are liable to be abused by being crushed and injected. Despite these recommendations significant amounts are being prescribed by general practitioners.

In practice, general practitioners find that patients request tablets for many reasons – either patients claim that they cannot tolerate the solution or that they find tablets easier to take – especially when large volumes of methadone have to be ingested. Patients also find tablets easier to transport, especially when travelling, and do not have to deal with dropped bottles or leaking bottle tops. More research is needed as to who would benefit from tablet formulations; in the meantime clinicians ought to be cautious when prescribing them to patients.

Buprenorphine for opioid maintenance

There is a growing body of evidence for buprenorphine for maintenance treatment of opioid dependence and that buprenorphine should now be considered an evidence-based addition to the range of pharmacological maintenance treatments. The goals of treatment are the same as those of methadone maintenance treatment: the reduction of illicit drug use and of associated risks and harms.

The effectiveness of buprenorphine maintenance treatment has been examined in a Cochrane review.[8] In comparison with placebo, there is evidence that buprenorphine is superior in terms of retention in treatment at low or moderate doses and at high doses. It is superior to placebo in terms of reduction in opioid positive urine tests at moderate doses and high doses but not at low doses. Three trials have examined reductions in use of benzodiazepines and/or cocaine, one showing that low dose buprenorphine does not reduce positive tests for cocaine or benzodiazepines, one showing that buprenorphine was inferior to placebo in relation to reducing benzodiazepine use, and one showing that buprenorphine was superior to placebo in relation to reducing cocaine use.

It is advisable to delay the first dose of buprenorphine until the patient is experiencing features of opioid withdrawal (this typically means at least eight hours after last heroin use, or 24–48 hours after last methadone use). Commence with an initial dose of 4–8 mg and increase the dose on each day for the next three to four days thereafter according to clinical response. Daily increases up to 4 mg/day are possible up to a maximum of 32 mg/day.

Transition to buprenorphine from heroin or low dose methadone (30 mg or below) can usually be accomplished with minimum complications, although restlessness, insomnia, and diarrhoea are commonly reported in the first one to three days. Some patients experience problems for up to two weeks.

Patients on higher doses wishing to transfer from higher dose methadone (over 30 mg) straight onto buprenorphine risk precipitated withdrawal. This can occur one to three hours after the first buprenorphine dose, peaking in severity over three to six hours and then gradually subsiding. Lofexidine can be used to alleviate symptoms. Induction from methadone doses over 30 mg should, ideally, be undertaken only in specialist settings by a clinician with the relevant experience. The dose of buprenorphine for maintenance prescribing is typically 8–32 mg/day.

Buprenorphine produces comparable outcomes to lower dose (e.g. 30–60 mg) methadone. Higher dose methadone maintenance treatment (>60 mg) appears more effective than buprenorphine, but adequate comparisons of higher dose (16–32 mg) buprenorphine with high dose methadone maintenance treatment (60–120 mg) are lacking.

Choosing between buprenorphine and methadone[5]

Current evidence suggests that buprenorphine and methadone are of similar efficacy in retaining patients in treatment and reducing heroin use. The decision as to which medication to use should be made in consultation with the patient. As with methadone, higher daily doses of buprenorphine (8–16 mg) are superior to lower doses, while doses in the region of 12–24 mg/day is preferable for maintenance treatment.[9]

Duration of maintenance treatment

A common question posed by clinicians treating drug users with methadone or buprenorphine maintenance is how long treatment should continue. Rigorous research is generally lacking and many longitudinal studies suffer from selection bias with the more problematic patients tending to leave early, meaning that the performance of the remaining patients appears to improve when in fact the reported outcome measures, such as continued heroin use, are diminishing owing to changes in the composition of the group rather than the accumulated impact of the treatment provided.

Some studies attempt to control for this and overall the finding is that the longer patients spend in maintenance treatment the more likely they are to benefit. The conclusion reached by Ward *et al.*[10] is that only a small number of patients will benefit from relatively short periods of methadone maintenance; these patients tend to have a short history of heroin use and significant social and psychological resources at their disposal which can be deployed in the recovery process. For the majority of entrants into treatment, it is more appropriate to have maintenance as a goal and to maximise retention rates so that the benefits of treatment are realised for both the individual and the community. There is no specifiable, optimal duration for methadone maintenance treatment. It is likely that this will be equally true for buprenorphine. The duration of maintenance should therefore be dictated by the needs of the patient rather than an artificially created end date.

Table 8.2 **Prescriptions of different formulations of methadone prescribed by England NHS GPs 2001/2**

Formulations	Number of items (% of total)
Methadone solution	113,199 (70%)
Methadone tablets 5 mg	33,460 (22%)*
Methadone 50 mg amps	10,000 (7%)

*Some of these prescriptions may be for reasons other than treatment of addiction.
From Prescribing Support Unit.

Data source: National Audit of controlled drug NHS prescribing prepared for the Shipman Inquiry by the Prescribing Support Unit.

Maintenance treatment involving injectable preparations

Two injectable products have been investigated, diamorphine (pharmaceutical heroin) and methadone. The recent Home Affairs review has recommended an expansion in the provision of injectable heroin to patients within the NHS;[11] if this is to happen considerably more needs to be known about who can benefit from this treatment, under what conditions it is best delivered, and what treatment outcomes should be expected. It is gratifying that a UK heroin trial is soon to begin.

Injectable heroin was provided in the early drug dependence clinics for treatment of heroin dependence, but this practice subsequently declined, with oral methadone becoming the dominant drug for maintenance treatment. Contrary to popular opinion the right for doctors to prescribe heroin has never disappeared, although to do so requires a special Home Office licence for the purposes of treating addiction. Few eligible doctors (eligibility usually implies a specialist addiction psychiatrist) have chosen to apply for this licence and even amongst those that have the necessary authority to prescribe heroin do so to only a small number of patients (around 600 in England 2002/03).

No such licence is required to prescribe methadone ampoules, and the amount of this drug prescribed is significantly more than heroin, even in primary care settings, where 7% of all methadone prescribed by general practitioners in England was in the injectable form (Table 8.2). Rationales for prescribing injectable drugs are that some patients continue to inject regularly when receiving oral methadone and that others are attracted into treatment only because injectable medications are available. Thus there may be some justification for injectable maintenance treatment in that it may be more effective as a 'bait' to capture users into treatment and as an 'adhesive' in retaining them into care and enabling change to occur.

Arguments for and against injectable preparations

Arguments for injectable prescribing are mainly centred on harm reduction: it decreases crime and provides a drug that is free from contaminants. Those opposed to this treatment point out that it perpetuates injecting behaviour and may postpone by years eventual abstinence from heroin use, and that it runs contrary to the duty of doctors to improve or maintain the physical health of their patients.[12]

Injectable methadone treatment is a world apart from oral methadone treatment. Whereas the drug itself is the same, the differences far exceed the similarities. These differences include the clear 'hit' or 'rush' that results from intravenous methadone (in contrast to oral methadone). When prescribing injectable opioids in clinical practice in the United Kingdom, a typical experience was described by Strang and colleagues:[13] 'The committed injector seeking a prescribed supply of injectable drugs would usually be quite amenable to moves between heroin and methadone in injectable form – in sharp contrast to the determined opposition which may be encountered to suggestions of moving from injectable methadone to its oral form.'

Methadone ampoules have a hedonistic appeal and black market value – especially the higher dose 30 mg and 50 mg preparations, which is similar to heroin when both drugs are compared in their injectable forms. A small number of patients might require prescriptions of injectable medications to keep them in treatment and/or ease the change from injecting the drug of dependence to taking a substitute orally.

Evidence for treatment with intravenous prescriptions of methadone 'wet amps'

Methadone ampoules are available only in the United Kingdom. Prescribing injectable methadone steadily increased to a mid-1970s peak after which the trend has been to move away from injectables with more reliance on oral methadone. In a survey of community pharmacies in England and Wales, 11% and 9.3% of all prescriptions were for tablets and injectable ampoules respectively.[14] These results included all community prescriptions and hence included hospital and GP prescribing. The amount of injectable methadone issued by general practitioners is small. A national survey of general practitioners prescribing of injectable methadone was conducted in 1999 by Beaumont and the results showed that of all 105 Health Authorities three quarters of them contained at least one practice from which injectable methadone was being prescribed, giving a total of 407 practices across England and Wales. When the survey drilled down to a smaller sample of individual prescribing doctors (n = 93) what emerged was that most (60%) general practitioners only prescribed injectable methadone to one patient, although 10 doctors prescribed to five or more patients. The results of this survey imply that prescribing of injectable methadone by general practitioners is only undertaken in exceptional circumstances and limited to one patient only in most cases.[15]

A recent trial comparing injectable methadone with oral methadone maintenance treatment at six months showed no significant differences in treatment outcome.[16] The trial did, however, establish that it was possible to set up supervised injecting clinics within an NHS service. The surprising conclusion of this supervised injectable service was how poor long-term injectors were in their injecting technique with many patients needing training in how to carry out safely a procedure they had been undertaking for many years.[17]

Evidence for prescribing heroin 'dry amps'

In recent years the use of heroin has been evaluated in a number of studies across Europe. The first of these was a Swiss uncontrolled feasibility study involving nearly 2,000 individuals.[18–20]

In another, smaller, randomised controlled trial (n = 51), oral methadone was compared with intravenous heroin. The outcome of the participants in the heroin group was significantly better after six months, though these positive effects could have been the result of the additional and mandatory psychosocial interventions in the group allocated to heroin.[21]

A larger multicentre, randomised trial (n = 539) in the Netherlands compared injectable or inhaled heroin with methadone alone and methadone plus heroin in patients who had been deemed treatment resistant. Heroin administration was supervised with no 'take-home' privileges allowed. At 12 months, the methadone plus heroin group had significantly better outcomes (defined at showing improvement in physical and mental health, and social domains) than methadone alone. At the end of the trial, 82% of the treatment responders in the experimental group deteriorated substantially in the two months after the planned discontinuation of the co-prescribed heroin. Despite the limitations of the study (self-report, no double blind possible, heroin group treated in newly established location with specially recruited staff) the study did provide evidence of the efficacy of prescribed heroin for patients who are resistant to other forms of treatment, though it may be difficult to replicate the intensity of the supervision in normal NHS practice.[22]

Other pharmacotherapies

There are a number of other pharmacotherapies that have been used for opioid treatment, though none of them have been as well researched as those described above.

Dihydrocodeine (DHC) is a minor opioid which produces less dependence than methadone. It may be useful at the tail end of methadone detoxification or for short-term (7–10 days) detoxification in well-motivated patients. It has little use for the long-term management of dependence and as yet there are only a few studies comparing DHC to other substitute medication. One such study carried out in Edinburgh audited the progress of 200 patients in substitution treatment in a primary care setting. There were no significant differences in patients prescribed methadone and those prescribed dihydrocodeine in terms of retention in treatment, death rate, and behaviour change.[25,26]

These findings were reported when DHC was compared to oral methadone in a randomised controlled trial in Scotland. There were no differences at 6 and 18 months in the two groups in terms of retention in treatment, criminal behaviour and injecting drug use (Roy Robertson, personal communication).

Many clinicians and the national clinical guidelines, however, continue to discourage the use of DHC. Large numbers of tablets are required (approximate milliequivalents 3 mg methadone = 30 mg dihydrocodeine), it has a short half-life, and is administered in tablet form making it an impractical opioid substitute.

Dihydrocodeine is not licensed for the treatment of drug users and the fact that it is in short-acting tablet form excludes supervised consumption and facilitates injection. Furthermore it cannot be dispensed on an FP10 (MDA) in England.

Morphine in slow release oral formulations suitable for once-daily dosing are now available for the management of pain and may also possess clinical utility for maintenance treatment for opioid dependence.[27–29]

Although morphine is likely to be beneficial as an alternative for patients who respond poorly to methadone, and has been tried for this purpose in several countries (Austria, Australia, United Kingdom),[30-32] quantitative assessments of patient outcomes and acceptability of morphine is impeded by the paucity of information regarding oral dose equivalence of methadone and morphine and the means by which patients should be transferred between these medications.

Mitchell *et al.*[33] have recently conducted a study that evaluated morphine as an alternative to methadone in patients who were finding that they experienced breakthrough craving on methadone maintenance. The study found that transfer to and from methadone was associated with few ill effects, in particular without any significant withdrawal symptoms. The final mean morphine: methadone ratio was found to be 4·6:1, though the range varied from 3·5:1 to 8:1 in the patients being studied. This study found that compared with methadone, morphine was associated with improved social functioning, weight loss, fewer and less troublesome adverse effects, greater drug liking, reduced heroin craving, an enhanced sense of feeling 'normal', and similar outcomes for unsanctioned drug use. Slow release morphine preparations could be considered as an alternative to methadone, but much more research is required in establishing which patients are best suited to this treatment, which has greater intrinsic risks of overdose and diversion than methadone.

Dextromoramide (Palfium™) has been suggested to have a role in the treatment of opioid addiction.

In one report, from the Netherlands, dextromoramide was used as an adjunct to methadone maintenance in hard-to-reach, entrenched drug users who continued to use heroin despite receiving prescribed methadone.[23] This was a highly structured treatment programme with patients having to collect daily prescriptions, with take-home weekend doses. The mean dose of dextromoramide was 30 mg, with a range of 15–50 mg, and they received a mean methadone dose of 75 mg (range 10–170 mg). Of note, even in this study, 13% of patients had their prescriptions stopped because of suspected sale of their dextromoramide. This study concluded that even a highly structured dextromoramide treatment programme is no 'permanent substitute for treatment with heroin'. At best dextromoramide can be seen as an adjunct to a methadone maintenance programme where patients who wish to experience the 'high' of heroin but are unable to obtain it, either through clinics or on the illicit market, instead receive prescribed dextromoramide.

Another study has shown that dextromoramide may be useful as an adjunct to treating craving in patients on a methadone maintenance programme. These patients were given between 5 and 10 mg dextromoramide besides their methadone. The results imply beneficial effects of a short-acting opiate on diminishing craving in opiate addicts who are difficult to stabilise with oral methadone maintenance.[24]

Relapse prevention

Naltrexone is a long-acting competitive opioid antagonist, which is effective when taken orally. It can be used to precipitate withdrawal in accelerated detoxification from opiates but its main use is for relapse prevention. The goal of naltrexone treatment is maintenance of abstinence from opioid drugs in previously dependent patients following detoxification. It is prescribed for oral use as a 50 mg tablet. The principle of treatment is that on establishing a dose of 50 mg per day, any ordinary amounts of opiates that are then taken are completely ineffective, the medication therefore acting as a strong deterrent to further use. This resembles disulfiram in alcohol abuse.

Since the mid 1990s some practitioners have used naltrexone implants though these products do not have a licence in the United Kingdom. A Cochrane review concluded that the evidence available did not allow an objective evaluation of naltrexone, but that it may be efficacious in highly motivated patients.[34] Probation-linked supervised naltrexone has been used as an alternative to custody in opiate misusing offenders;[35] providing there is a 50 mg dose each day, treatment can be given twice or three times a week.

General practitioners can prescribe naltrexone, although it is wise first to ensure that there are no opioids in the patient's system (which usually means commencing treatment 7–10 days after last opiate use) and that there is normal liver function before commencement. There is little to guide the clinician as to the length of treatment on naltrexone and, therefore, until the evidence is clear it is probably wise to tailor the length of treatment on the outcome in individual patients.

There are no controlled studies of naltrexone implants or the newer preparation, naltrexone depot.

Conclusion

There are several options available to the practitioner when prescribing treatment for opioid dependence. Practitioners would be well advised to start with treatments that are well used and well researched. Detoxification should be a primary goal for all opioid addicts, but practitioners may quickly become aware that maintenance stands the best chance of keeping many individuals away from crime and illicit drugs. More controversial and less common treatments such as injectable methadone or dihydrocodeine should not be prescribed without serious consideration of their suitability.

It is essential that practitioners read Chapter 9 on the practicalities of opioid treatment prescribing. Even when a method of treatment is decided upon there are many issues that need to be addressed in order to tailor the treatment to an individual patient. Whatever the treatment chosen, prescribing should be tailored to the needs of the individual, and prescribing practices should reflect the evidence base that currently exists; this evidence base should also be expanded through the evaluation and research of other interventions.

Further reading

ACMD (2000). *Reducing drug related deaths*. Ontario: Health Canada, 2002. www.hc-sc.gc.ca/hecs-sesc/cds/publications/methadone_treatment/toc.htm

Carnwath T, Smith I. *Heroin Century*. London: Routledge, 2002.

Ward J, Mattick R, Hall W. *Methadone Maintenance Treatment and Other Opioid Replacement Therapies*. The Netherlands: Harwood Academic Publishers, 1998.

Jameison, Beals, Lalonde & Associates Inc. *Methadone Maintenance Treatment*. Literature review for the Office of Canada's Drug Strategy. Ontario: Health Canada, 2002.

Ford C, *et al*. (Ed). Guidance for the Use of Buprenorphine for the Treatment of Opioid Dependence in Primary Care. London: RCGP, 2003.

References

1. Amato L, Davoli M, Ferri M, Ali R. Methadone at tapered doses for the management of opioid withdrawal. In: Cochrane Collaboration. *Cochrane Library*. Issue 3, Chichester: John Wiley, 2004.

2. Mattick R P, Hall W. Are detoxification programmes effective? *Lancet* 1996; **347**: 97–100.

3. Gowing L, Ali R, White J. Buprenorphine for the management of opioid withdrawal. In: Cochrane collaboration. *Cochrane Library*. Issue 3, Chichester: John Wiley, 2004.

4. Gowing LR, Farrell M, Ali RL, *et al*. α_2–Adrenergic agonists in opioid withdrawal. *Addiction* 2002; **97**: 49–58.

5. Mattick RP, Breen C, Kimber J, Davoli M. Methadone maintenance therapy versus no opioid replacement therapy for opioid dependence. In: Cochrane Collaboration. *Cochrane Library*. Issue 4. Chichester: John Wiley, 2002.

6. Farrell M, Ward J, Mattick R, Hall W, *et al*. Methadone maintenance treatment in opiate dependence: a review. *BMJ* 1994; **309**: 997–1001.

7. National Treatment Agency for Substance Misuse. *Methadone Dose and Methadone Maintenance Treatment. Briefings for Drug Treatment Providers and Commissioners*. Research into practice briefing. London: NTA, 2004.

8. Mattick RP, Kimber J, Breen C, Davoli M. Buprenorphine maintenance versus placebo or methadone maintenance for opioid dependence. In: Cochrane Collaboration. *Cochrane Library*. Issue 3. Chichester: John Wiley, 2004.

9. Ling W, Charuvastra C, Collins J F. *et al*. Buprenorphine maintenance treatment of opiate dependence: A multicenter, randomized clinical trial. *Addiction* 1998; **93(4)**: 475–86.

10. Ward J, Mattick R, Hall W. How long is long enough? Answers to questions about the duration of methadone maintenance treatment. In: *Methadone Maintenance Treatment and Other Opioid Replacement Therapies*. The Netherlands: Harwood Academic Publications, 1998; 265–305.

11. Select Committee on Home Affairs. *Third Report. The government's drugs policy: is it working?* 2002. London: HMSO, 2002.

12. Zador D. Injectable opiate maintenance in the UK: is it good clinical practice? *Addiction* 2001; **96**: 547–53.

13. Strang J, Gossop M. The 'British System': visionary anticipation or masterly inactivity? In: *Heroin Addiction and Drug Policy: the British System*. Oxford: Oxford University Press, 1994; 342–51.

14. Strang J, Sheridan J, Barber N. Prescribing injectable and oral methadone to opiate addicts: results from the 1995 national postal survey of community pharmacies in England and Wales. *BMJ* 1996; **313**: 270–2.

15. Beaumont B. Survey of injectable methadone prescribing in general practice in England and Wales. *Int J Drug Policy* 2001; **11**: 35–42.

16. Strang J, Marsden J, Cummins M, *et al*. Randomised trial of supervised injectable versus oral methadone maintenance report of feasibility and 6 month outcome. *Addiction* 2000; **95**(11); 1631–54.

17. Cummins M. The supervised injecting clinic: a drug clinic's experience of supervising the intravenous self-administration to prescribed injectable methadone. In: Tober G, Strang J. (Eds). *Methadone Matters. Evolving Community Methadone Treatment of Opiate Addiction*. London: Martin Dunitz, 2003; pp 119–128.

18. Farrell M, Hall W. The Swiss heroin trials: testing alternative approaches. *BMJ* 1998; **316** (7132): 639.

19. Wodak A. Prescribing heroin: nothing else to fear but fear itself? Illicit drug policy based on punitive measures has failed, and it is time to seek a health care approach. *Med J Austr* 1998; 168: 590–1.

20. Ali R, Auriacombe M, Casas M, *et al*. *Report of the External Panel on the Evaluation of the Swiss Scientific Studies of Medically Prescribed Narcotics to Drug Addicts*. Geneva: World Health Organization, 1999.

21. Perneger T V, Giner F, Del Rio M, Mino A. Randomized trial of heroin maintenance programme for addicts who fail in conventional drug treatments. *BMJ* 1998; 317: 13–18.

22. van den Brink W, Hendriks V M, Blanken P, *et al*. Medical prescription of heroin to treatment resistant heroin addicts: two randomised controlled trials. *BMJ* 2003; **327** (7410): 310–12.

23. Van Brussel G H A, Buster M, van Der Woude D H. Two mangoes in 1979: Evaluation report dextromoramide treatment for long-term heroin addicts. Zorgstad (available at: www.zorgstad.amsterdam.nl/gemeente/GGGD/mangoes.htm).

24. De Vos J W. Ufkes J G. Craving patterns in methadone maintained treatment with Dextromoramide as adjuvant. *Addictive Behaviours* 1999; **24** (5):707.

25. MacLeod J, Whittaker A, Robertson J R. Changes in opiate treatment during attendance at a community drug service: findings from a clinical audit. *Drug and Alcohol Review 1998*; **17** (1): 19–25.

26. Banbery J, Wolff K, Raistrick D. Dihydrocodeine: a useful tool in the detoxification of methadone maintained patients. *J Subst Abuse Treat* 2000; **19**: 301–5.

27. Fischer G, Presslich O, Diamant K, *et al*. Oral morphine sulphate in the treatment of opiate dependent patients. *Alcoholism* 1996; **32**: 35–43.

28. Mitchell T B, White J M, Somogyi A A, Bochner F. Comparative pharmacodynamics and pharmacokinetics of methadone and slow-release oral morphine for maintenance treatment of opioid dependence. *Drug and Alcohol Dependence* 2003; **72**: 85–94.

29. Kraigher D, Ortner, R, Eder H, *et al*. Slow release of morphine hydrochloride for maintenance therapy of opioid dependence. *Wiener Klinische Wochenschrift* 2002; **114**: 904–10.

30. Brewer C. Recent developments in maintenance prescribing and monitoring in the United Kingdom. *Bulletin of the New York Academy of Medicine* 1995; **72**: 359–70.

31. Dyer K R, White J M. Patterns of symptom complaints in methadone maintenance patients. *Addiction* 1997; **92**: 1445–55.

32. Sherman J P. Managing heroin addiction with a long-acting morphine product (Kapanol). *Med J Australia* 1996; **165**: 239.

33. Mitchell T, White J, Somogyi A, Bochner F. Slow release oral morphine versus methadone: a crossover comparison of patient outcomes and acceptability as maintenance pharmocotherapies for opioid dependence. *Addiction* 2004; **99**: 940–45.

34. Kirchmayer U, Davoli M, Verster A. Naltrexone maintenance treatment for opioid dependence. In: Cochrane Collaboration. *Cochrane Library.* Issue 4. Oxford: Update Software, 2001.

35. Brahen L S, Brewer C. Naltrexone in the criminal justice system. In: *Treatment Options in Addiction, Medical Management of Alcohol and Opiate Abuse.* London. Gaskell, 1993; 46–53.

CHAPTER 9

Practical aspects of methadone treatment

Clare Gerada

Introduction

This chapter will explore the practical issues in administering methadone in order to avoid potentially dangerous consequences, while ensuring that individual patients are prescribed the dose that suits their situation.

How does methadone work?

Methadone mixture is seen as the gold standard for treatment of opioid dependence as it has low addictive potential, low potential for injection when prescribed as 1mg/ml solution and relatively low 'street' value if diverted onto the illicit market.[1,2] Methadone is a synthetic opioid and has been the mainstay of substitute treatment for over 30 years.

Methadone works predominantly by binding itself to opioid receptors in the brain, where, if given in sufficient quantities, it blocks the effects of other opioid drugs, such as heroin, thereby preventing the unpleasant side effects of withdrawal and avoiding the same euphorogenic effects. It is nearly completely absorbed across the gastrointestinal tract with a bioavailability of more than 80%. Methadone is stored extensively in the liver and secondarily in other body tissues, but not 'in the bones' – a common urban myth amongst drug users and doctors.[3] The amount in the bloodstream is kept relatively constant by the slow release of methadone from tissues, which helps account for its long half-life.[4]

Steady state occurs after an interval of five times the elimination half-lives, which is approximately five to ten days, although, in some patients, it can take longer.[5] The extent of plasma binding is high – approximately 90%.

The advantages of methadone include:

▶ It is taken orally, which avoids the risk of injecting use.

▶ It has a long half-life, which means only a single daily dose is required for most patients.

▶ It accumulates in the body, which means steady state blood level is achieved easily.

▶ It effectively suppresses opioid withdrawal symptoms, which increases comfort/ compliance amongst patients.

▶ It develops cross-tolerance (or blockades) to the effects of illicit opioid use, which decreases use of illicit opioids during maintenance.

▶ It has no serious long-term side effects when used on a long-term basis.

Methadone itself is addictive, in that it produces dependence and a recognised withdrawal syndrome, but less so than heroin. Nevertheless, many users complain bitterly about symptoms that may go on for weeks, even months in some cases after stopping methadone. Methadone is less potent and it has a long duration of actions, which avoids the need for regular 'topping-up', which is characteristic of shorter acting opioids.

Main problems with methadone

▶ Constipation

▶ Lethargy and depression

▶ Loss of libido

▶ Weight gain, more likely to be related to increased well being rather than the calories in methadone itself

▶ Dental problems, even with sugar free preparations

▶ Nausea

▶ Sweating, due to histamine release

▶ Menstrual disturbances

The importance of tolerance

Despite its advantages, like all opioids methadone is dangerous to anyone who is not tolerant to opioids and a single dose of around 30–40 mg can cause life-threatening respiratory depression.[6] An opioid-tolerant person, however, can function normally at doses that can be fatal to a non-tolerant person. Opioid tolerance is a complex process of neuroadaptation and even experienced opioid users can be at risk of toxic methadone effects.[7] It is essential, therefore, to estimate an individual's opioid-dependence and level of tolerance before starting methadone treatment and again after a period of abstinence lasting more than a few days.

Tolerance develops more quickly to some effects of opioids than others. For example, tolerance develops quickly to the euphoric effects, whereas tolerance to gastrointestinal effects (e.g. constipation), sedation, or respiratory depression is slower to develop. This can be potentially fatal if users start to ingest increasingly greater amounts of opioids for its euphoric effect. In the case of methadone, tolerance development is incomplete, so the respiratory depressant effects of other agents such as alcohol, sedatives and other opiates, or acutely excessive methadone may not be completely blocked even in a person stabilised on methadone maintenance doses.

Tolerance testing in primary care

Observing a patient after a first dose of methadone may not be sufficient to establish a level of tolerance. Often it can be inferred only that the dose given is not a significant overdose. Careful dose induction, starting with a low dose and increasing gradually over the course of several days, is preferable and should provide reasonably confident grounds for identifying non-tolerant patients and adjusting their dose (or even reviewing the appropriateness of methadone treatment) accordingly.[8] See Tables 9.1 and 9.2.

Table 9.1 **Approaches to the assessment of methadone tolerance**

Naloxone challenge test	Not generally used in primary care setting although practitioners working in specialist services may undertake this test. Based on the observation that the greater the degree of opioid dependence, the less naloxone is needed to cause a certain intensity of withdrawal syndrome. The naloxone challenge test is claimed to provide a quantitative assessment of the degree of opioid dependence[9]

continued over

Clinical assessment using history taking and examination	May be supplemented by questionnaires and obtaining corroborative evidence from previous doctors or dispensing pharmacists
Tolerance testing	Involves observing the effects of methadone administered, and is the most direct and least ambiguous way of assessing methadone tolerance, though it carries the significant risk of overdose if the patient overestimates their use of illicit heroin or other opioids

Table 9.2   **Subjective and objective characteristics at various doses of methadone**

Overdose	Respiratory depression, pinpoint pupils unreactive to light, snoring giving way to shallow respirations, bradycardia and hypotension, varying degrees of reduced consciousness and coma
Overmedication	Sedation, small pupils, itching, low blood pressure, flushing, depressed respiration, cognitive decline, spasticity
Comfort range	Comfortable, neither withdrawing nor intoxicated
Subjective withdrawal	Craving, anxiety, dysphoria, irritability, fatigue, insomnia, myalgia, anorexia, nausea, stomach cramps, restlessness, hot and cold feelings
Objective withdrawal	Dilated pupils, sweating, gooseflesh, muscle twitching, diarrhoea and vomiting, running nose and eyes, sneezing, yawning, fever, tachycardia, high blood pressure

Methadone deaths

Most methadone-associated deaths have been reported in individuals with little or no tolerance to opioids.[10] Although many fatalities during methadone induction involve the use of alcohol and benzodiazepines in conjunction with methadone, the level of methadone tolerance plays an important role in the risk of fatal overdose. The major risk factors are starting the patient on too high a dose of methadone (although there does not appear to be a unique fatal concentration of methadone) and not using daily supervised dispensing.

The risk of death during methadone induction has been calculated as nearly sevenfold greater than the patient's risk of death prior to entering methadone maintenance treatment,[11] and nearly 98 times greater for new patients than patients who have been safely receiving methadone for more than two weeks.[12] There are inherent risks associated with starting patients on methadone treatment. Deaths usually occur during the first three to ten days of treatment,[13] at home during sleep, many hours after peak serum methadone level has occurred.

Deaths in the first two weeks of treatment have been associated with doses in the range of 25–110 mg/day, although most tend to fall within the range of 40–60 mg/day. A significant proportion of methadone-related deaths involve individuals who were in poor health, and had other diseases, particularly HIV, hepatitis, and other infections, which may have contributed to their death. Heroin users who have a lower tolerance to opioids are at greater risk of methadone toxicity. Polydrug use is also an important factor in many deaths in methadone treatment.

The risk of death is greatest in the first two weeks of methadone maintenance treatment. See Box 9.1.

Box 9.1 **Risk factors in starting methadone**

✓ first presentation or where drug and alcohol history is unclear

✓ initial dose over 30 mg

✓ concomitant use of other drugs, especially benzodiazepines and alcohol

✓ general health of the patient, especially respiratory disease, hepatitis, and HIV

✓ intolerance to opiates

Methadone induction

Testing for tolerance is the first stage of initiating a patient safely onto methadone. Dose induction involves reaching steady-state plasma methadone levels. Prior to steady state, it is important clinicians understand that half of each day's dose remains in the body and is added to the next day's, producing rising serum methadone levels even without any increase in dose.[14] Until steady state is reached, any dose increase should be made with caution. See Figure 9.1 and Box 9.2.

With methadone treatment, it may take up to 12 half-lives before steady state is reached.

During methadone induction, patients may be in mild withdrawal towards the end of the dosing interval, so doses should not automatically be increased based on how the patient feels at 12 hours or more after dosing. Instead, patients should be asked how they felt at three to eight hours after the last dose, and if they were relatively comfortable no increase is needed. See Table 9.3.

Figure 9.1 **Serum methadone levels take on average 4–5 days to reach steady state**

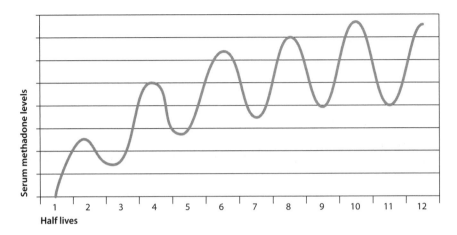

Reproduced with permission of J Thomas Payte

Table 9.3 **Improving safety during induction**

Good clinical assessment	Use of corroborative evidence such as urine tests, and examination of veins for evidence of injecting drug use
	Contact previous prescribers
	Contact previous dispensing pharmacist
	Contact previous prison doctor
Dose with caution: 'start low, go slow'	Review regularly in the early stages of dose induction

Induction dose recommendations

Given that it can take four to five days until steady state is reached and that it has been shown that methadone's half-life can result in an accumulation of methadone and a resulting overdose one or two weeks after treatment begins it is important that the clinician proceeds with care during the induction stage. Since there is no exact formula to guide the clinician in calculating opioid tolerance the recommendation for methadone induction is to 'start low and go slow'.

Table 9.4 gives different examples of international induction regimes.

Authorities in various countries have produced guidelines to cover the induction stage. Most give starting doses of methadone of 20–30 mg. These are summarised in Table 9.4.

Methadone induction

✓ Start low, go slow

Table 9.4 **Induction dosing guidelines**

Methadone dose range	Country
Initial dose not to exceed 30 mg or 40 mg total in the first day	USA[15]
Initial dose 10–20 mg if tolerance low or uncertain; 25–40 mg if opioid tolerance established	UK [clinical guidelines]
Initial dose 10–20 mg if opioid tolerance low or uncertain; 25–40 mg if tolerance high	Europe[16]
15–30 mg/day during the first 3 days (which represents time to 87.5% of steady state)	Canada[17]

Factors affecting response to methadone

Body weight, age, sex, individual differences in metabolism and excretion rate, certain physiological or pathological states, and other drugs, in particular enzyme inducers, can all influence the rate of methadone metabolism. Flexibility in dosing is required to stabilise patients in whom methadone's effects can be so variably altered.

The most notable physiological state associated with changes in methadone metabolism is pregnancy. Pregnancy is associated with lower than expected methadone plasma levels in the third trimester. Liver disease is common in methadone maintenance patients owing to hepatitis infection or in some cases alcohol dependence. Liver disease may result in a slowing of the rate of elimination of methadone and such individuals should be dosed with care to avoid toxicity.[18,19]

Some drugs have been shown to influence the amount of methadone present in blood plasma by speeding up the elimination of methadone from the body. Rifampicin, phenytoin, barbiturates, benzodiazepines, carbamazipine, and disulfiram have all been associated with lowering of plasma methadone levels and onset of withdrawal symptoms in methadone maintained patients. Concurrent use of fluvoxamine and desipramine have been associated with higher plasma levels and increased risk of toxicity.[20]

Box 9.2   **Summary of methadone induction**

> ✓ Death can occur owing to lack of tolerance
>
> ✓ Methadone blood concentrations can take a week to reach a steady state
>
> ✓ The use of other CNS depressant drugs, for example heroin, benzodiazepines, alcohol, etc. in significant concentrations can reduce the quantity of methadone needed for a fatal dose.
>
> ✓ The presence of significant natural disease can increase the toxic potential of methadone

Therapeutic drug monitoring

Measuring plasma levels of methadone to determine peaks and troughs are used in clinical practice though rarely used in day-to-day practice. Monitoring of methadone dose is not a necessity in the management of patients, since careful clinical follow up of objective signs and subjective symptoms is sufficient for dose titration. The clinician might find monitoring useful however, in selected situations, for example when dosages much in excess of 100 mg/day are prescribed and it is feared that such dosages might lead to very high methadone concentrations and cardiac toxicity. Kim Wolff, a psychopharmacologist at the National Addiction Centre in London describes a number of indications where plasma methadone monitoring would be useful in clinical practice in Box 9.3.

Injectable preparations

The 1999 Clinical Guidelines place prescribing of injectables within the specialist domain and emphasise that when a clinician embarks on such a form of treatment it should be against a background of a long and persistent history of injecting drug use, and that in all cases there should be clear goals that can be assessed at defined periods. Means should exist to supervise and monitor, in a clinical setting, the administration of the drug in the early stages of treatment, and at stages where concern over clinical progress arises. Where pharmacy dispensing occurs, it should be daily to reduce the risk of diversion. Where evidence of diversion exists, daily-supervised forms of medication should be re-established.

Box 9.3 **Plasma methadone monitoring: an aid to dose assessment, monitoring compliance and exploration of drug interaction**

Reason for requesting plasma measurement

Assessment of compliance with methadone

✓ Monitor take-home medication

✓ Monitor prescription of ampoules

✓ Suspect 'double-scripting'

Change in dose regime

Patient complaining of withdrawal despite high dose

Change in clinical state, for example, pregnancy

Chronic liver disease

During methadone induction, especially where higher doses may be required

Concomitant use of additional drugs that may inhibit or enhance methadone metabolism

Adapted from: Kim Wolff, In: *Methadone Matters*, Strang J. and Tober G. p 75

In the absence of demonstrated significant superior outcomes from this form of treatment, and in the recognition of the greater inherent dangers and the cost burden of such prescriptions, doctors should review and audit outcomes against set performance standards. In all cases the further away from established practice the greater the responsibility of the doctor to ensure prescribing is safe and that mechanisms are in place to minimise risk to the patient. Injectable drugs should be considered as a possible 'second line' treatment where well-supported oral methadone treatment in appropriate doses is unsuccessful.[21]

There are no simple criteria for prescribing injectables, but a complex clinical decision based on the suitability of each individual patient. Prescribing injectable drugs has costs (prolonged dependence, collusion with drug culture, problems of misuse, diversion) and so the benefits (health gain, reduced criminality, engaging more entrenched users) must be clear.

The general goals of treatment using injectable preparations are those of other forms of substitute prescribing for treatment of opioid dependence: the reduction of illicit heroin use, of injecting and other risk behaviours, and of associated harms. The focus differs from oral methadone maintenance in terms of selection

of patients. As there is considerable evidence supporting oral methadone maintenance, the use of injectable drugs is considered mainly for those who have failed
to benefit from optimal oral treatment, or who have not been attracted or retained
in treatment by oral methadone maintenance programmes.

It is unlikely that many general practice surgeries or pharmacists will have the
facilities for supervised ingestion of injectable prescriptions.

Once on injectable preparations it is unlikely that the patient will voluntarily
switch to oral preparations, so it is important that the clinician makes a decision
to prescribe carefully and consistently. For those who feel that injectable preparations have a role in the management of injecting drug users, Sarfraz and Alcorn
have suggested the following clinical guidance including eligibility criteria (see
Box 9.4): [22]

Box 9.4   **Clinical guidance for injectable prescriptions**

Objective evidence of:

✓ Opioid dependence

✓ Injecting for several years

✓ Current intravenous opioid use

✓ Previous unsuccessful treatment including detoxification, oral methadone or
   residential rehabilitation. Most clinicians would require previous unsuccessful
   treatment with oral methadone at adequate dosages

✓ Unwillingness or inability to stop injecting

✓ No evidence of severe mental health problems (affective disorder, psychotic
   illness, cognitive impairments) which may reduce compliance or increase risk
   to self or others

✓ No use of alcohol or other psychoactive drugs in amounts that would severely
   affect physical or cognitive state

✓ No medical contraindications to intravenous administration including anti-
   coagulant treatment, DVT, subacute bacterial endocarditis, pregnancy

✓ Demonstrated ability to cooperate with the services including reliable
   attendance, examination, and urinalysis

Should general practitioners prescribe injectable preparations? Of course the
question is a rhetorical one, as general practitioners already do prescribe this
drug, and judging by prescribing data for 2002/03 GPs are prescribing relatively

large amounts: 100,000 50 mg methadone ampoules were prescribed by English GPs, representing 7% of all methadone preparations.

Beaumont,[23] a general practitioner in north London, carried out a survey of all 105 health authorities in England and Wales in 2001 and found that three-quarters of these health authorities have at least one practice from which methadone ampoules were prescribed. Not surprisingly, when the prescription patterns were examined in more detail it emerged that a very small number of general practitioners were prescribing to a relatively small number of patients. Sixty per cent of the GPs were prescribing to only one patient and 93 GPs who were prescribing methadone were treating only 211 patients. Most of these GPs were merely continuing a prescription on behalf of or initiated by a specialist service rather than initiating the treatment themselves. Dr Ford, a general practitioner in north London and her co-researcher Ryrie have identified four broad categories that influenced general practitioners' decisions to prescribe injectable preparations to their patients. These are: the patient's previous treatment experience, in particular limited success both with detoxification and oral preparations; individual need such as injecting users presenting with serious health and social problems; the level or otherwise of existing provision, such as an unwillingness to prescribe and/or insufficient provision of injectable preparations by local specialist services; and finally, as a result of a direct request from another agency such that a local non-statutory agency advocating on behalf of individual patients who they believe would benefit from an injectable prescription.[24]

However, whilst a small number of experienced GPs do prescribe injectable preparations most feel it is not an appropriate treatment to be given by GPs in a general practice setting. A national survey of general practitioners engaged on the RCGP Certificate in Drug Misuse, in England (Strang *et al.* unpublished, Royal College of General Practitioners Conference 2001), indicated that, whereas there was substantial acceptance of the appropriateness of oral methadone maintenance in primary care settings, this was not the same for injectable substitute prescribing. Over half of all GPs reported oral methadone maintenance was either 'very appropriate' or 'somewhat appropriate' in the management of dependent opioid users in their practice. Ninety-three per cent of GPs, however, reported that they considered injectable methadone prescribing to be 'not at all appropriate' and a further 6% considered it only 'somewhat appropriate' in a primary care setting. It is likely that there would be an even greater proportion of GPs who consider injectable heroin prescribing as 'not at all appropriate'. Clearly, therefore, a small number of GPs are skilled enough and have the systems in place to commence and monitor injectable prescribing, although this prescribing should be seen as the exception rather than the rule and GPs should embark on this form of treatment with great care.

Supervised consumption and dispensing frequency

Ensuring that patients take substitute drugs under supervision at pharmacies or specialist treatment agencies has many advantages and is recommended by the 1999 Clinical Guidelines and by the ACMD report on reducing drug related deaths. Supervised consumption has been part of methadone treatment services since the 1960s, especially in the United States and Australia where take-home doses are the exception rather than the norm. The impetus in the United Kingdom behind the recommendation of supervised consumption was the increasing concern about the number of drug related deaths and increasing concerns about 'leakage' of methadone onto the illicit market, possibly causing the increase in drug related deaths.

Roberts *et al.* have reported on a supervised consumption scheme in Glasgow, where the number of participating pharmacists has risen from 20% (43/212) in 1994 to 80% (173/215) in 2003.[25] The number of pharmacists involved in providing supervised consumption in a pioneering shared care scheme in Berkshire is 76%.[26] From these experiences the benefits of supervised consumption are:[27]

▸ introduction of a routine as a result of the requirement for daily, personal attendance at the pharmacy

▸ assistance in compliance and avoidance of exceeding a daily dose

▸ daily contact between pharmacist/client and a health professional

▸ the opportunity to increase dosage safely

▸ reduction in diversion onto illicit market, including where patients are coerced into selling their drug soon after leaving the pharmacist

▸ an opportunity to monitor progress

▸ increased opportunities for communication between other carers.

In addition to these advantages, when asked, patients support supervised consumption.

A study sought views from three groups: new patients referred for assessment and treatment; the consensus view of the Methadone Alliance (a national users' forum); and the consensus view of a local service users' forum. All three groups expressed the view that supervised consumption had an important place in methadone treatments. Users understood the need for daily supervision of methadone and were generally willing to accept it. Users' views support the introduction of flexible methadone prescribing regimens incorporating supervised consumption. Privacy in pharmacies and the possibility of moving away from supervision are important elements in an acceptable programme. Supervised consumption is an important component of safe, effective and responsible methadone prescribing.[28]

There are problems with supervised consumption. At the very least there are cost implications of providing a safe and confidential area for ingestion and fees payable to the pharmacist for providing this service. It has been suggested that strict supervision programmes can discourage people from staying in treatment and that doctors should be allowed to use their clinical judgement so that treatment plans meet the patients' needs rather than adopting a uniform approach for all.[29] Confidentiality can be a problem, particularly in busy small pharmacies, and problems may arise where the pharmacists offer a needle exchange scheme and the patient/client is making use of this. Despite these problems, when used correctly the advantages of supervised ingestion far outweigh the disadvantages and patients can gain considerable benefit from the stabilising influence of daily attendance at a community pharmacist.

Whether or not supervised consumption is available, initial prescriptions should specify dispensing on a daily basis. As treatment progresses, gradually decreasing dispensing frequencies can reward clinical improvement. Similarly, deterioration in response to treatment would indicate resumption of daily dispensing.

Tests of compliance – urine and hair testing

Urine drug testing provides a snapshot of recent drug use and is an essential adjunct for initial assessment and monitoring progress. The advantage of urine testing is that it provides an objective means of monitoring drug use that can be used for evaluating progress. The disadvantages are that the procedure communicates to the patients from the outset that they cannot be trusted. It is humiliating for both staff and patient to undergo supervised collection and it is a relatively inaccurate measure of drug use as the sample can be subject to manipulation or sample substitution. Testing is also expensive. There is no research evidence that urinalysis improves the outcome for the patients.

Oral fluid and saliva testing is being increasingly used and is much more acceptable to staff and patients, but there are concerns about the accuracy of some of the tests.

Analysis of hair is more expensive but records use over time, a centimetre sample from the head represents approximately one month's growth. The use of hair testing for compliance or monitoring purposes is rare in NHS practice. The reader is advised to consult with the references listed under further reading for more information.

Split dosing

At any dose, if a patient is clinically overmedicated several hours after dosing but experiences withdrawal before the next dose is due, then splitting the daily dose of methadone would seem appropriate. In such cases, increasing the once-a-day dose will not make the dose last longer and would elevate only the peak level not the trough level, so can result in overmedication during the early hours but continued opioid withdrawal later.[30]

Using on top

For many patients heroin use does not come to a complete stop when they commence methadone maintenance treatment. A significant number continue to use additional heroin.

Best *et al.* found that 71% of a cohort of patients on methadone maintenance for a mean of over three years had been using heroin on at least one occasion in the three months before interview, and 31% on a daily basis.[31] Similarly Ball and Ross found that 29% of methadone treatment patients had used heroin intravenously in the month before interview and Iguchi *et al.* reported that three months into treatment 54% of patients failed to submit an opiate-free urine specimen.[32, 33] Many users also 'top-up' their prescription with additional methadone acquired through the illicit market, and up to 25% of one sample had taken non-prescribed methadone six months after entering a methadone maintenance programme.[34]

So what influences the individual to continue with illicit drug use, and what should be the response of the primary care practitioner in the further management of the patient? Perhaps the most important factor that determines the frequency and amount of additional use is the dose of methadone being prescribed. Studies have shown a dose related association with increasing doses of methadone associated with reducing additional heroin use.

Dose, however, is not the whole story; some researchers have failed to find a clear association between methadone dose and reduced heroin use.[35] Factors other than methadone dose are important. Patients who receive ancillary services and greater levels of counselling and support during treatment show markedly greater improvements in retention and outcome than those who received methadone alone.[36] The important message is that successful treatment should not be seen as exclusively related to prescribing a biological substitute, but that its impact on continued heroin use is modified significantly by psychosocial factors such as individual motivation, treatment affiliation, commitment, additional support, education, and opportunities for employment.

Given the relatively high prevalence of non-prescribed methadone use and the associated risks, it may be necessary for prescribers to review polices regarding methadone dispensing management to ensure that patients are neither tempted to sell their prescriptions nor to supplement their prescribed dose through the 'grey' market of diverted methadone.

Summary of predictors of retention in methadone maintenance (better retention linked to better outcomes)

Patient characteristics and retention

Predicting outcomes in treatment can be difficult. 'No single characteristic or set of characteristics can fully predict those who will do well or poorly in treatment.'[37] Some patient characteristics and some early treatment results are associated with better outcomes. See Table 9.5.

Table 9.5 **Patient characteristics and retention**

Age	Older age predicts greater retention in treatment and is the characteristic most consistently associated with better outcome. Older users are also more likely have a drug related death from overdose
Gender	There is conflicting evidence from studies on gender as a predictor of outcome or retention. It is further complicated by the finding that men are more likely to have non-using partners than women – and hence are more likely to be supported during their treatment
Criminal history	Patients who have an extensive criminal history have more problems in remaining in treatment and do not do so well when they leave. This is complicated by the confounder that those more likely to commit crimes are more likely to be incarcerated and then more likely to use protective supports on leaving prison and more likely to become embroiled in a drug taking lifestyle
Opioid use	Patients who have a longer and heavier history of opioid use do less well if they leave methadone maintenance treatment
Psychological adjustment	Severe psychological symptomatology predicts lower retention rates
Employment	Employment at entrance to treatment is predictive of longer retention in treatment, although employed users are also more likely to have fewer psychosocial problems, which is also predictive of a more favourable outcome

continued over

Living with partner/family	Patients who have better social support do better in methadone maintenance
Alcohol use	High level of alcohol use is negatively associated with retention and overall treatment outcome
Polydrug use	Polydrug use is predictive of shorter stays in treatment and worse outcome. Drug use other than heroin is associated with riskier behaviours and poorer psychological functioning

Treatment characteristics and retention

According to research reviewed by Ward *et al.*[20] longer retention in treatment is associated with improved post-treatment outcomes including reduced opioid use and reduced criminal activity. Many studies have confirmed that a longer length of time in treatment increases reductions in criminal behaviour and also increases socially productive behaviour (e.g. employment, school, homemaking). The caveat, as Ward *et al.* state is that the benefits of methadone maintenance treatment 'continue only as long as patients remain in treatment.' Consequently, as Joseph *et al.* have stated, 'it may be necessary for patients to remain in treatment for indefinite periods of time, possibly for the duration of their lives.'[38] See Table 9.6.

Table 9.6   **Factors that improve retention rates**

Methadone dose	Patients on higher doses stay in treatment longer and patients who are maintained on low doses due to the philosophy of the treatment agency as opposed to clinical need tend to drop out of treatment
Treatment philosophy	Short-term maintenance philosophy associated with poorer retention
Ancillary services	Medical, psychological and financial services provided during treatment associated with better retention. Mandatory compared to optional counselling associated with poorer retention rates
Clinic accessibility	Accessible services predictive of better outcome
Take home methadone doses	Provision of more take home doses associated with increased retention
Rapid assessment	Having a rapid assessment as opposed to a slow assessment process associated with better subsequent retention into treatment

Urinalysis and monitoring of drug use during treatment	Recent research suggests that programmes with a 'non-punitive' approach to illicit drug use are more likely to meet the needs of patients
Contingency contracting	The use of negative consequences such as reductions in methadone dose or even discharge from the services as a response to illicit drug use has been associated with losing patients from treatment

Alcohol

Concurrent use of opioids and alcohol is very common, and alcohol dependence is more common amongst drug users than the general population. Many patients continue to use alcohol even after starting methadone replacement. Prevalence rates for the incidence of alcohol abuse in treatment populations have been reported to be between 20 and 50%.[39,40]

Concurrent use of methadone and alcohol places the patient and staff at increased risk. For the patient, the added complications of excessive alcohol can negatively affect the process of recovery and increases the risk of serious morbidity and mortality. These patients also have increased levels of anxiety and depression and are more likely to continue to abuse a range of illicit drugs compared to those without a drinking problem. For staff, concomitant alcohol use makes it difficult to establish an effective therapeutic relationship, and consultations are often marked by aggression and confrontation.

There is the added dilemma of continuing to prescribe hepatotoxic drugs and possible hasten serious liver damage. Excessive alcohol use in methadone maintenance patients is commonly associated with poorer treatment outcomes and can be a contributory factor in treatment failure. It is important for the clinician to tackle the issue of alcohol consumption in all patients presenting for treatment and to provide specific interventions and treatment to prevent alcohol-related deterioration.

Cocaine

There are high rates of cocaine use in patients on methadone maintenance programmes, both before admission and during treatment. Patients who use cocaine are more likely to have a negative outcome, are more likely to leave treatment early and are more likely to take part in criminal activities. There is also consistent evidence that methadone treatment reduces the frequency of cocaine use. Among the National Treatment Outcome Research study (NTORs) sample, significant reductions in the frequency of crack cocaine and cocaine powder use were found between intake and one-year follow up in both reduction and maintenance programmes, with use reduced to less than half the pre-intake levels.

The best predictors of reduced cocaine use following methadone treatment initiation are reduced heroin use and reduced injecting. Methadone patients who also use cocaine have greater treatment needs and the treatment objectives may need to be amended to deal with this additional drug problem. At the very least it is important to discuss the negative impact of cocaine on future progress with the patient and to try and reduce this use as much as possible.

Conclusion

There is plentiful research and many useful guidelines that will help a doctor decide the best treatment for opioid dependent patients. There is also much onus on a doctor's own judgement. Of paramount importance is that caution is exerted during induction and that treatment is subsequently tailored to the individual patient's needs. There should not be a set formula for methadone prescription; a doctor must establish the best level of methadone dose for each patient with clear goals for the treatment and rigorous analysis of the risks that each patient represents. The prescription of any drug is perhaps the pinnacle of responsibility for a primary care clinician in the treatment of addiction and this responsibility should not be taken lightly.

Further reading

Tober G, Strang J. (Eds). *Methadone Matters. Evolving Community Methadone Treatment of Opiate Addiction*. London: Martin Dunitz, 2003.

Ward J, Mattick R, Hall W. *Methadone Maintenance Treatment and Other Opioid Replacement Therapies*. The Netherlands: Harwood Academic Publishers, 1998.

Methadone Drug Interactions booklet (available at: http://www.atforum.com/mdi_booklet.shtml).

National Treatment Agency for Substance Misuse. Injectable heroin (and injectable methadone). Potential roles in drug treatment. Full Guidance Report 2003 (available at: www.nta.nhs.uk).

References

1. Farrell M, Ward J, Mattick R, *et al.* Methadone maintenance treatment in opiate dependence: a review. *BMJ* 1994; **309**: 997–1102.

2. Gossop M, Marsden J, Stuart D, *et al.* Methadone treatment practices and outcome for opiate addicts treated in drug clinics and in general practice: results from the National Treatment Outcome Research Study. *Br J Gen Pract* 1999; **49**: 31–4.

3. Humeniuk R, Ali R, White J, Hall W, Farrell M. *Proceedings of Expert Workshop on the Induction and Stabilisation of Patients onto Methadone*. Monograph Series No 39. Adelaide, South Australia: Commonwealth Department of Health and Aged Care, 2000 (available at: www.health.gov.au).

4. Borg L. Kreek M J. The pharmacology of opioids. In Graham A W, Schulz T K, Mayo-Smith M F, Ries R K, Wilford B B. (Eds). *Principles of Addiction Medicine*. Chevvy Chase, M D: American Society of Addiction Medicine, 2003; 141–55.

5. Eap C B, Bourquin M, Baurmann P. Inter-individual variability of the clinical pharmacokinetics of methadone: implications for the treatment of opioid dependence. *Clin Pharmacokin* 2002; **41(14)**: 47–54.

6. Harding-Pink D. Opioid toxicity. *Lancet* 1993; **341**: 66–6.

7. Department of Health. *Drug Misuse and Dependence: Guidelines on Clinical Management*. London: DoH, 1999.

8. Bell J, Caplehorn J M, McNeil D R. The effect of intake procedures on performance in methadone maintenance. *Addiction* 1994; **89**: 463–72.

9. Judson B A, Goldstein A. Uses of naloxone in the diagnosis and treatment of heroin addiction. In: Coper J R, Altman F, Brown B S, Czechowicz D. (Eds). *Research into the Treatment of Narcotic Addiction: State of the Art*. Washington, D.C.: National Institute on Drug Abuse, 1983.

10. Buster M, van Brussel G. Is methadone more likely to kill you than heroin? *Euro-Methwork* 1996; Nov: 9.

11. Caplehorn J R M, Drummer O H. Mortality associated with New South Wales methadone programme in 1994: lives lost and saved. *Med K Aust* 1999; **170(3)**: 104–9.

12. Karch S B. Stephens B G. Toxicology and the pathology of deaths related to methadone: retrospective review. *West J Med* 2000; **172**: 11–14.

13. Zador D, Sunjic S. Deaths in methadone maintenance treatment in New South Wales, Australia 1990–1995. *Addiction* 2000; **95(1)**: 77–84.

14. Wolff K, Sanderson M, Hay A W M, Raistrick D. Methadone concentrations in plasma and their relations to drug dosage. *Clin Chem* 1991; **37(2)**: 205–9.

15. Federal Register. Opioid drugs in maintenance and detoxification treatment of opiate addiction; final rule. 2001 (Jan 17); **66(11)**: 4085, 42 CFR Part 8.

16. Vester A, Buning E. European Methadone Guidelines. Amsterdam, The Netherlands: *Euro-Methwork* 2000 (available at: www.q4q.nl/methwork/).

17. Health Canada. *Methadone Maintenance Guidelines*. Toronto, Ontario: College of Physicians of Ontario, 2001 (available at: www.cpso.on.ca).

18. Kreek M J. Factors modifying the pharmacological effectiveness of methadone, In: Cooper J R et al. (Eds). *Research on the Treatment of Narcotic addiction: State of the Art. National Institute of Drug Abuse Research Monograph Series*. Washington, D.C.: Government Printing Offices, 1983; 95–114.

19. Leavitt S B. The methadone dose debate continues. *Addiction Treatment Forum* 2003; **12(1)**: 1, 3 (available at: www.atforum.com).

20. Ward J, Mattick R, Hall W. The use of methadone during maintenance treatment: pharmacology, dosage and treatment outcome. In: Ward J, Mattick R, Hall W. (Eds). *Methadone Maintenance Treatment and Other Opioid Replacement Therapies*. The Netherlands: Harwood Academic Publishers, 1998; 205–35.

21. National Treatment Agency. *Injectable Heroin (and Injectable Methadone): Potential Roles in Drug Treatment*. London: National Treatment Agency, 2003 (available at: www.drugs.gov.uk).

22. Sarfraz A, Alcorn R J. Injectable methadone prescribing in the United Kingdom: current practice and future policy guidelines. *Substance Use and Misuse* 1999; **34**: 1709–21.

23. Beaumont B. Survey of injectable methadone prescribing in general practice in England and Wales. *Int J Drug Policy* 2001; **12(1)**: 91–101.

24. Ford C, Ryrie I. Prescribing injectable methadone in general practice. *Int J Drug Policy* 1999; **10**: 39–45.

25. Roberts K, Hunter C. A comprehensive system of pharmaceutical care for drug misusers *Harm Reduction Journal* 2004; 1: 6 (available at: http://www.harmreductionjournal.com/content/1/1/6).

26. Management and Treatment of Substance Misuse in Berkshire (2001) (locally called 'The purple guidelines' is available in PDF at: www.berkshire.nhs.uk/mentalhealth/professional/documents/sub_misuse_contents.pdf).

27. Roberts K. Supervised consumption of methadone in a community pharmacist. In: Tober G, Strang J. (Eds). *Methadone Matters, Evolving Community Methadone Treatment of Opiate Addiction*. London: Martin Dunitz, 2003; 211–21.

28. Stone E, Fletcher K. User views on supervised methadone consumption. *Addiction Biology* 2003; **8(1)**: 45–8.

29. Ford C. SMMGP, Advice on SCMGs Document, Dec 2000 (available at: www.smmgp.demon.co.uk/html/scmg/scmg01d.htm).

30. Tenore P L. Guidance on optimal methadone dosing. *Addiction Treatment Forum* 2003; **12(3)**: 1, 6–7 (available at: www.atforum.com).

31. Best D, Gossop M, Stewart D, *et al.* Continued heroin use during methadone treatment: relationship between frequency and use of reasons reported for heroin use. *Drug and Alcohol Dependence* 1999; **53**: 191–5.

32. Ball J C, Ross A. *The Effectiveness of Methadone Maintenance Treatment*. New York: Springer-Verlag, 1991.

33. Iguchi M Y, Belding M A, Morral A R, *et al.* Reinforcing operants other than abstinence in drug abuse treatment; an effective alternative for reducing drug use. *J Consulting and Clin Psychol* 1997; **65**: 421–8.

34. Best D, Harris J, Gossop M, *et al.* Use of non-prescribed methadone and other illicit drugs during methadone maintenance treatment. *Drug and Alcohol Review* 2000; **19**: 9–16.

35. Saxon A J, Wells E A, Fleming C, *et al.* Pre-treatment characteristics, program philosophy and levels of ancillary services as predictors of methadone maintenance treatment outcome. *Addiction* 1996; **91**: 1197–209.

36. McLellan A T, Arndt I, Metzger D, *et al.* The effects of psychosocial services in substance abuse treatment. *JAMA* 1993; **269**: 1953–9.

37. Strain E C. Methadone dose during maintenance treatment. In: Strain EC, Stitzer M L. (Eds). *Methadone Treatment for Opioid Dependence*. Baltimore: Johns Hopkins University Press, 1999; 62–85.

38. Joseph H, Stancliff S, Langrod J. Methadone maintenance treatment (MMT): A review of historical and clinical issues. *The Mount Sinai Journal of Medicine* 2000; **67(5, 6)**: 347–64.

39. Hunt D E, Strug D L, Goldsmith D S, *et al.* Alcohol use and abuse: Heavy drinking among methadone clients. *Am J Drug and Alcohol Abuse* 1986; **12**: 147–64.

40. Chatham I R, Rowan-Szal G, Joe G W, *et al.* Heavy drinking in a population of methadone maintenance clients. *J Studies on Alcohol* 1995; **56**: 417–22.

CHAPTER 10

Benzodiazepines use, misuse and management

Clare Gerada and Chris Ford

IN THIS CHAPTER

Introduction || *Benzodiazepine misuse* || *Dose* || *Reasons for non-therapeutic use* || *Problems associated with benzodiazepine use* || *Management of benzodiazepine abuse in illicit drug users* || *Dispensing* || *Follow up* || *Conclusion*

Introduction

Benzodiazepines are the most commonly used hypnotics/anxiolytics and are used in clinical practice for the treatment of anxiety, insomnia, seizures, skeletal muscle spasticity, alcohol withdrawal, and panic disorder and may also be used to sedate patients prior to surgery or to manage the adverse effects of some forms of chemotherapy.

When first introduced into clinical practice in the 1960s they were thought to have distinct advantages over other hypnotics, in particular barbiturates: an improved safety profile, greater anxiety reduction in therapeutic dose, and no physical dependence potential. It is the last claim that has subsequently been shown to be untrue. During the 1970s and '80s benzodiazepine prescribing by doctors increased dramatically, reaching a peak in 1979, but has fallen ever since. Even today there are around 1–1.5 million long-term users, with women outnumbering men by a ratio of 2:1. Most are prescribed for 'therapeutic' use.[1]

A survey carried out in Maine, USA, found that one in five females of 40 years and over received a prescription for benzodiazepines in 2002.[2] Most worrying about this survey was that the fastest increase in prescriptions issued for benzodiazepines was in the 18–19-year-old age group.

Patients with dual diagnosis are more likely than those with severe mental illness alone to be prescribed benzodiazepines. Five-year prevalence of benzodiazepine use for persons with and without substance misuse disorder was 63% compared with 54% for schizophrenia, 75% compared with 58% for bipolar disorder, 66% compared with 49% for major depression, and 48% compared with 40% for other psychiatric disorders. Differences were statistically significant over 5 years.[3]

Benzodiazepine use by illicit drug users is so common that taking them may be deemed ubiquitous in this group of patients. General practitioners are often 'persuaded' to start or continue prescribing benzodiazepines to patients undergoing opioid substitution treatment; paradoxically some doctors are perhaps more comfortable prescribing benzodiazepines than methadone where the latter is clearly indicated. It is important that clinicians understand that there is little evidence for the value of substitute prescribing of benzodiazepines in illicit opioid users – no evidence is not the same as negative evidence.

Whilst short-term prescribing may have a role in supporting drug users to control their intake of these drugs and stabilise their lives, the benefits of long-term prescriptions are less certain and the risks are clear.

This chapter deals predominantly with non-therapeutic use of benzodiazepines by illicit drug users (and not dependent users for whom there is other guidance available, including that contained within the *British National Formulary*) and gives suggestions for management.

Benzodiazepine misuse

Within the illicit drug user population, benzodiazepines are the drugs most frequently used in combination with opioids and are rarely their sole drug of misuse. Ninety per cent of users at drug treatment centres reported taking benzodiazepines in a one-year period;[4] about half injected their benzodiazepines.[5] A two-year American treatment outcome study found that 15% of heroin users also used benzodiazepines daily for more than one year, and 73% more often than weekly.[6] Studies indicate that from 5% to as much as 90% of methadone users are also regular users of benzodiazepines.[7]

It is not only drug users who misuse benzodiazepines; between 3 and 41% of problematic drinkers report that they also misused benzodiazepines at some time, often to moderate intoxication or withdrawal effects.[8] Medical prescriptions, often from general practitioners, are the main source of supply for people who misuse benzodiazepines – with some of these drugs being diverted onto the illicit market for resale.

Dose

Unlike therapeutic users who tend not to exceed the recommended dosages, illicit drug users can take extraordinarily high doses, becoming tolerant to the sedative effects of the drugs. Use of over 1,000 mg has been reported and some addicts claim to consume even higher daily doses.[9]

Reasons for non-therapeutic use

The reasons that illicit drug users give for taking benzodiazepines often conflict, even in the same user, and typically there will always be newer or more compelling reasons given to justify why they take these drugs. For example, some claim to take them for relaxation or to achieve hypnosis, whereas others take them to obtain a 'rush' or 'buzz'. See Box 10.1.

Box 10.1   **Reasons given by drug users for taking benzodiazepines**

Sometimes used as primary drug of use

✓ Improve mood/treat depression

✓ Rapid onset of effect (good buzz)

✓ Hypnotic/anxiolytic/relaxant effects

Frequently used in combinations with other drugs

✓ Enhancing the subjective effects to give a better 'high', for example with alcohol, antihistamines, and opioids, particularly methadone

✓ Avoiding withdrawal symptoms as cross-tolerance with alcohol and other hypnotics

✓ Self-medication for drug adverse effects: 'come-down' from crack cocaine and amfetamines; anxiety/insomnia; opiate withdrawal

Iatrogenic addiction: 'Doctors have prescribed me these drugs for years ... so why not now?'

As potential drugs of abuse, short-acting benzodiazepines (such as temazepam and lorazepam) seem to be preferred by illicit drug users because of the rapidity of their effect (see Box 10.2). In general, drug users prefer benzodiazepines with rapid onset of action, a high potency, brief duration of action, high purity, and water solubility (for intravenous use). Highly lipophilic drugs, such as diazepam, and drugs with short half-life and high potency, such as lorazepam, are the most likely to be associated with misuse. Non-generic forms and drugs of higher dose in one tablet tend to have higher street value than generic forms.[10]

Box 10.2   **Rate of onset of different benzodiazepines (and benzodiazepine-like drugs) after oral use**

✓ **Very rapid**: zolpidem, flunitrazepam

✓ **Rapid**: diazepam, desmethyldiazepam,* midazolam,* temazepam (gel caps), nitrazepam, zopiclone, lormetazepam, clonazepam

✓ **Intermediate:** alprazolam, temazepam (tabs), flurazepam, triazolam,* lorazepam, chlordiazepoxide, promethazine, diphenhydramine

✓ **Slow**: oxazepam, prazepam,* halazepam,* loprazolam

* Not available in UK or not in oral form in UK

Problems associated with benzodiazepine use

The widespread use of benzodiazepines is a major clinical problem. The illicit use of the drug is linked to higher rates of needle sharing, higher levels of polydrug use, an increased chance of injecting during methadone maintenance, higher levels of criminality, and poorer social functioning, though there is no evidence for increased risk for prescribed use.[11] The overall clinical picture of benzodiazepine users is of a more risky, distressed, and chaotic lifestyle.

When used alone, benzodiazepines carry an extremely low risk of acute toxicity. Benzodiazepines, however, are commonly used with other drugs, and these drugs can enhance the toxic effects of benzodiazepines. Benzodiazepines interact synergistically with other central nervous system depressants, including alcohol and opioids, and fatal overdoses can occur if taken together.

Mortality and morbidity

A review of emergency department admissions in the United States found that in 2002, 100,784 drug abuse related attendances involved benzodiazepines and that patients between the ages of 26 and 44 had the highest rate of benzodiazepine-involved attendances. Those aged 18 to 19 showed the fastest growing trend with a tripling of attendances between 1995 and 2002. Nearly half of these attendances were as a result of suicide attempts.[12] Using medical examiner data regarding drug deaths for 2002, the Maine study found that the prevalence of drug deaths due to benzodiazepines, either alone or in combination, was 10% and the number of deceased with benzodiazepine toxicology was 34%. See Box 10.3.

Box 10.3   **Complications of high dose benzodiazepine use**

Fatal overdose if used with other CNS depressants such as methadone

Psychomotor retardation – especially after initial administration or with sudden increase in dose

Memory impairment

Paradoxical disinihibition

Depression

Neonatal dependence and withdrawal if used in pregnancy

Emotional blunting, drugged driving, hip fractures and falls (especially in the elderly), liver failure, fits on withdrawal

Benzodiazepine use increases the risks of

✓ road traffic accidents

✓ falls amongst the elderly

✓ accidental overdose and death

✓ polypharmacy complications

✓ memory impairment

Tolerance and dependence

Tolerance to all the actions of benzodiazepines can develop, although at variable rates and to different degrees. Tolerance to the hypnotic effects tends to develop rapidly, noticed as a reduced efficacy in the relief of insomnia. Tolerance to the anxiolytic effects seems to develop more slowly than tolerance to the hypnotic effects; they lose their efficacy after four or six months of continuous use.[13] Dosage escalation often maintains the cycle of tolerance and dependence. Dependence on benzodiazepines can occur after as few as two months' continuous use, though short-acting, high potency drugs, such as lorazepam, cause dependence sooner than longer-acting drugs such as chlordiazepoxide (Librium™) and diazepam.

Withdrawal

Withdrawal effects from therapeutic dosages of benzodiazepines are similar to anxiety symptoms.[14] The withdrawal syndrome from the abrupt stopping of high dose use can be severe, including life-threatening delirium.[15] The time frame of the emergence of acute withdrawal symptoms corresponds to the half-life of the particular drug taken. The severity of the withdrawal symptoms generally depends on the amount of the original dosage and the rate at which the dosage is reduced, so that protracted withdrawal symptoms are seen in users who have taken benzodiazepines for long periods and in high dosages. See Box 10.4.

Box 10.4   **Features of benzodiazepine withdrawal syndrome**

Psychological symptoms: anxiety, insomnia, and other sleep disturbances, depression, phobias, and paranoid thoughts; perceptual disturbances (de-realisation, abnormal body sensations, and heightened sensitivity to sound or light)

Physical symptoms: headache, pain, stiffness, fatigue, tremor, sweating

Major complications : rare and usually from acute withdrawal, but include withdrawal fits (1–2% especially if high dose is stopped abruptly), psychosis, paranoia, and confusion

Management of benzodiazepine misuse in illicit drug users

Most of the literature on management of 'ordinary-dose' benzodiazepine dependency relates to patients prescribed these drugs for psychiatric disorders (mainly anxiety and depression) who tend not to have concurrent drug misuse problems.[16] This literature is more extensive than the literature relating to use by illicit drug users. The advisability of applying standard benzodiazepine withdrawal guidelines to illicit drug users is affected not only by clinical criteria, but also by the need to avoid abuse and diversion potential of the prescribed medication.

It is largely unknown how addictive benzodiazepines are in drug using populations and which patients in particular develop problems with them. Williams *et al.* found, in a detoxification unit, that benzodiazepine withdrawal symptoms emerged in only half of opioid addicts reportedly using concurrent benzodiazepines and the dose of diazepam required to stabilise patients who did exhibit withdrawal symptoms was unrelated to claimed use, at a mean level of 40 mg/day.[17]

Beyond a few descriptive accounts of clinical services, there is a paucity of literature to guide clinicians on the best management of these patients. Most general practitioners dealing with opiate users will encounter patients who are dependent on these drugs and will be called on to make clinical decisions with respect to management. There are no controlled studies of additional benzodiazepine prescribing in illicit drug users to guide the clinician,[18] much of the current practice is based on opinion rather than evidence, and there is little agreement on how to withdraw from these drugs. It is also unknown which patients may or may not benefit from replacement treatment. Short-term prescribing of benzodiazepines may have some benefit in supporting drug users in controlling their intake of benzodiazepines and stabilising their lives.

The benefit of long-term prescribing of benzodiazepines to drug users is more questionable and of uncertain benefit and may actually be harmful in some sub-groups of patients, but helpful in others.[19] Long-term use of more than 30 mg daily may cause cognitive impairment.[20]

Practical management

The following guidance is drawn from the 1999 National Clinical Guidelines on drug misuse and from advice drawn from primary care experts in the field to assist their colleagues in the management of benzodiazepine dependence.[21-24]

Phases of treatment

It is probably best to think of the management of benzodiazepine dependence in the same manner as any other addiction, bearing in mind that in a small minority of patients maintenance prescribing may be advisable:

1. assessment
2. conversion
3. dose induction
4. detoxification
5. follow up
6. the case for maintenance.

Assessment

It is important that the clinician assesses the patient to determine the degree of dependence, previous attempts at withdrawal (including previous fits), presence of co-existing alcohol dependence, and the presence of depression, anxiety, and insomnia.

Conversion

It is useful first to change all the benzodiazepines into a single preparation. This is best done by converting all other benzodiazepines to the equivalent of diazepam, making this change all in one go. Rarely, if the patient is very anxious, this conversion can be done over a 1—2 week period. See Box 10.5.

Box 10.5 **Conversion of equivalent benzodiazepines**

Valium™	diazepam 10 mg
Restoril™	temazepam 20 mg
Mogadon™	nitrazepam 10 mg
Ativan™	lorazepam 1 mg
Librium™	chlordiazepoxide 20–30 mg
Dalmane™	flurazepam 30 mg
Rohypnol™* not on NHS prescription)	flunitrazepam 1 mg

Source: *British National Formulary* (www.BNF.org)

Dose induction

Detoxification can start at much lower doses than the patient has reported. For example, with a reported use of 200 mg daily, detoxification can start at 60 mg or even less without ill effect and, occurring quickly, without fits.[25]

Others have shown that even where patients report very high benzodiazepine use (equivalent to 140 mg per day), detoxification can start safely (that is without causing fits) at 40% of reported daily consumption, with rapid daily reductions thereafter.[26]

For very high users, for example over 500 mg per day, initial inpatient treatment may be required. See Box 10.6.

Review after two weeks

If the patient is experiencing withdrawal symptoms the dose can be increased by increments of diazepam 5–10 mg, up to a maximum of 60 mg.

Other drugs that can be used for symptomatic relief

All patients should be offered advice about sleep hygine, and if insomnia continues to be a problem use a non-benzodiazepine hypnotic for a short period (for example two weeks).

Box 10.6 **Dose induction**

1. The aim of dose induction is that the patient should not be intoxicated, 'stoned', or drowsy during the day.

2. Aim at the lowest dose possible.

3. Start at 10–30 mg daily of diazepam. Higher doses are rarely required, though if 'street use' is very high (for example over 100 mg diazepam/day) it may be necessary to prescribe 2 × 10 mg three times/day (60 mg) and reduce to 10 mg three times/day within six weeks.

4. It may be advisable, whatever the daily dose, to suggest the patient takes it in two instalments, reserving a dose for night time use.

▶ Sedating anti-depressants should be used only if there is underlying depression and not for sleep alone and must be used with extreme care as they, particularly amitriptyline and dosulepin (previously known as dothiepin hydrochloride), have been frequently found as an additional drug in drug-related deaths.

▶ There are increasing reports of misuse with the 'z' drugs such as zopiclone. They provide no added value above standard benzodiazepines, are much more expensive and NICE do not recommend their use. Zopiclone works on the same receptor site as benzodiazepines and has a similar potential to produce dependence and misuse.[27]

Detoxification from benzodiazepines

There are a number of studies of discontinuation schedules ranging from several days to several weeks or even discontinuation over many years and again these studies are almost all within non-drug using populations. Short term (less than six months) prescribing of 30 mg daily or less may have some benefit in supporting drug users to control their intake.[28]

Where studies look specifically at drug using populations it appears that relatively low-dose short-acting benzodiazepines should suffice in the majority of individuals. Without a doubt, supportive psychological interventions should be used as an adjunct to treatment and the rate of detoxification should be such that it minimises the risk of illicit use or of withdrawal fits.

Box 10.7 contains a suggested regimen from the Royal College of General Practitioners Drug Training Unit.

Box 10.7   **Detoxification regimen for benzodiazepine dependence**

1. Reduction by an eighth of the daily dose per fortnight would be a reasonable approach.

2. Reduction can be quicker if shorter use.

3. When the patient reaches a dose of 20 mg or less, it should be possible to reduce by 1 mg every 1–2 weeks.

4. When down to 5 mg reduce by 0.5 mg every 2 weeks. (NB can use ½ or ¼ of 2 mg tablet or oral solution of diazepam 2 mg/5 l or 5 mg/5ml).

5. Reduction may need to be slower if experiencing withdrawals.

6. While reducing, suggest counselling, support groups, relaxation techniques, and herbal teas, all of which can be helpful.

7. Continue support and relapse prevention after completion of detoxification.

Maintenance

Maintenance prescribing occurs more commonly in opioid maintenance patients than might seem advisable and is the area where general practitioners are most likely to feel the pressure to prescribe. Greenwood published results from her clinical treatment service in Edinburgh where dramatic reductions in illicit opioid use and risk behaviour were accomplished by a treatment regime that included maintenance benzodiazepine prescribing to methadone maintained patients.[28] However, others have shown that maintenance prescribing of benzodiazepines has not been shown to have any definite medical value (unlike methadone) and is rarely justified.

There may be some justification in providing low dose maintenance prescribing to those with alcohol problems who have become detoxified from alcohol using benzodiazepines and who find it difficult to remain abstinent unless they are on a small dose of benzodiazepines. In these cases the clinician should weigh the risks and benefits of on the one hand maintaining abstinence from alcohol and on the other of substituting one addiction (alcohol) for another (benzodiazepines). The balance may be tipped in favour of benzodiazepines in these patients if they have additional risks such as hepatitis C where continuing to drink will increase health risks. In these situations it would be prudent to restrict prescribing to no more than 30 mg diazepam per day. It may be useful for patients with hepatitis C to use a non-hepatic metabolised benzodiazepine such as lorazepam.

There are also a few people who have a long-term opioid and benzodiazepine problem and do not stabilise on opioid substitution medication alone and who are too dependent on benzodiazepines to withdraw successfully.

More contentious are the patients who are self-medicating to improve their mood or improve their coping skills and where it may seem overly punitive to stop their treatment. One emerging indication used by treatment services for longer-term prescribing of benzodiazepines is for the treatment of agitation produced when withdrawing from stimulants. Withdrawal from cocaine is one situation where the clinician needs to balance the merits of prescribing benzodiazepines against the risks of addiction or diversion. See Box 10.8.

Box 10.8 **The pros and cons for maintenance or long-term prescribing of benzodiazepines to drug misusers**

For	Against
Stabilising influence of managed substitute medication avoiding the need to obtain from illicit sources	Promoting dependence
	Risk of erratic or dangerous usage
	Benzodiazepines use associated with worse outcomes in some studies
Can be used as bait to treatment	Prescribing can set unsatisfactory precedent
Failure of repeated attempts to stop	Risk of diversion especially with fast-acting drugs such as flunitrazepam.
May be a mechanism of controlling illicitly obtained benzodiazepines	High risk of dependency and some tolerance
	Coming off benzodiazepines reported to be more difficult than opiates
Effective symptomatic treatment in patients with poor coping skills	After long-term use, usually withdrawal symptoms sometimes prolonged
	Risk of withdrawal symptoms increasing with length of use
	Withdrawals worse if high doses have been used
	Benzodiazepines prescribed for oral use may be injected
	Evidence of cognitive damage from high dose use (> 30 mg diazepam) over a long period
	Risk of diversion onto illicit market as they have a definite 'sellable' potential

The clinician should consider maintenance prescribing only if:

▶ the goals of the prescribing have been established for

- stabilisation of lifestyle
- stabilisation of drug use
- patients able to remove themselves from the illicit drug market

▸ benzodiazepines are taken daily and the person is dependent on these benzodiazepines

▸ at least two positive urine drug screens confirm the presence of benzodiazepines.

(Remember that if benzodiazepines are taken regularly they can stay in urine for three to four weeks.)

Dispensing

1. Prescribe for daily dispensing at the start of treatment, during the period of stabilisation, and continue daily if on daily prescribing of other substitute prescribing. Discuss dispensing with the pharmacist; they may dispense daily if requested on the prescription.

2. As yet in England, benzodiazepines cannot be written on an FP10 (MDA) but it is hoped that in the near future this will be possible. At the present time therefore they need to be written or computer generated separately for instalment dispensing. It is possible to write benzodiazepines on instalment prescriptions in both Scotland and Wales.

3. If prescriptions have been lost or the drugs have been used before the next prescription is due they should not be repeated. Remember the risk of fits is small and it is not for the doctor to collude with inappropriate drug use.

Follow up

As with other drugs of addiction, benzodiazepine dependence has a high risk of relapse. Protracted withdrawal symptoms may occur, especially if high doses are used and/or there is pre-existing co-morbidity. Rates of relapse can be reduced by ensuring that any other addiction problem is optimally managed and with relapse prevention treatments. The National Treatment Outcome Research Study examined the risk of relapse of benzodiazepine use in patients on a methadone prescription and found that the rate of use had decreased from 34% at intake into the study to 12% at four to five years' follow up. Amongst residential patients the percentage using at the start was 44% and this fell to 13% at follow up.

Conclusion

Benzodiazepine use is a large problem in the drug using population. Though they are often used to reduce anxiety, help sleep or counter the negative effects of other drugs, they are nevertheless addictive and commonly subject to abuse and diversion.

Clinicians need to decide how to address benzodiazepine use. To ignore the problems or to steadfastly refuse to offer any substitute prescribing is not the solution. Short-term prescribing of benzodiazepines in drug users may help to stabilise their drug use and their lifestyle. Long-term prescribing of benzodiazepines to drug users is more difficult. We need to consider all the potential harms weighed against the potential gains and to use long-term prescribing in selected patients only. We need to think carefully about the goals that we hope to achieve *before* starting a prescription of benzodiazepine, even before giving a prescription for a short-term reducing dose. We should be more reluctant to prescribe benzodiazepines than opioid substitutes, since the evidence base for the latter is far more robust. The practitioner needs to explain to the patient the unwanted effects of benzodiazepines, such as the cognitive impairment from long-term high dose use, its addictive properties, the withdrawal symptoms and emotional suppression, and the development of a learning deficit/reduced coping ability.

Further reading

Seivewright E N. (Ed). The case for substitute prescribing. Benzodiazepines. In: *Community Treatment of Drug Misuse: More than Methadone.* Cambridge: Cambridge University Press, 2000.

References

1. Ashworth M, Gerada C, Dallmeyer R. Benzodiazepine: addiction and abuse. *Drugs: Education, Prevention and Policy* 2002; **9(4)**: 389–97.

2. Song M, Mugford J, Gressitt S. Maine benzodiazepine study group annual report 2003. A white paper summarizing the survey of the 2002 data and proceedings of the First Annual Maine Benzodiazepine Study Group Conference, 2003 (available at: www.noemaine.org/benzo/benzo.htm).

3. Clark R, Haiyi X, Brunette M. Benzodiazepine prescription practices and substance abuse in persons with severe mental illness. *J Clin Psychiatry* 2004; **65**: 151–5.

4. Perera K M H, Tulley M, Jenner F A. The use of benzodiazepines among drug addicts. *Br J Addiction* 1987; **82(5)**: 511–15.

5. Strang J, Griffiths P, Abbey J, Gossop M. Survey of use of injected benzodiazepines among drug users in Britain. *BMJ* 1994; **308 (6936)**: 1082.

6. Dumont R L. Abuse of benzodiazepines: the problems and the solutions. A report of a committee of the Institute for Behaviour and Health, Inc. *Am J Drug Alcohol Abuse* 1988; **14 (1)**: 1–69.

7. Iguchi M Y, Griffiths R R, Bickel W K, *et al*. Relative abuse liability of benzodiazepines in methadone-maintained populations in three cities. In: Harris L S. (Ed). *Problems of Drug Dependence*, 1988: proceedings of the 50th Annual Scientific Meeting, the Committee on Problems of Drug Dependence, Office of Science, 1989. DHHS publication no. (ADM) 89–1605.

8. Ciraulo D A, Sands B F, Shader R I. Critical review of the liability for benzodiazepine abuse among alcoholics. *Am J Psychiatry* 1988; **145**: 1501–6.

9. Strang J, Griffith P, Abbey J, *et al*. Survey of use of injected benzodiazepines among drug users in Britain. *BMJ* 1994; **308**: 1082.

10. Parran T. Prescription drug abuse. A question of balance. *Med Clin North Am* 1997; **81 (14)**: 967–78.

11. Drake S, Swift W, Hall W, Ross M. Drug use, HIV risk-taking, and psychosocial correlates of benzodiazepine use among methadone maintenance clients. *Drug Alcohol Depend* 1993; **34**: 67–70.

12. Demographic characteristics of benzodiazepine involved ED visits. 1995–2002 (available at: DAWNinfo.samhsa.gov/).

13. Marriott S, Tyrer P. Benzodiazepine dependence. Avoidance and withdrawal. *Drug Saf* 1993; **9 (2)**: 93–103.

14. Busto U, Sellars E M, Naranjo C A, *et al*. Withdrawal reaction after long-term therapeutic use of benzodiazepines. *New Engl J Med* 1986; **315 (14)**: 854–9.

15. Ashton H. Toxicity and adverse consequences of benzodiazepines use. *Psychiatric Annals* 1995; **25 (3)**: 158–65.

16. Ashton H. The treatment of benzodiazepine dependence. *Addiction* 1994; **89 (11)**: 1535–41.

17. Williams H, Oyefeso A, Ghodse A H. Benzodiazepine misuse and dependence among opiate addicts in treatment. *Irish J Psychol Med* 1996; **13**: 62–4.

18. Seivewright N. *Community Treatment of Drug Misuse: More than Methadone*. Cambridge: Cambridge University Press, 1999, 70–9.

19. Darke S. The Use of benzodiazepines amongst injecting drug users. *Drug & Alcohol Review* 1994; **13 (1)**: 63–9.

20. Seivewright N. Theory and practice in managing benzodiazepine dependence and abuse. *Journal of Substance Misuse* 1998; **3**: 170–7.

21. Department of Health. *Drug Misuse and Dependence: Guidelines on Clinical Management*. London: DoH, 1999.

22. Ford C. Use and abuse of benzodiazepines by polydrug users. In: Beaumont B. (Ed). *Care of Drug Users in General Practice*. Abingdon: Radcliffe Medical Press, 2004.

23. Guidance on Good Practice in Prescribing Benzodiazepines to Drug Users in Primary Care. SMMGP Production (available at: www.smmgp.co.uk).

24. Seivewright N, Dougal W. Withdrawal symptoms from high dose benzodiazepines in poly drug users. *Drug & Alcohol Dependence* 1993; **32**: 15–23.

25. Scott R T A. The prevention of convulsions during benzodiazepine withdrawals. *Br J Gen Pract* 1990; **40**: 261.

26. Harrison M, Busto U, Naranjo C A. Diazepam tapering in detoxification for high dose benzodiazepine abuse. *Clin Pharmacol Therapeutics* 1984; **36 (4)**: 527–33.

27. National Institute for Clinical Excellence. *Zaleplon, Zolpidem and Zopiclone for the Short-term Management of Insomnia*. Technology Appraisal Guidance 77. London: NICE, April 2004 (available at: www.nice.org.uk/pdf/TA077quickrefguide.pdf).

28. Greenwood J. Six years' experience of sharing the care of Edinburgh drug users. *Psychiatric Bulletin* 1996; **20**: 8–11.

CHAPTER 11

Central nervous system stimulants

Clare Gerada and Chris Ford

IN THIS CHAPTER

Cocaine || *Amfetamines* || *Methamfetamine* || *Khat*

Cocaine

The Royal College of General Practitioners have recently published clinical guidance aimed at the primary care practitioner working with cocaine users. This chapter should be seen alongside this document.[1]

Prevalence

Cocaine use, in all its forms, is increasing in England and general practitioners should be aware of this. Many of the skills used in general practice are helpful and must not be forgotten. Whereas there is a large evidence base to support the use of methadone for the treatment of opioid addiction, no effective substitute drug treatment exists for cocaine although many have been tried. This does not mean that there is nothing the clinician can do to help cocaine users, and this chapter will explain what role a health professional can play.

Whilst the numbers of cocaine users is on the increase it does not yet approach the levels of use in the United States. By the middle of the 1980s it was estimated that around one tenth of the US population had used cocaine. Although cocaine misuse has featured among UK treatment populations for decades, it has rarely been the prime focus. Many working in the drugs field have waited for the impending 'crack-epidemic' since the 1980s at a time when the crack scene exploded in America. Services prepared themselves and learning exchanges to the United States were arranged. Stories about 'crack-babies' appeared in the news and the British population waited for the invasion. For almost 20 years nothing happened. Crack cocaine was certainly being used, but was largely contained to a small population mainly in inner cities such as London and Manchester. However, we cannot be complacent as we are now seeing year on year increases in the numbers of cocaine users in this country. Not only has the latest British Crime Survey shown an increase in cocaine use but also the amount of crack cocaine seized in London has quadrupled between 2003 and 2004, while heroin seizures halved over the same period. It is uncommon now to come across drug users who *do not* use cocaine and its use places great challenges on treatment services.

The proportion of new referrals to English drug treatment services reporting any cocaine use rose from 7% to 24% between 1998 and 2001, while the proportion reporting cocaine as their main drug of use rose from 3% to 8%. The British Crime Survey 2002/3 showed that nearly 5% of people between 16 and 24 years of age had used cocaine in the last year, an increase from 1% in 1996 [2] (see Box 11.1).

Box 11.1   **Use of cocaine 2002–2003** [3]

Prevalence of cocaine use (16–24 years)			
PERCENTAGE USED	16 – 19	20 – 24	16 – 24
Cocaine			
Last year	3.0	6.4	4.7
Last month	1.3	2.5	1.9
Crack			
Last year	0.4	0.5	0.5
Last month	0.1	0.3	0.2
Estimate of last year drug users (16–24 year olds)			
NUMBER WHO HAVE USED	BEST ESTIMATE	LOW ESTIMATE	HIGH ESTIMATE
Cocaine	270,000	229,000	317,000
Crack	27,000	16,000	46,000
Estimate of the number of drug users (16–59 year olds)			
	BEST ESTIMATE	LOW ESTIMATE	HIGH ESTIMATE
Cocaine			
Last year	642,000	578,000	714,000
Last month	275,000	234,000	324,000
Crack			
Last year	63,000	44,000	88,000
Last month	28,000	17,000	47,000

What is cocaine?

Cocaine is a powerful stimulant that directly affects the brain. The Inca people worshipped the coca bush as a plant of divine origin. It was extracted in pure form around the 1860s and first appeared on the commercial market in the mid 1880s in the form of extracts of coca-leaf. The best known of these extracts was Vin Mariani, a coca wine product that was produced in France before 1870. This beverage was closely followed by the development of other products, one of which evolved to become Coca-Cola (although the product no longer contains cocaine). In the early 1900s cocaine was the main stimulant drug used in most of the tonics/elixirs that were being produced. Cocaine is available for medicinal use and is indicated as a local anaesthesia for some eye, ear, and throat procedures. Within the illicit world, cocaine is used either in its powdered form (cocaine hydrochloride) or in its alkaloid form, commonly called crack. The term crack refers to the noise made when the crack 'rocks' are heated in order to be smoked, it is the later formulation of cocaine that most general practitioners are now familiar with as its use becomes increasingly common amongst our drug-using patients.

Cocaine purity and price

To get from the highlands of Columbia to the user, cocaine passes through many hands, and is diluted at each stage to increase profit. For that reason, the average gram 'wrap' is usually between 20 and 65% actual cocaine. The rest is probably cornstarch, vitamin C powder, sugar, talcum powder, baby milk powder, or local anaesthetic (to simulate the numbing effect).

At the time of writing (2004) the price for powder cocaine in the United Kingdom is upwards of £40 per gram, whereas crack is more expensive at between £5 and £20 per rock depending on the size and purity and very much on the area of the country.

Patterns of cocaine use

The frequency of cocaine use varies considerably. 'Recreational' use is relatively common with individuals taking the drug only occasionally (often 'snorting'). This is often in association with social activities and includes weekend use. Daily use occurs, as does heavy and intermittent use or 'bingeing'. Binges tend to take the form of repeated dosing with the drug, often in escalating amounts over a period of hours or days, terminating in a 'crash' with exhaustion and depressive symptoms. Cocaine may be used in association with other drugs such as alcohol or heroin. The injecting of heroin together with cocaine ('speedballing' or 'snowballing') is a highly dangerous practice that is becoming more prevalent.

See Boxes 11.2 and 11.3.

Box 11.2   **Different patterns of cocaine use**

Recreational user	Infrequent user, shares with friends and tends not to have a regular pattern of use. This group tends to run into problems only if use escalates
Binge user	Actively seeks crack cocaine, will buy increased quantities. Social activities are dominated around cocaine purchase and use. Probably experiences several physical or psychological problems including withdrawal phenomena. This person may present for help
Chronic high-dose user (sometimes associated with dependent use)	Will consume as much as possible and may demonstrate life-threatening use. Values and activities centred on use and relationships and work affected by this use. Person will experience severe psychological and physical problems

Routes of use

Cocaine is well absorbed via the mucous membranes and is often taken via the intranasal route or dabbed directly on to the gums. After intravenous or smoking routes peak concentrations are reached within minutes (five to ten) and after around 60 minutes if taken intranasally. Effects diminish after as little as one hour after ingestion.

Box 11.3   **Routes of use**

✓ **Snorting:** most commonly snorted in its hydrochloride powdered form

✓ **Piping:** most commonly smoked through a pipe; glass pipes, tin cans, and water bottles are used. This is the quickest route of absorption

✓ **Injecting:** cocaine hydrochloride is soluble in water and hence can be injected. Crack cocaine must be reconverted back to its salt form to become soluble

✓ **Chasing:** like heroin, crack cocaine can be heated on tin foil and the vapour 'chased'

✓ **Smoking/chipping:** this involves flaking small amounts of cocaine or crack into the top of a tobacco cigarette to form a 'joint'. Typically less cocaine is ingested through this route

Effects and complications of cocaine use

The transition from cocaine powder to crack cocaine has changed the face of cocaine usage. Crack cocaine is a purer, more volatile form of cocaine and is much more potent in its effects, its addictive potential, and its withdrawal symptoms on cessation of use. The faster the absorption the more intense the 'high' and the faster the effect wears off. After inhalation, crack cocaine reaches peak plasma concentrations in a matter of seconds, with its peak effects or 'rush' arising after a few minutes and then decreasing rapidly, producing a deep depression or 'crash'. The main effects are to increase sense of wellbeing, energy, and alertness and to reduce appetite and need for sleep. See Table 11.1.

Table 11.1 **Effects of cocaine use**

Short-term effects of cocaine	Increased energy Decreased appetite Mental alertness Increased blood pressure Increased pulse rate Increase in core body temperature, decreased heat perception and impairment of sweating and skin blood flow Dilated pupils Talkativeness and restlessness Increased self-confidence Volatile train of thoughts – appearance of being manic Wavering judgement
Long-term effects of cocaine	Dependence Irritability Mood disturbances Restlessness Paranoia Auditory hallucinations Tactile hallucinations (false sensation of touch such as insects crawling under the skin – formication) Loss of libido Insomnia Suicidal thoughts or attempts Regular intranasal use: chronic rhinitis, reduced sense of smell, nosebleeds, septal perforation Smoking: severe exacerbation of asthma, acute lung injury ('crack-lung')
Other	The crack cocaine scene is one of violence, with high rates of gun crime, whilst crack cocaine misuse in women is strongly associated with prostitution

As with all psycho stimulants, cocaine use has many physical and psychiatric effects, some of which can be serious and life threatening. Because of cocaine's stimulant effects on the noradrenergic system, heavy use carries significant risks of cardiovascular complications, including angina, myocardial infarction, and stroke.

Sudden death of users can occur on the first use or unexpectedly thereafter, even with low doses. Deaths are often as a result of cardiac arrest or seizures following respiratory depression.

Cocaine powerfully constricts blood vessels. This leads to a massive rise in blood pressure soon after the drug is taken, with a risk of stroke. One study has shown that the risk of a heart attack is increased 23-fold in the hour following cocaine use.[4]

In long-term users, surges in blood pressure can lead to a build-up of atheroma, so that a regular cocaine user as young as 25–30 years without any other risk factor can develop triple vessel coronary artery disease as a result of cocaine use. Reports from the United States suggest that as many as one in four myocardial infarctions in people aged 18–45 are linked to cocaine use. Dissection of the aorta has also been reported in cocaine users.[5]

As with all psycho stimulants, cocaine may cause seizures or unmask epilepsy. Brain perfusion deficits and associated neuropsychological compromise (such as deficits in attention, concentration, new learning, visual and verbal memory, and word production) may be persistent. Tics, stereotypes of speech or movement, ataxia, and disturbed gait may occur, which may disappear after the drug use is stopped.

Psychiatric effects are common. Psychotic episodes, especially involving paranoid delusions together with increase in aggressive and violent behaviour are the risks of heavy binge use. Confusion and aggressive behaviour may develop and in such a state, which some term 'excited delirium', violent behaviour may ensue and the individual may require restraint and detention prior to treatment. During such restraint, however, sudden deaths have been reported.

The symptoms usually resolve over hours or days of stopping the cocaine use but may be more persistent. Cocaine use can lead to impairments in brain function through decreased perfusion and multiple small ischaemic infarcts. This may affect the ability of the individual to take part in treatment successfully.

Cocaine use appears to increase the risk of the transmission of HIV, not only through the potential for sharing of needles, but through increased sexual activity and loss of sexual inhibition.

Dependence

A central descriptive characteristic of any dependence syndrome is the desire (often strong, sometimes overpowering) to take the drug in question. There is some debate about the presence or otherwise of a cocaine dependence syndrome. Whatever the academic answer, cocaine causes psychological dependence, sometimes leading to profound psychological addiction, produced by high doses of cocaine, which can cause euphoric excitement. Tolerance occurs, but true physical dependence has not been confirmed: no stereotypical withdrawal syndrome occurs when the drug is discontinued. For some users the tendency to continue taking the drug is strong and there does appear to be a cluster of physiological, behavioural, and cognitive phenomena in which the use of cocaine takes on a much higher priority for a given individual than other behaviours that once had greater value.

Diagnostic guidelines for dependence

International Code of Diseases (ICD-10) gives the following diagnostic criteria for cocaine dependence. A definite diagnosis of dependence should usually be made only if three or more of the following have been experienced or exhibited at some time during the previous year:

▶ a strong desire or sense of compulsion to take cocaine

▶ difficulties in controlling cocaine-taking behaviour in terms of its onset, termination, or levels of use

▶ a physiological withdrawal state when cocaine use has ceased or been reduced, as evidenced by the characteristic withdrawal syndrome for cocaine, or use of the same (or a closely related) substance with the intention of relieving or avoiding withdrawal symptoms

▶ evidence of tolerance, such that increased doses of cocaine are required in order to achieve effects originally produced by lower doses (clear examples of this are found in cocaine-dependent individuals who may take daily doses sufficient to incapacitate or kill non-tolerant users)

▶ progressive neglect of other pleasures or interests because of cocaine use

▶ increased amount of time necessary to obtain or take the substance or to recover from its effects

▶ persisting with cocaine use despite clear evidence of overtly harmful consequences, such as depressive mood states consequent to periods of heavy substance use, or drug-related impairment of cognitive functioning; efforts should be made to determine that the user was actually, or could be expected to be, aware of the nature and extent of the harm.

Narrowing of the personal repertoire of patterns of cocaine use has also been described as a characteristic feature.

It is an essential characteristic of the dependence syndrome that either cocaine taking or a desire to take cocaine should be present; the subjective awareness of compulsion to use drugs is most commonly seen during attempts to stop or control substance use.

Cocaine use and other drug/alcohol use

Cocaine users often take other sedative drugs to terminate an episode of use and alleviate withdrawal effects. These additional drugs are typically cannabis, alcohol, benzodiazepines, and heroin. There is evidence that combining alcohol and cocaine can cause more harm on the user than either drug taken separately, especially to the cardiovascular system, and increase the overall morbidity and mortality associated with cocaine use. There is a potentially dangerous interaction between cocaine and alcohol. The combination increases the euphoric effects of cocaine through the production in the liver of cocaethylene, a long-acting ethyl homologue of cocaine, which may increase the risk of sudden death. Alcoholics Anonymous in the United Kingdom has recorded a significant increase in the number of members discussing their cocaine use at regular meetings.

Cocaine use and pregnancy

The risk of premature birth, stillbirth, poor growth for gestational age, and central nervous system damage are reported consequences of maternal cocaine use during pregnancy, mainly related to the powerful vasoconstrictor effects of cocaine on placental vessels, although the evidence for this is conflicting. With respect to direct teratogenic effects on the foetus, dozens of studies over the past decade now indicate that the pharmacological impact of cocaine has been greatly exaggerated, that other factors are responsible for many of the long-term effects found in the infants of heavy cocaine users.

Many cocaine-using women do not maintain adequate nutrition, do not attend antenatal care classes, and use other drugs that could themselves be harmful, including alcohol and tobacco. The child exposed intrauterine to cocaine, given proper parenting and educational support, may well develop normally with a bright-future. Supporting cocaine-exposed children and their family is an important task for all health professionals who deal with children.[6]

Treatment for cocaine users

Given the diversity of the cocaine-using population, and the differing needs of each group of users, it is clear that service interventions should be provided at a range of levels to meet the gradations of need. There are likely to be a number of key principles of service provision including:[7]

- easy access to services (including opening times and location)

- multiple points of entry

- person-centred and timely and shared assessment procedures

- information and support services when required

- specific pharmacological/psychological and psychosocial interventions when required

- effective referral procedures and protocols to ensure an integrated approach to providing treatment and care (including specialist mental health and detoxification services where necessary)

- support for children of psychostimulant users when appropriate

- access to social care and accommodation.

It is important that general practitioners and other primary care professionals are aware of the signs of problem stimulant use, so that they can engage the person in treatment, give information, and make appropriate referrals. GPs are often the first point of contact for drug users, especially stimulant users. It is equally important for this contact to be as productive as possible, that GPs adopt a non-judgmental attitude, and have basic knowledge about stimulants and their complications. General practitioners can provide basic healthcare needs for stimulant users including assessment of physical health with assessment of injection sites if appropriate. Mental health assessment is vital in the case of stimulant drug users and GPs should be able to carry out a basic assessment and arrange for onward referral as necessary.

Health promotion advice is of particular importance in this area given the potential cardiac complications of cocaine use in a population with high rates of cardiovascular disease.

The possible treatments for cocaine misuse and the evidence of their effectiveness have been the subject of reviews conducted by a number of academics. To date, most of our knowledge about treating cocaine use comes from the United States, following an increase in cocaine use in the 1980s. Overall, there is no evidence to strongly support any single treatment (either symptomatic or substitute). The focus of research has been on symptomatic medications that relieve withdrawal, rather than medications that provide a substitute for cocaine. Controlled trials have mostly focused on desipramine and other antidepressants.

A systematic review examining the use of antidepressants examined 18 randomised controlled studies, which concluded that there was no evidence for supporting the clinical use of antidepressants in the treatment of cocaine dependence. Carbamazepine has also been recommended, although there is currently no evidence to support its use in the treatment of cocaine dependence.[6] A systematic review of the five randomised controlled trials of the drug found no evidence to support its use with cocaine users. Another systematic review addressing the use of dopamine agonists concluded that current evidence does not support the clinical use of these. Finally, an American study suggests that combining disulfiram with buprenorphine can reduce cocaine misuse in heroin users who also use cocaine, although the evidence is weak.[8]

Given that there is no pharmacological bullet it is important that the clinician and the patient do not lose hope: there is more to treatment than medication. The National Treatment Agency offers encouragement by saying: 'Treating patients with crack dependence is neither extraordinarily difficult nor does it necessarily depend on totally new skills.'[9]

Non-pharmacological interventions

Drug-free psychosocial interventions such as counselling, provided on a non-residential basis, are the most cost-effective options for patients with few complicating problems. Patients with multiple needs tend to benefit from intensive residential rehabilitation and (if they stay long enough) do better there than in community-based drug counselling.[10] Intensive rehabilitation programmes can be provided just as effectively on a day-care basis.

Behavioural therapies, in particular contingency management approaches, are used in the United States and are gaining acceptance and usage in the United Kingdom. The treatment involves using rewards for adhering to certain behaviours and has been demonstrated to be effective in cocaine dependence, including in those who are methadone-maintained opiate addicts. Cognitive behavioural therapy has also been shown to be effective in cocaine misusers and those in methadone maintenance programmes.[10]

In 1999, the results from the National Institute on Drug Abuse's Collaborative Cocaine Treatment study were published.[11] This US study aimed to determine the most effective psychosocial therapy for cocaine dependence and compared individual drug counselling therapy plus group drug counselling (GDC), cognitive therapy plus GDC, supportive–expressive counselling plus GDC, and GDC alone over six months. Individual drug counselling plus GDC, which incorporated a 21-step philosophy, was the most effective in reducing cocaine use. The authors proposed that the success of the individual therapy might have been because it focused on stopping current drug use.

Harm reduction

There are a number of principles of safer drug use that can be discussed with the drug user to reduce harm related to crack cocaine use. These include general advice to use glass pipes, to reduce amounts in one sitting, not to share needles when injecting, to switch from injecting to other routes, not to share pipes or straws, and to practise safer activity.

Cocaine vaccine

A 'cocaine vaccine' could be a promising immunotherapeutic approach to treating cocaine dependence. It induces the immune system to form antibodies that prevent cocaine from crossing the blood–brain barrier to act on receptor sites in the brain. Studies in rats show that cocaine antibodies can block cocaine from reaching the brain and prevent reinstatement of cocaine self-administration. A successful phase 1 trial of a human cocaine vaccine has been reported.[12] The most promising application of a vaccine is to prevent relapse to dependence in abstinent users who voluntarily enter treatment. Any use of a vaccine to treat cocaine addicts under legal coercion raises major ethical issues and if done at all should first undergo careful clinical trials and be implemented only after significant experience is obtained from using the vaccine in voluntary settings.

Amfetamines

Amfetamines – as with other psycho-stimulants – boost energy, improve mood and (in the short-term) decrease appetite.

There are three basic types of amfetamine: laevoamfetamine, dextroamfetamine, and methylamfetamine. The most widely available form on the black market is a white crystalline powder containing both laevoamfetamine and dextroamfetamine in equal proportions. It is commonly called 'amp', 'speed', 'whizz', or 'sulph'. The purity of amfetamine powder seizures has remained fairly stable over the years at around 8.6%, with caffeine the most common adulterant found in amfetamine powder. Other substances include methamfetamine, MDMA, cocaine, ketamine, ephedrine, phenacetin and selegiline.[13]

Amfetamine was first synthesised in 1887 and has been used to treat a number of conditions, including narcolepsy and attention deficit disorder in children. In the past it was used to treat depression – sometimes combined with barbiturates. Use of the drug in non-therapeutic situations is widespread yet there is little research to guide the clinician with respect to effective treatments.

Amfetamine, commonly called 'mother's little helper' when used by women, is often used at parties and social events. Amfetamine is a powerful central nervous system stimulant, used recreationally for the euphorogenic effects as well as 'functionally' to ward off fatigue and increase energy and capacity for physical activity. It can improve performance on some simple tasks, increase activity levels, and produce anorexia. The liability of amfetamines to abuse is thought to be primarily related to their euphoric effects. However, their dependence and abuse are viewed as resulting from a process in which multiple interacting factors (social, psychological, cultural, and biological) influence drug-using behaviour.[14]

Amfetamines have been abused almost since their introduction. The ease of synthesis from inexpensive and readily available chemicals makes widespread amfetamine dependence and abuse possible. Two major epidemics of amfetamine dependence and abuse were widely recognised in the 1960s and 1990s. These epidemics, in particular the latter, affected many developed and developing countries around the world, especially North America, Europe, Far East Asia, and Australia. Of 180 million people worldwide consuming drugs in the late 1990s, 29 million were taking amfetamine-type stimulants.[15] This figure was larger than the number of people consuming cocaine and opioids combined. An Australian multi-city study looking at injecting drug users found that amfetamines were the drugs most commonly first injected (45.8%); almost half of the 872 sample had used amfetamines in the month prior to the interview (94.4% of whom had injected).[16]

Routes and patterns of amfetamine use are complex and changeable and vary amongst different socio-economic groups.

Amfetamine use can be oral (tablets), intravenous (crushed tablets), intranasal (powder) or smoked as amfetamine base.

On average, regular users make the transition to injecting after about two years.[17] Once users begin injecting they are unlikely to return to snorting or swallowing. Most first time users and recreational users swallow the drug and these users tend not to approach treatment services. Taken intravenously, the abuse potential of amfetamines is comparable to that of heroin or cocaine.[18] Injecting of amfetamine is associated with more frequent use, higher risk of dependence, poorer social function, and psychological morbidity.

The World Health Organization has classified the patterns of amfetamine use as:[19]

1. Instrumental use: amfetamines are exploited by the users to achieve desired goals, such as to improve concentration and ward off fatigue.

2. Sub cultural/recreational use: amfetamine stimulant properties are exploited to allow the user to remain active for longer periods in social/recreational settings, such as at music and dance events.

3. Chronic use: for several reasons, such as craving, tolerance, and withdrawal, some amfetamine users turn into chronic users to relieve unwanted effects of abstinence.

The Diagnostic and Statistical Manual of Mental Disorders, Fourth Edition (DSM-IV) describes the following 10 amfetamine psychiatric related disorders:

1. amfetamine-induced anxiety disorder

2. amfetamine-induced mood disorder

3. amfetamine-induced psychotic disorder with delusions

4. amfetamine-induced psychotic disorder with hallucinations

5. amfetamine-induced sexual dysfunction

6. amfetamine-induced sleep disorder

7. amfetamine intoxication

8. amfetamine intoxication with delirium

9. amfetamine withdrawal

10. amfetamine-related disorder not otherwise specified.

Death in amfetamine users is rare but where it has occurred, it is usually attributable to accidents, cerebrovascular haemorrhages, acute cardiac failure, and suicide.[20] The development of tolerance and dependence to the psychological and physiological effects of amfetamines are less pronounced than that for opioids but it is still well established. Cessation of amfetamine use in a tolerant individual is associated with both physical and psychological withdrawal symptoms.

Treatment for amfetamine users

There are proportionately far more occasional and recreational users of amfetamine than of heroin and it is likely that the general practitioner will come across non-dependent, non-problematic users in the course of their work. For these patients, simple explanations and techniques used in brief intervention in alcohol use may suffice.

Even at the dependent, heavier end of use, most amfetamine users have no contact with treatment services. This may be because services are designed for opiate users; it may also be because of the nature of a user's habits. Three-quarters of amfetamine users surveyed in an Australian study had tried to reduce their use without professional assistance. Of these, 93% successfully reduced their amfetamine use and 83% were satisfied with the outcome.[21] For heavier use the treatment of amfetamine dependence is similar to that of other stimulants, with a strong reliance on general measures and psychosocial treatments rather than the magic bullet of substitute medication.

Pharmacological treatments

As with treatment for cocaine users, the overall research evidence on treatments for amfetamine dependence is limited. A number of potential treatments have been studied. Fluoxetine, amlodipine, imipramine, and desipramine appear to have very limited benefits for amfetamine dependence. Fluoxetine may decrease craving in the short term and imipramine may increase the duration of adherence to treatment. A further systematic review on treatments for amfetamine psychosis found limited evidence on effectiveness. The results of two studies among amfetamine users show that agitation and some psychotic symptoms may abate within one hour of an antipsychotic injection.[22] Dexamfetamine sulphate (Dexedrine™) is the most frequently studied drug for amfetamine users. It has been prescribed in England and Wales for the treatment of primary amfetamine use.

The proponents of oral amfetamine substitution therapy argue that:

1. There is a need for an appropriate intervention for amfetamine users, and that current treatment modalities for illicit drug users are irrelevant to their needs, in that they are orientated primarily to opioid users or relief on abrupt withdrawal.[23]

2. Oral amfetamine substitution can allow stabilisation of patients on a dose that causes neither withdrawal nor craving, and thereafter a subsequent gradual dose reduction and eventual cessation.

3. Needle sharing by amfetamine users makes amfetamine prescribing an important public health approach to the prevention of infectious diseases, a potential that may outweigh the risks associated with prescribing.

However, there are a number of reasons why amfetamines should not be prescribed, citing issues concerning dependence, toxicity, psychosis, neurotoxicity, diversion, difficulties in monitoring illicit use, and the failure of previous attempts of amfetamine substitution. In addition, many amfetamine users are not regular users, and therefore there is a serious risk of increasing drug use and endangering further instability.

Nevertheless, despite the paucity of evidence with respect to the efficacy of substitute prescribing,[24] general practitioners are prescribing large quantities. This prescribing, although not being in the same order as methadone prescribing to opiate addicts, nevertheless represents the next most prevalent prescribing practice in the community management of addiction, with an estimated 900–1,000 addicts currently being prescribed amfetamine.[25]

The 1999 Clinical Guidelines suggest that there may be a limited place for the prescription of dexamfetamine sulphate 5 mg in the treatment of amfetamine abuse, although this should be initiated only by specialists. There is no research to guide the clinician with respect to dose and duration of prescription. Daily dispensing is recommended and it is generally advisable to avoid long term prescribing. Injecting behaviour, illicit drug use, mental state, blood pressure, weight, and urine should all be monitored regularly, although the Department of Health guidelines suggest that prescribing should be restricted to particular groups:

▸ primary amfetamine users

▸ injecting users

▸ heavy, dependent use for more than three months, that is more than 1 g per day or on more than three days a week

▸ evidence that use is escalating and increasing tolerance and craving

and that they are not prescribed in the following cases:

▸ polydrug use

▸ history of mental illness

▸ hypertension or heart disease

▸ pregnancy.

Community management

Seivewright and others have offered advice as to the appropriate management of amfetamine abuse, based on their own clinical service. To this effect, Seivewright has developed a treatment policy within his community service, which has been developed pragmatically over a number of years.[26] Most amfetamine users receive counselling alone. This includes all individuals whose amfetamine use is short-term and/or occasional (e.g. weekends) and those in whom there is no convincing evidence or indications for pharmacological treatments. Nearly all such users take the street powder by ingestion or snorting. This form of amfetamine tends to be very impure, sometimes as little as 5% active ingredient. For heavier users, more specific behavioural techniques are used, to try to reduce use to fewer days per week.

The next category of users is those dependent individuals, who may have even moved on to injecting. For these an initial trial of symptomatic drugs are used but for those where their use is causing serious mental health problems or where use is heavy and through the injecting route then substitute amfetamines are used. See Table 11.2.

What ever the course of action with respect to prescribing amfetamines to patients, general practitioners should be mindful of the risks of diversion and of perpetuating an otherwise transient habit. The clinician must be clear that the benefits of such prescribing outweigh any risks and that their reasoning for pre-scribing is well documented and clear.

Table 11.2   **Community management options**

Treatment	Indication
Counselling alone	Short-term use, less than 6 months Occasional use Not injecting
Counselling plus limited course of symptomatic medication: fluoexetine, diazepam, nitrazepam	Inability to tolerate withdrawal effects
Counselling plus dexamfetamine sulphate prescribing	Heavy daily use Severe direct health or social problems Other approaches failed but highly motivated to avoid illicit use

Methamfetamine

Special mention should be made of methamfetamine. This is a powerful variant of amfetamine that is becoming an extremely serious and growing problem in parts of the world, particularly the Asian subcontinent, Australia, and the United States and there is now an enormous illicit production of this drug in many countries, particularly the Asian-Pacific region and United States. In the Asian subcontinent, especially Thailand, it has replaced heroin as the number one drug of abuse, and brings with it many worse problems, such as violence. Illicit manufacture of methamfetamine is a global problem with far-reaching political, public health, and clinical problems and implications. Methamfetamine has many names, including 'ice', 'crystal' and 'glass'. It comes in both powder and rock form and reports of its availability in the UK have just begun to surface.

Just as 'crack' represents a highly purified form of cocaine, 'ice' is a very pure smokable form of methamfetamine. It is made up of large, usually clear crystals of high purity and is smoked in a glass pipe like crack cocaine. The smoke is odourless, leaves a residue that can be resmoked, and produces effects that may continue for 12 hours or more.

The effects of methamfetamine are similar to other stimulants, in particular amfetamine (see Table 11.3). It releases high levels of dopamine. It has hedonis-tic and performance-enhancing effects, reduces fatigue and appetite, increases alertness, and enhances mood. It has a high abuse and dependence potential.

The main negative effects are raised blood pressure, sweating and insomnia, and more serious mood disorders, including depression, anxiety, and psychosis. See Table 11.4.

Increased HIV and hepatitis B and C transmission are likely consequences of increased methamfetamine abuse, particularly in individuals who inject the drug and share injection equipment. Research also indicates that methamfetamine and related psychomotor stimulants can increase the libido in users, in contrast to opiates, which actually decrease the libido. Long-term methamfetamine use may be associated with decreased sexual functioning, at least in men. Additionally, methamfetamine seems to be associated with rougher sex, which may lead to bleeding and abrasions. The combination of injection and sexual risks may result in HIV becoming a greater problem among methamfetamine abusers than among opioid and other drug abusers, something that already seems to be occurring in California.[27]

Like other stimulants, methamfetamine can be taken orally or intranasally (snorting the powder), by intravenous injection, and by smoking. Immediately after smoking or intravenous injection the user experiences an intense sensation or 'rush' that lasts only a few minutes and is described as extremely pleasurable. Oral or intranasal use produces euphoria but not a 'rush'. Users may become addicted very quickly and use it with increasing frequency and in increasing doses. As with other stimulants, methamfetamine is often used in a binge and crash pattern. As tolerance for methamfetamine occurs, the pleasurable effects disappear within minutes before the drug concentration in the blood falls significantly. Users therefore try to maintain the high by bingeing on the drug.

Table 11.3 **Effects of methamfetamine**

Short-term/acute effects	Long-term/chronic effects
Increased attention	Dependence and addiction
Decreased fatigue	**Psychosis:**
Decreased appetite	Paranoia
Euphoria	Auditory and tactile hallucinations
	Mood disturbance (depression, anxiety, suicide ideation)
'Rush'	Repetitive mood activity
Increased respiration	
Increased blood pressure	Stroke
Hyperthermia	Weight loss
Anxiety	
Acute psychotic symptoms	

Table 11.4   **Differences between methamfetamine and cocaine**

Methamfetamine	Cocaine
Man-made	Plant-derived
Smoking produces a high that lasts for 8–24 hours	Smoking produces a high that lasts 20–30 minutes
50% of the drug is removed from the body in 12 hours	50% of the drug is removed from the body in 1 hour
Has some limited medical use	Used as a local anaesthetic

Treatment for methamfetamine abuse

At the time of writing the most effective treatments for methamfetamine addiction are cognitive behavioural interventions aimed at modifying the person's thinking, expectancies, and behaviours and at increasing skills in coping with life stresses.

As with amfetamine addiction, many pharmacological treatments have been tried but they do not hold up to rigorous research. The current pharmacological approach is borrowed from experience with the treatment of cocaine addiction. As with cocaine treatment, no single pharmacological agent has been found to be successful or efficacious in clinical trials, although antidepressant medication may be helpful in dealing with the depressive symptoms.

Khat

Clinicians working with communities from Africa may come across patients who use khat (*Catha edulis*). Khat has been known as a plant drug for centuries on the Horn of Africa and the Arabian peninsula. The plant contains the psychotropic substances cathine and cathinione, which when chewed have stimulating effects, similar to those of amfetamines. The leaves rapidly lose their effects when dried out. As a plant drug, khat is not subjected to international control and is regarded and handled as a fresh product when flown from growing areas to Europe. Many countries such as France and Sweden have, however, placed khat under domestic drug control.

Use

The chewing of khat is a cultural tradition in Ethiopia, Somalia, and Yemen. It is often done in large social groups, generally of adult males, led by a guest who socialises with members of that community. The groups often discuss topics of interest, listen to local music or poetry, and solve individual or group disputes or conflicts. Drinks, mainly water, black tea, and Coca-Cola are often served during the session. Because of existing cultural and religious barriers, these communities are not able to access other social events enjoyed by non-Muslim communities: khat use is seen as the only acceptable socialising entertainment available to them.

Misuse[28]

Elderly khat users still adhere to and observe these traditional patterns in the United Kingdom. New trends and patterns of excessive khat use are developing among younger people. These new trends have been identified within the countries of common use and beyond their borders as well.

To cope with their deepening social problems (i.e. unemployment, poor housing, racism after civil war, cultural alienation etc.) a number of young khat users have been exposed to the probable risks of excessive khat chewing. In these situations, young people chew on a regular basis, for extended periods, with khat use becoming part of a sense of exclusion, inactivity, boredom, and despair. Living under similar social conditions a number of Somali women have developed the habit of khat chewing. Chewing more than two sessions a week, late-night sessions, chewing in congested environments, and poor diet are all recognised as features of excessive use.

Health risks

Khat chewing is not physically or mentally addictive, but excessive and prolonged use could lead to health risks (i.e. oral cancer, dental problems, acute constipation, and loss of sexual drive in men). Acute loss of appetite, lack of ample rest, and lack of regular exercise could also lead to more serious consequences. As with other stimulants, chewers may use sleeping pills or sometimes alcohol to help sleep at the end of a session.

Further reading

Donmall M, *et al. National Cocaine Treatment Study. The effectiveness of treatments offered to cocaine/crack users.* University of Manchester Drug Misuse Unit and Community Health Sheffield NHS Trust, 1995.

Gossop M, *et al.* Changes in crack cocaine after drug misuse treatment: 4–5 year follow-up results from the National Treatment Outcomes Research Study (NTORS). *Drug and Alcohol Dependence* 2002; **66**: 21–8.

Simpson D D, *et al.* A national evaluation of treatment outcomes for cocaine dependence. *Archives of General Psychiatry* 1999; **56**: 507–14.

References

1. Royal College of General Practitioners. Guidance for working with cocaine and crack users in primary care, RCGP Drug and Alcohol Misuse Training Programme RCGP, Sex, Drugs and HIV Task Group. SMMGP, 2004.

2. Simmons J, Dodd T. (Eds). Home Office Statistical Bulletin. Crime in England and Wales 2002/2003. London: ONS, July 2003.

3. Condon J, Smith N. Prevalence of drug use: key findings from the 2002/2003 British Crime Survey Findings 229. London: Home Office, 2003.

4. Mittleman M A, Mintzer D, Maclure M, *et al.* Triggering of myocardial infarction by cocaine. *Circulation* 1999; **99**: 2737–41.

5. Quereshi A I, Suri M F K, Gutermann L R, Hopkins L N. Cocaine use and the likelihood of non-fatal myocardial infarction and stroke; data from the third National Health And Nutrition Examination survey. *Circulation* 2001; **103**: 502–6.

6. Buehler B A. Cocaine: how dangerous is it during pregnancy? *Nebr Med J* 1995; **80(5)**: 116–17.

7. Scottish Advisory Committee on Drug Misuse: Psychostimulant Working Group Report 10/06/02 (available at: www.scotland.gov.uk/library5/health/pwgr-02.asp).

8. Lima M S, Soares B G O, Reisser A A P, Farrell M. Pharmacological treatment of cocaine dependence: a systematic review. *Addiction* 2002; **97(8)**: 931–49.

9. Research into Practice no. 1a. Drug Services' Briefing, Treating Cocaine/Crack Dependence (Aug 2002) (available at: www.nta.nhs.uk/publications/research_briefing1a.htm).

10. Simpson D, Joe W G, Broome K M. A national 5-year follow-up of treatment outcomes for cocaine dependence. *Arch Gen Psychiatry* 2002; **59(6)**: 538–44.

11. Crits-Christoph P, Siqueland L, Blaine J, *et al.* Psychosocial treatments for cocaine dependence: National Institute on Drug Abuse Collaborative Cocaine Treatment Study. *Arch Gen Psychiatry* 1999; **56(6)**: 493–502.

12. Hall W, Carter L. Ethical issues in using a cocaine vaccine to treat and prevent cocaine abuse and dependence. *J Med Ethics* 2004; **30**: 337–340.

13. Drug Abuse Trends. Issue 27 April – June 2004. The Forensic Science Service. Drugs Intelligence Unit, 2004.

14. Jaffe J H. Amphetamine (or amphetamine-like)-related disorders. In: Kaplan H I, Sadock B J. (Eds). *Comprehensive Textbook of Psychiatry*. 7th ed. Baltimore: Williams & Wilkins, 2000; 971–82.

15. United Nations Office for Drug Control and Crime Prevention. *World drug report 2000*. Oxford: Oxford University Press, 2000.

16. Loxley W, Carruthers S, Bevan J. *In the Same Vein: First Report of the Australian Study of HIV and Injecting Drug Use*. Perth: NCRPDA, Curtin University of Technology, 1995.

17. Darke S, Cohen J, Ross J, *et al.* Transitions between routes of administration of regular amphetamine users. *Addiction* 1994; **89**: 1077–83.

18. Kramer J C, Fischman V S, Littlefield D C. Amphetamine abuse: pattern and effects of high doses taken intravenously. *J Am Med Assoc* 1967; **201**: 305–9.

19. World Health Organization. *Amphetamine-type stimulants*. Geneva: World Health Organization, 1997.

20. Kalant H, Kalant O J. Death in amphetamines users: Causes and rates. *Canadian Med Assoc J* 1975; **112**: 299–304.

21. Hando J, Topp L, Hall W. Amphetamine-related harms and treatment preferences of regular amphetamine users in Sydney, Australia. *Drug and Alcohol Dependence* 1997; **46**: 105–13.

22. Srisuraponont M, Jarusuraisin N, Kittirattanapaiboon P. Treatment for amphetamine dependence and abuse. (Cochrane Review). In: *The Cochrane Library*, Issue 3, 2004, Chichester, UK: John Wiley & Sons, Ltd.

23. Mattick R, Darke S. Drug replacement treatments: is amphetamine substitution a horse of a different colour? *Drug and Alcohol Review* 1995; **14**: 389-4.

24. National Centre for Education and Training on Addiction. *Models of intervention and care for psycho stimulant users*. Commonwealth of Australia: Monograph Series No 32, 1998.

25. Strang J, Sheridan J. Prescribing amphetamines to drug misusers: data from the 1995 national survey of community pharmacies in England and Wales. *Addiction* 1997 **92(12)**: 833-8.

26. Seivewright N. treatment of non opiate misuse. In: *Community Treatment of Drug Misuse: More than Methadone*. Cambridge: Cambridge University Press, 2000 129-130.

27. National Institute on Drug Abuse. Research Report Series Methamphetamine Abuse and Addiction. Re NIH Publication Number 02-4210 January 2002.

28. A harm reduction approach to khat chewing based on development work with the Somali communities in the UK, Ahmed Suleman Omar/Kujog 1997 (available at: www.drugtext.org/library/articles/suleman.htm).

CHAPTER 12

Alcohol

Clare Gerada

IN THIS CHAPTER

Introduction ‖ Current terminology ‖ Prevalence of different drinking patterns in the population ‖ Alcohol consumption and primary care ‖ Vulnerable drinking, vulnerable groups ‖ Risks and harms associated with excess alcohol use ‖ Beneficial effects of alcohol ‖ Costs of alcohol misuse ‖ Recognising the heavy drinker ‖ Treatment ‖ Alcohol withdrawal syndromes ‖ Drugs that aim to promote abstinence or attenuate drinking behaviour: what works? ‖ Psychological interventions ‖ Women and drinking ‖ The elderly and drinking

Introduction

Most adults drink and the majority of them drink sensibly. It would be true to say, however, that across the United Kingdom every general practitioner, practice nurse, and pharmacist will encounter at least two patients per day where the reason for the consultation is related to the person's alcohol use. Whether the patient or the health professional recognises this is another matter.

Alcohol is used by most of the population and is responsible for more physical, psychological, and social harm than all the other drugs mentioned in this book put together (including tobacco). Perhaps because it is 'Britain's favourite drug' the potential for harm is often ignored or minimised by users, and is all too often relegated to low down on the list of lifestyle concerns by doctors and receives little interest when services compete for funding. It is also telling that the new general practice contract quality and outcomes framework ignores alcohol detection or intervention despite its relevance to the range of physical and mental health problems that are within the framework.

The UK government has recently published a long-awaited alcohol strategy consultation document.[1] Whereas many of the aims in the strategy are laudable, especially in its attempts to reduce the link between binge drinking and crime, it still fails to address the rising tide of alcohol problems and the fact that we are increasingly becoming the 'alcoholics of Europe'.

Current terminology

The terminology used to describe drinking patterns is complex and at times confusing. There is no definition of binge drinking or what constitutes risky drinking levels on a single occasion. Table 12.1 summarises the different terms used.

Table 12.1 **Definitions used for alcohol consumption**

	Men	Women
Light	1–14 units/week	1–10 units/week
Moderate	15–21 units/week	11–14 units/week
Heavy	35–50 units/week	22–35 units/week
Very heavy	>50 units/week	>35 units/week
Sensible	<21 units/week 3–4 units/day with 2 drink-free days per week	<14 units/week 2–3 units/day with 2 drink-free days per week
Hazardous	Very heavy and binge drinkers whose drinking poses a considerable risk to their own or others' health (Royal College of Physicians)	
Harmful or problem drinking	Clear evidence that alcohol is responsible for or substantially contributes to physical or psychological harm, including impaired judgement or dysfunctional behaviour which may lead to disability or have adverse consequences for interpersonal relationships	
Binge or heavy episodic	**Adults** 10+ units on a single occasion (RCP) 8+ units (Health Education Authority, HEA) **Young** 5 drinks in a row on 3+ occasions in past 30 days	**Adults** 7+ units in a single sitting (RCP) 6+ units (HEA) **Young** 5 drinks in a row on 3+ occasions in past 30 days
Alcohol dependence	3 or more of the following present at some time during the previous year: a strong desire or compulsion to drink; difficulty controlling drinking; a physiological withdrawal state on stopping or reducing alcohol use; evidence of tolerance; progressive neglect of other pleasures or interests; persisting use of alcohol despite clear evidence of harm. (ICD-10) See Chapter 1	

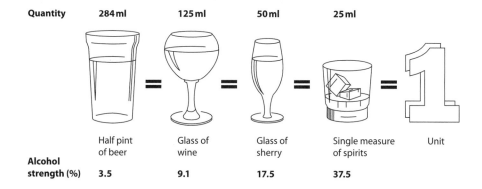

Quantity	284 ml	125 ml	50 ml	25 ml	
	Half pint of beer	Glass of wine	Glass of sherry	Single measure of spirits	Unit
Alcohol strength (%)	3.5	9.1	17.5	37.5	

Alcoholic strength (expressed by volume) varies from about 2 to 5% for beers to 10 to 15% for table wines and 35 to 55% for spirits. Other constituents (congeners) are added to contribute to the flavour.

Prevalence of different drinking patterns in the population

Since the middle of the 20th Century, levels of alcohol consumption in the United Kingdom have been rising. The General Household Survey 2000/01 estimates that 29% of men and 17% of women were 'non-sensible' drinkers and that 21% of men and 10% of women were drinking in binges at least once in the previous week. Thirty-nine per cent of men and 23% of women exceeded the 1995 Department of Health safe drinking limits on at least one day per week (Figures 12.1 and 12.2).

In 2004, the United Kingdom was placed in the middle of the range for alcohol consumption compared with other European countries. Whereas consumption has fallen over recent years in most of the wine-producing countries, British alcohol consumption continues to rise. If present trends continue, the United Kingdom will rise to near the top of the consumption league within the next ten years. See Figure 12.3.

Alcohol consumption and primary care

About one in five individuals consulting primary care drink more than the recommended amount. Problem drinkers are twice as likely to consult their GP than the average patient. See Figure 12.4.

Figure 12.1 **Prevalence of drinking habits in population:[1] alcohol consumption in the UK 1900–2000**

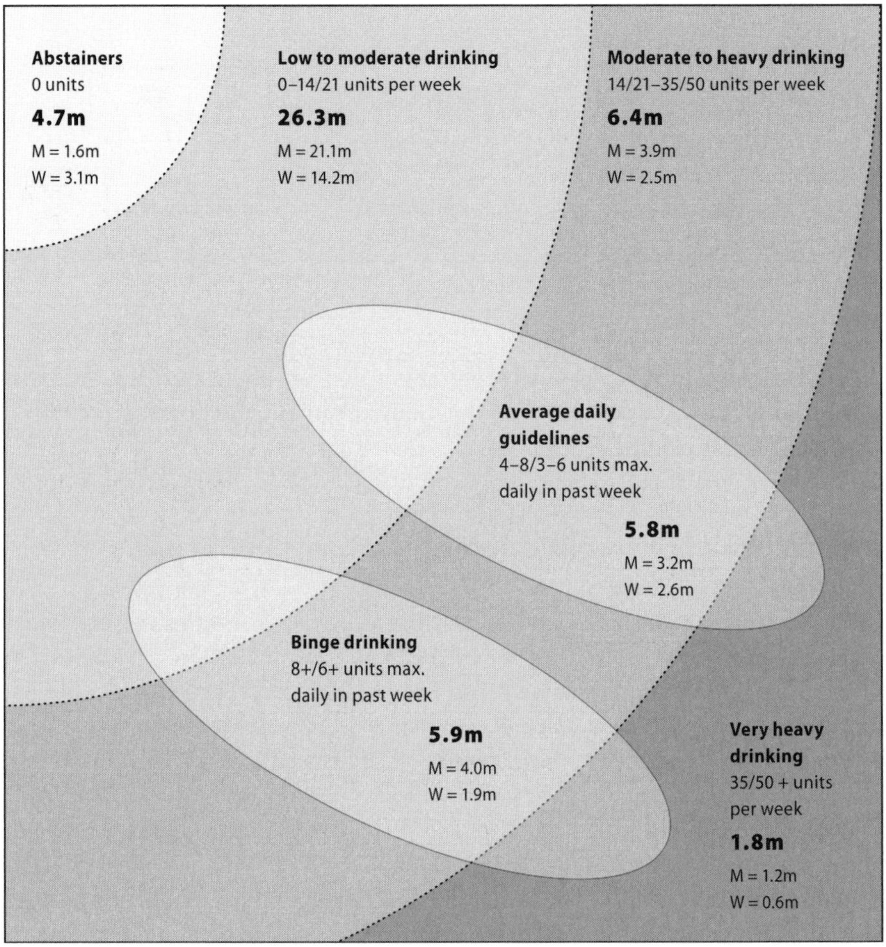

Abstainers
0 units

4.7m

M = 1.6m
W = 3.1m

Low to moderate drinking
0–14/21 units per week

26.3m

M = 21.1m
W = 14.2m

Moderate to heavy drinking
14/21–35/50 units per week

6.4m

M = 3.9m
W = 2.5m

Average daily guidelines
4–8/3–6 units max.
daily in past week

5.8m

M = 3.2m
W = 2.6m

Binge drinking
8+/6+ units max.
daily in past week

5.9m

M = 4.0m
W = 1.9m

Very heavy drinking
35/50 + units per week

1.8m

M = 1.2m
W = 0.6m

Source: Cabinet Office – Prime Minister's Strategy Unit

Vulnerable drinking, vulnerable groups

Two drinking patterns are particularly likely to lead to harm: binge drinking and chronic drinking.

Binge drinkers

Binge drinking has been blamed for the massive increase in inner-city violence – especially on Friday and Saturday nights. 'Happy hour' and cheap alcohol deals

Figure 12.2 **Per capita consumption of 100 per cent alcohol**

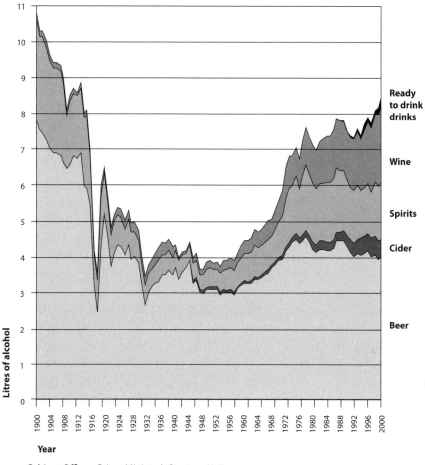

Source: Cabinet Office – Prime Minister's Strategy Unit

have been blamed on promoting bring drinking. Binge drinkers and those who drink to get very drunk are likely to be aged less than 25 years old. They are more likely to be men, although women's drinking has been rising fast over the past ten years. Binge drinkers are at increased risk of accidents and alcohol poisoning. The impacts on society are visible in, for example, high levels of attendance at emergency departments related to alcohol. Nearly six million people have drunk more than twice the daily recommended amount in the past week. Binge drinking in men makes them more likely both to be a victim of violence and to commit violent offences. There can also be a greater risk of sexual assault. Binge drinking has been 'blamed' on women, where women, with their increasing participation in heavy drinking, now no longer act as a restraint on men.

Figure 12.3   **Alcohol consumption in the world: litres of pure alcohol per inhabitant, 1999**

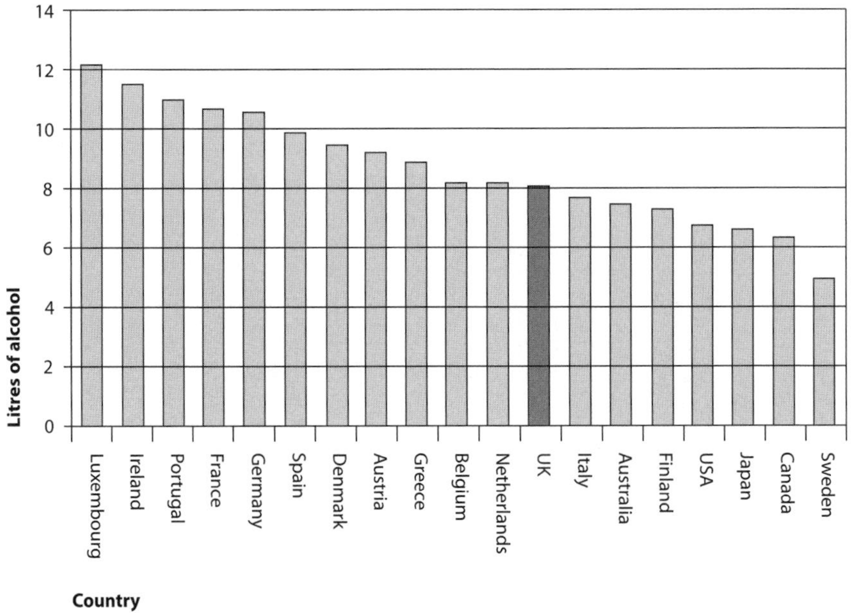

Source: Cabinet Office – Prime Minister's Strategy Unit

Chronic drinkers

These drinkers are more likely to be aged over 30, around two-thirds are men, and they are the group most likely to present to primary care services. They are at increased risk of a variety of health harms such as cirrhosis (which has nearly doubled in the past 10 years), cancer, and haemorrhagic stroke; they are also at higher risk of premature death and suicide. If chronic drinkers come into contact with the criminal justice system, it is more likely to be through crimes such as domestic violence and drink driving. The impacts on society are less visible but are reflected in effects on their families, lost productivity, and costs to the health service. It is estimated that 1.8 million drinkers consume more than twice the recommended weekly guidelines.

Alcohol-related harms may also be experienced by a range of vulnerable groups such as ex-prisoners, street drinkers, those who suffered abuse as children, children of those who misuse alcohol, and young drinkers. As well as alcohol problems they are more likely to experience a whole range of other problems, such as mental illness, drug use, and homelessness, and so have multiple needs.

Figure 12.4 **Alcohol consumption in general practice patients[2]**

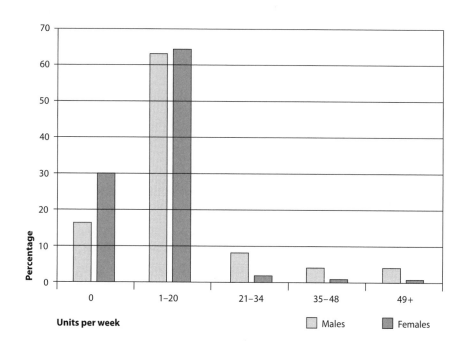

Drug users

A significant number of those with drug problems are also misusing alcohol. The National Treatment Outcome Research Study found that almost half of those being treated by drug services were drinking at excessive levels.[3] The study also found that the treatment drug users received did not impact on their alcohol problem, which was largely ignored by treatment services. Alcohol may substitute for opiates when the heroin user begins to detoxify.

Prison population

Both alcohol and drugs are a great problem for offenders before they enter the criminal justice system. Among male prisoners, 58% of remand and 63% of sentenced prisoners were drinking hazardously before going to prison, whereas 50% of remand and 43% of sentenced prisoners had a drug problem.[4]

Risks and harms associated with excessive alcohol use

The complications of excessive alcohol use are protean and affect every organ and system within the body. A full discussion of the effects and complications is beyond the scope of this book and only a brief summary is therefore included.

A useful framework for conceptualising the harms involve the four-L model:

▸ **Liver**: for example, health problems, in particular liver cirrhosis, hypertension, stroke, gastritis

▸ **Lover**: for example, domestic violence, family breakdown

▸ **Livelihood**: for example, loss of job, debt

▸ **Law**: for example, drink driving, arrest for disorderly conduct, involvement in road traffic accidents.

A less well recognised but common consequence of excessive alcohol use is hypertension. It is estimated that up to 30% of 'essential hypertension' is in fact related to alcohol consumption. Blood pressure generally improves with reduction or abstinence. The primary care practitioner would do well to enquire about alcohol consumption in any newly diagnosed hypertensive or any patient where the hypertension is difficult to control. Alcohol is also a factor in a number of cancers, especially those where alcohol has a direct effect, such as the oropharynx, oesophagus, and stomach. It appears to be a predisposing factor in breast cancer. See Table 12.1.

Beneficial effects of alcohol

Regular consumption of two drinks a day for men and one drink a day for women decreases the risk of arteriosclerosis and associated disorders; this beneficial effect is irrespective of the type of alcohol consumed.

Costs of alcohol misuse[1]

The annual cost of alcohol misuse includes:

▸ expenditure of £95m on specialist alcohol treatment

▸ over 30,000 hospital admissions for alcohol dependence syndrome

▸ up to 22,000 premature deaths per annum

▸ at peak times, up to 70% of all admissions to accident and emergency departments

Table 12.1 **Estimates of proportion of deaths attributable to alcohol from various conditions[5]**

Condition	Attributable death (%)
Cancer oesophagus	14–75
Cancer liver	15–29
Cancer female breast	3–4
Hypertension	5–11
Chronic pancreatitis	60–84
Acute pancreatitis	24–35
Falls	23–35
Drowning	30–38
Fire injuries	38–45
Suicide	27–41
Assault	27–47

▶ up to 1,000 suicides

▶ 1.2m violent incidents (around half of all violent crimes)

▶ 360,000 incidents of domestic violence (around a third) linked to alcohol misuse

▶ increased antisocial behaviour and fear of crime – 61% of the population perceive alcohol-related violence as worsening

▶ up to 17m working days lost through alcohol-related absence

▶ between 780,000 and 1.3m children affected by parental alcohol problems

▶ increased divorce – marriages where there are alcohol problems are twice as likely to end in divorce.

See Figure 12.5.

Recognising the heavy drinker

The health professional is central to the identification and treatment of alcohol problems. Many of these patients are unrecognised, however, either because of

Figure 12.5   **Alcohol-related harm**

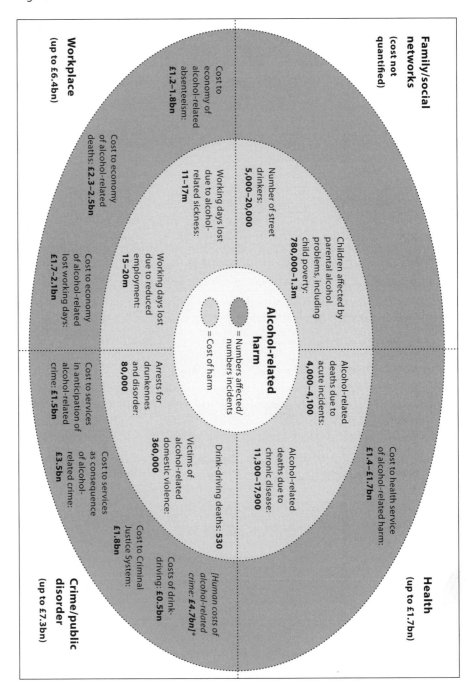

*Source: Cabinet Office[1]

clinician factors (lack of confidence in managing alcohol misuse, belief that treatment is pointless) or patient factors (hiding their habit or lack of insight). At the very least primary care practitioners should be aware of the high prevalence of alcohol problems amongst their patients and have a high index of suspicion in frequent attendees, and those with conditions such as hypertension, anxiety, depression, and upper gastrointestinal problems. Patients with all of these diagnoses have a very high probability that excessive alcohol intake is a causative factor. Asking about drinking consumption and patterns of intake should become part of most consultations. See Box 12.1.

Box 12.1   **Useful questions**

Leading questions:

✓ Have you or others ever been concerned about your drinking?

✓ We often find that people's drinking, eating, and smoking habits have effects on their health; I'd like to ask you some questions about them

Questions where dependence is suspected:

✓ Do you crave alcohol?

✓ Have you been unable to stop drinking once you have started?

✓ Do you skip meals because you are drinking?

✓ Do you notice your hands shaking in the morning?

✓ Do you ever feel the need to have a drink in the morning to settle your nerves?

✓ Have you ever felt guilty about your drinking?

Screening for alcohol problems[6]

A number of screening tools are available to identify current or potential alcohol problems among patients.[7] Several standardised screening questionnaires, such as the Alcohol Use Disorders Identification Test (AUDIT),[8] the CAGE (see Box 12.2),[9] and the Michigan Alcoholism Screening Test (MAST),[10] and its derivatives (e.g. the Brief MAST can identify alcohol problems among current drinkers) exist.[11,12] Laboratory tests, such as the test for the liver enzyme gamma-glutamyltransferase (GGT), may also reveal the presence of unsuspected alcohol problems.[13] Nothing, however, can replace the astute clinician.

Box 12.2   **The CAGE Questionnaire**

---

1. Have you ever felt you should Cut down on your drinking?

2. Have people ever Annoyed you by criticizing your drinking?

3. Have you ever felt bad or Guilty about your drinking?

4. Have you ever had a drink first thing in the morning to steady your nerves
    or to get rid of a hangover? (eye-opener?)

Two positive answers indicate a high likelihood of alcohol dependency

---

Reproduced with permission from the American Medical Association

Treatment

It is beyond the scope of this book to give guidance as to the basic assessment, medical management, and detoxification of patients with alcohol misuse problems. The reader can obtain this information from sources listed in *Further reading*. Chapter 22 describes the treatment of coexisting alcohol dependence and anxiety.

Management of alcohol detoxification (assisted withdrawal)

Many alcohol withdrawal episodes take place without any medical or pharmacological treatment and are self-managed. In those patients where detoxification is a planned medical or nursing intervention, the balance between giving medication unnecessarily and giving sufficient to minimise withdrawal symptoms appropriately has to be struck.

Consideration should also be given to prevention of complications, such as seizures and delirium tremens (DTs), during each withdrawal episode and also in future withdrawal episodes. Successive episodes of alcohol withdrawal are associated with increased withdrawal severity and rate of complications; post-detoxification support should maximise the opportunities for remaining abstinent.

With appropriate shared care and support general practitioners can safely provide alcohol detoxification to patients in community settings, and perhaps this can be part of an enhanced service offered (as defined in the nGMS contract) by the practice. Appropriate patients for community detoxification are those with good support at home, where there are no serious concomitant physical or psychological problems, where there is no previous history of severe alcohol withdrawal, in particular delirium tremens, and where the patient is committed to attending for frequent reviews, certainly daily at the start of treatment.

The clinician must be prepared to review the patient daily or on alternate days for at least the first seven days (once stable this can be by telephone review) and should be available during the detoxification should complications arise.

Partnership with a local pharmacist and support through a shared care or community alcohol nurse are also important aspects for successful treatment.

The specific regimen used will differ for individual patients, but is based on a rapidly reducing dose of benzodiazepines, together with the administration of thiamine and symptomatic treatment for muscle pains, insomnia, and where necessary prophylactic anti-epileptic medication. In some cases small doses of a major tranquilliser may be necessary to alleviate symptoms of agitation or severe restlessness.

It is important to advise the patients to maintain their fluid intake and that, if they experience severe vomiting, or if the carer is concerned as to the level of confusion or consciousness, the detoxification programme is terminated and medical assistance sought.

What detoxification treatment to use

Benzodiazepines[14]

Benzodiazepines are the drug of choice for the treatment of acute alcohol withdrawal. The most important consideration is not which benzodiazepine to use, but to ensure that adequate doses are administered early in the course of withdrawal. Early treatment coupled with close and regular monitoring appears to be effective in avoiding prolonged withdrawal, sedation-related morbidity, and extra resource utilisation.

The British Association for Psychopharmacology has recently reviewed the use of benzodiazepines in alcohol withdrawal and concludes that they all appear to be equally efficacious in reducing signs and symptoms of withdrawal. Particular drugs can be used to suit different circumstances, for example, lorazepam or oxazepam in liver failure. Longer-acting benzodiazepines, such as diazepam, may be more effective in preventing seizures and delirium, but this needs to be weighed against their accumulation in the elderly and in those with marked liver disease.[15]

Medication is typically given for seven to ten days. Alcohol withdrawal severity varies widely and the amount of benzodiazepine required for symptom amelioration can also vary. There is no fixed standardised dose for all patients, but a typical regimen for covering uncomplicated withdrawal is 20–40 mg four times daily of chlordiazepoxide, reducing over seven days. Additional medication can be given for symptomatic relief of symptoms for a further two to three days to be used as required.

Typical regimens are suggested in the British National Formulary and the clinical guidelines.

Box 12.3   **Diary of a home detoxification**

Paul, aged 43 years, is an electrician. He admits to drinking at least four cans of extra strong lager a day for the past 3 years. He has a history of alcohol dependence for about 12 years since the break up of his first marriage. His last alcohol-free day was 12 months ago when he tried a home detoxification but failed as he found the withdrawal symptoms too unbearable. Of note, he did not have any major withdrawal features, in particular any fits. He wants to try again but with the help of medication. His new girlfriend is keen to help him and to monitor his medication.

Four cans of extra strong lager (9% vol) 440 ml / can = approx. 15 units.

Week before: see the patient with girlfriend. Ask patient to begin to reduce alcohol intake and to stock up on soft drinks at home.

12 hours before detoxification: stop drinking.

Day 1: ask the patient to present on the morning of the first day of the detoxification (preferably early in the week). Breathalyse patient, if breath over 50 micrograms / 100 ml alcohol postpone detoxification. If not commence the detoxification programme. Give prescription to carer asking her to dispense medication daily or ask pharmacist to dispense daily. On no account should the patient be responsible for his own medication. Commence thiamine 100 mg qds and Vitamin B Strong 30 mg / day for duration of detoxification.

Drug regimen varies but the following is frequently used:

Day 1 • chlordiazepoxide 30 or 40 mg qds

Day 2 • review either face to face or by telephone – speak to patient and carer; chlordiazepoxide 20 or 30 mg qds

Day 3 • review face to face: chlordiazepoxide 20 or 30 mg tds

Day 4 • review either face to face or by telephone – speak to carer and patient; chlordiazepoxide 20 mg tds

Day 5 • chlordiazepoxide 20 mg bd

Day 6 • review face to face: chlordiazepoxide 10 mg bd

Day 7 • consider continuing 10 mg nocte for following 3–7 nights

Day 14 • review face to face; consider starting acamprosate

Day 28 • review face to face: relapse prevention; stop thiamine

Chlormethiazole

Although chlormethiazole has been shown to be superior to placebo, its use in outpatient settings is no longer recommended principally because of the greater risk of respiratory depression if alcohol is drunk, and because of its addictive potential and 'street value'.[16] The 1999 Clinical Guidelines advise against using chlormethiazole in patients where there is a history of addiction and where there may be risks of diversion.

Carbamazepine

Whereas in the United Kingdom benzodiazepines are the most widely used pharmacotherapy for alcohol withdrawal, carbamazepine alone is used elsewhere in the world and might be a first-line alternative to benzodiazepines. Carbamazepine appears to be effective throughout the range of alcohol withdrawal symptoms including severe ones, and is not contraindicated in liver failure.

Alcohol withdrawal syndromes

The hallmarks of withdrawal are a continuum of signs and symptoms, ranging from tremulousness to full blown delirium tremens. At one time, alcohol withdrawal was divided into stages.[17] Since the full spectrum of symptoms varies greatly and overlaps in duration and over time, however, it is perhaps more clinically helpful to define a set of signs and symptoms ranging from mild to major symptomatology.[18] Seizures can occur with any severity level of withdrawal.

Mild withdrawal

Heavy dependent drinkers can experience tremors ('shakes') within 24 hours after the last drink (usually within five to ten hours, so the morning after night's sleep). Tremor can be accompanied by other symptoms, such as nausea, diarrhoea, and decreased appetite, and signs such as raised pulse and sweating. One to three days after the last drink users can develop grand mal seizures, most occuring within 48 hours after the last drink. These can be the prelude to major withdrawal syndrome.

Moderate withdrawal

Moderate withdrawal is an intermediate position along the continuum with the hallmark of hallucinations but an otherwise clear sensorium. Seizures, hallucinations, and delirium tremens are considered major phenomena.

Major withdrawal

About three to ten days from the last drink, about 5% of dependent drinkers develop delirium tremens. This is characterised by agitation, disorientation, high fever, sweating, paranoid delusion, and visual hallucinations. This is a medical emergency and should be managed by urgent admission to hospital. The symptoms may persist for up to two weeks.

A description of the various alcohol withdrawal syndromes follows.

Hangover

Hangover is often overlooked in classifications of alcohol withdrawal, perhaps because it occurs so commonly after acute alcohol exposure. It is the mildest form of withdrawal, occurring within several hours of cessation. It consists of a period of psychomotor impairment that follows an acute exposure to inebriating quantities of alcohol. Severity of hangover symptoms is a risk factor for subsequent alcohol dependency, perhaps because individuals prone to severe hangover develop a pattern of relieving symptoms by further drinking, known as an 'eye-opener'.[19]

Alcohol withdrawal tremor

Barring additional alcohol intake, the chronic drinker develops increasing tremors and craving for alcohol during the first 8–12 hours of observation, which peaks at 24–48 hours. The patient may also experience insomnia, tachycardia, anxiety, and nausea at this stage. The drinker may calm 'the shakes' at this point by consuming additional alcohol.

Alcohol withdrawal hallucinations

Alcohol withdrawal hallucinations are noted as early as 24 hours after the last drink and last approximately as long. They occur in about a quarter of cases and are usually visual but less frequently will be auditory or combined auditory and visual.[20]

Delirium tremens

Delirium tremens is a severe, life-threatening complication of alcohol withdrawal. It is rarely seen in primary care. It is characterised by increasingly pronounced disorientation, agitation, and autonomic stimulation, with hypertension, tachycardia, hyperthermia, and profound diaphoresis. Mortality rates of up to 20%

have been noted in the past but have improved gradually with better recognition and treatment. Onset typically occurs approximately 48 hours after cessation of drinking. The mild tremor and lucid hallucinations of early withdrawal give way to delirium and agitation. The patient begins to pull at imaginary objects or at his or her clothing and sheets. Death can occur through hyperthermia and dehydration.

Alcohol-related seizure

Alcohol is a common cause of adult convulsions. Alcohol itself may also exacerbate other existing conditions, such as epilepsy. To add to the complexity, chronic alcohol abusers have an increased frequency of structural alterations secondary to repeated head injuries.[21,22]

Predicting the severity of withdrawal

It is difficult to predict the severity of withdrawal, though the pattern of previous withdrawals can be an important indicator. A past history of fits, hallucinations, and delirium tremens may be a guide to a probably severe withdrawal and hence the need for inpatient detoxification. Repeated episodes of alcohol withdrawal may lead to an increase in the severity of subsequent episodes and a lower seizure threshold through a process known as kindling.[23] Individuals who have had five or more alcohol detoxifications have a greater risk of withdrawal seizures.[24]

Vitamin deficiency

Vitamin deficiency in alcoholism is common and multifactorial in origin. There is a particular need to replenish thiamine stores owing to its critical role as a cofactor for metabolic enzymes and the risk that thiamine deficiency may lead to Wernicke's encephalopathy. The role of thiamine supplementation in 'healthy uncomplicated' alcohol dependent patients undergoing detoxification is unclear. Based on clinical practice, current recommendations where symptoms of withdrawal are not severe are that oral thiamine 100 mg qds should be given until withdrawal is complete, reducing to 100 mg bd for up to one month.[25]

Drugs that aim to promote abstinence or attenuate drinking behaviour: what works?

There are a range of drugs that have been studied as potential alcohol attenuating agents (drugs that aim to moderate alcohol consumption, promote abstinence, and/or prevent relapse) with conflicting evidence of effectiveness.[26,27]

Disulfiram (Antabuse™)

Disulfiram causes an accumulation of acetaldehyde, and hence flushing, nausea and vomiting, palpitations, and difficulty in breathing. This drug was popular in the treatment of alcohol dependence around 20 years ago and was claimed to work by negative reinforcement produced by these unpleasant effects caused by drinking whilst on the drug. There is little evidence of significant effects of disulfiram when compared with placebo in double-blind trials. It may have an effect when combined with psychosocial treatment, family involvement, supervision, or coercion. There is no evidence to support the efficacy of disulfiram implants and these are now rarely used.[28]

Naltrexone

Naltrexone is an opioid agonist that is licensed in the United States and some European countries for treatment of alcohol dependence, but not in the United Kingdom (but it can be prescribed). Like acamprosate, naltrexone is used to maintain abstinence as an adjunct to psychosocial intervention.

The evidence for effectiveness is mixed. Although there is some evidence of a reduction in alcohol consumption and relapse in naltrexone-treated subjects, compliance is a problem, with high drop-out rates. Nausea appears to be the main problem and seems to be related to the frequency and level of alcohol consumption. Naltrexone also has adverse effects on liver function and has limited value in patients with severe liver disease.[29,30] The principal contraindication is coexisting opiate addiction, which therefore rules it out as a treatment of choice in patients with dual addictions. As for acamprosate, it is not clear how long to prescribe naltrexone for, and the trials tend to be short in duration, for example 12 weeks.

Acamprosate

Several randomised controlled trains have been conducted and most show a 10–15% increase in abstinence and reduced levels of drinking and relapse compared with placebo.[31] In a meta-analysis conducted for the Health Technology Board of Scotland by Slattery *et al*, available on: http://docs.scottishmedicines.org/docs/pdf/Alcohol%20Report.pdf, acamprosate was shown to be effective compared with placebo. The recent UK multicentre trial of acamprosate, however, showed no difference between acamprosate and placebo and had a lower completion rate (35%) than most other trials.[32]

Acamprosate does not have hypnotic, anxiolytic, or antidepressant effects. It is safe to use in the absence of severe liver or renal disease. Adverse effects include diarrhoea, headache, nausea, and pruritus. Compliance may be an issue as the dose is generally two tablets (300 mg each) three times a day. In view of the fact that not everyone benefits from acamprosate, there have been several attempts to define the characteristics of a 'responsive' alcohol-dependent patient. As yet there is no clear evidence to suggest which type of patient may benefit although it has been suggested that a classical, primary type of alcohol-dependent patient appears more likely to benefit than one with a psychiatric or organic disorder or with social problems or one that is an episodic drinker.[33]

Lithium™

There are limited studies on the effects of lithium in primary alcoholics without comorbid mood disorders. There is evidence that lithium is not efficacious in the treatment of the core symptoms of alcohol dependence. There is minimal evidence for the efficacy of lithium for the treatment of alcohol-dependent symptoms in patients with comorbid depression.

Psychological interventions

Over the past decade there has been considerable emphasis on brief and minimal interventions (less than five minutes sessions) in the treatment of non-dependent and dependent drinkers. Brief interventions have been found effective for helping non-alcohol-dependent patients reduce or stop drinking, for motivating alcohol-dependent patients to enter long-term alcohol treatment, and for treating some alcohol-dependent patients. Research indicates that brief intervention for alcohol problems is more effective than no intervention[34–37] and often as effective as more extensive intervention.[38]

Brief interventions are designed to be carried out in general healthcare settings – including general practice and accident and emergency departments – and generally restricted to four or fewer sessions, each session lasting from a few minutes to one hour, and delivered by health professionals who do not specialise in addictions treatment. It is most often used with patients who are not alcohol dependent, and its goal may be moderate drinking rather than abstinence.[39,40]

The content and approach of brief intervention vary depending on the severity of the patient's alcohol problem. Although the approaches used in brief intervention are similar for alcohol-dependent and non-alcohol-dependent patients, the goal of brief intervention for alcohol-dependent patients is abstinence.

The recently published alcohol strategy contains a commitment by the government to improving early identification of alcohol problems and the announcement of the development of a number of pilot schemes to test how best to use a variety of models of targeted screening and brief intervention in primary and secondary care. The strategy also acknowledges the importance of training for medical and nursing staff.

The nGMS contract provides an opportunity to improve the care of people with alcohol misuse problems through an enhanced service. Whereas some areas may choose to implement the National Enhanced Service it is felt that most localities will look to a locally enhanced scheme to increase the quality and range of alcohol interventions provided in primary care settings including developing some GPs with a special interest in the field.

As little as five minutes advice from a health professional can significantly reduce drinking six months later in a non-dependent drinker.

Brief intervention involves the following elements:

Feedback: assessment and evaluation of the problem

Responsibility: emphasising that drinking is their choice

Advice: explicit advice on changing drinking behaviour

Menu: offering alternative goals and strategies

Empathy: the role of the counsellor is vital.

Follow up

The healthcare professional continues to follow up on the patient's progress and provide ongoing support. Follow up may take the form of telephone calls from office staff, repeat office visits, or repeat physical examinations or laboratory tests.

Timing

Much of the research investigating the relationship between an individual's readiness to change and actual behaviour change is based on studies of smoking cessation. Research findings have been applied to reducing drinking.[41] Individuals are most likely to make behaviour changes when they perceive that they have a problem and when they feel they can change. Some patients may not be ready to change when brief intervention begins, but may be ready when they experience an alcohol-related illness or injury. Because a patient's readiness to change appears to be a significant predictor of changes in drinking behaviour it is important to assess patients' readiness to change when beginning a brief intervention. For patients with little motivation to change, Heather and colleagues found that motivational interviewing was more effective than specific instructions.[42]

Motivational interviewing with problem drinkers

Miller has described an alternative approach to dealing with problem drinkers who are not ready to change their addictive behaviour.[43] The traditional approach is to assume that the patient is not motivated and 'in denial' and this usually results in the adoption of a confrontational approach by the counsellor or clinician; such confrontation might be characterised by an attempt on the part of the counsellor to label the drinker and to prescribe the best course of action. If the patient has not yet decided to embark on any course of action the natural response will be to resist such exhortation.

Motivational interviewing gives an alternative strategy for the clinician, which addresses the motivational balance of the patient. Behaviour continues when the perceived advantages of changing are outweighed by the perceived disadvantages. Success happens when the clinician is able to shift this balance and this is best done, according to Miller, through the use of a series of self-motivational statements so that there is a recognition that their behaviour causes problems, that they are able to express concerns about this behaviour and its consequences, and they expressed an intention to change their behaviour and have an optimistic belief about such change. The key principles of motivational interviewing are described as:

▸ a de-emphasis on labelling, or using such terms as alcoholic or addict

▸ assertion that the definition of the problem and a decision to change rests with the patient

▸ that responsibility for any course of action rests with the patient

▸ that identification of a discrepancy between where the patient is and where they want to be, or between what they are doing now and how they perceive themselves, is an uncomfortable state likely to result in change.

The goals of motivational interviewing are to increase self-esteem and self-efficacy, as these are associated with positive changes; to increase dissonance and direct it towards behaviour change. The strategies likely to enable the clinician to reach these goals are: reflective listening, the expression of accurate empathy, affirmation of the patient's difficulties and achievements, and identification of how the patients perceive and can solve their problems through the use of open questions.

The practice of motivational interviewing has been the subject of several studies and clinical trials and has been shown to be associated with reductions in drinking when compared with a confrontational approach, greater compliance with treatment than a standard approach, and similarly improved drinking outcomes (reduced levels of consumption) when compared with cognitive behavioural therapy and twelve-steps treatment programmes. It can equally be used with opioid users.

Women and drinking

The levels of drinking in women are rapidly increasing in almost all Westernised societies. Young women and women working in male-dominated environments are more likely to drink heavily and to have drinking problems. Women appear to be more influenced by the drinking patterns of their partners than by their peer group, although women who drink heavily are likely to mix with men who drink heavily and be more tolerant of their partners' drinking patterns. Women who have multiple roles (family, marriage, employment) appear to have a lower risk of problem drinking, as though it would be difficult to juggle different roles if alcohol were a significant part of the woman's life.

It is estimated that over 20% of pregnant women worldwide consume alcohol.[44] Current research suggests that alcohol intake of seven or more standard drinks (one standard drink = 13.6 grams of absolute alcohol) a week during pregnancy places the fetus at significant risk of the negative effects of ethanol.[45]

Risk factors associated with problem drinking in women

▸ strong family history

▸ behavioural disorder in childhood

▸ early use of illicit drugs

▸ depression

▸ divorced/separated

▸ heavy-drinking partners

▸ working in a male dominated environment.

Sex differences

The ways in which women and men metabolise alcohol differ significantly. After consuming a given dose of alcohol adjusted according to body weight, women have higher blood alcohol levels than men. The higher proportion of body fat in women, changes in alcohol absorption with the menstrual cycle, and differences in the relative amount of gastric alcohol dehydrogenase contribute to this disparity.[46] These differences may explain the 'telescoping' phenomenon of alcohol use disorders in women: women experience a more rapid progression to alcoholism and its medical complications than men despite lower levels of consumption.[47]

Alcoholic liver disease

The telescoping phenomenon is most evident in the rates of alcoholic liver disease in women compared with men. A prospective study of more than 13,000 men and women over 12 years found that women have a higher risk of liver disease for any given level of alcohol intake compared with men.[48] This study estimated the relative risk of cirrhosis in women who consumed 28 to 41 drinks a week to be 16 times higher than that of non-drinking women. For the same level of alcohol consumption, men were estimated to have one-third the risk of cirrhosis of women.

Breast cancer

A recent meta-analysis of six large, prospective cohort studies demonstrated a correlation between alcohol use and breast cancer risk.[49] Women who consumed, on average, two and a half to five drinks a day had a 40% higher incidence of breast cancer than non-drinkers. Importantly, this study also found a dose-response relationship between alcohol consumption and breast cancer risk: the risk was elevated by 9% for each 10 g (about one drink) increase in alcohol intake a day for increases of up to 60 g a day; this effect persisted even adjusting for possible confounders such as age, diet, smoking, menarche, parity, and menopause.

Osteoporosis

Alcohol consumption influences the incidence of hip fractures among women. One study showed that women younger than 60 years who consumed two to six drinks per day had an increased risk of hip and forearm fracture.[50] This increased risk may be due to a greater incidence of falling and to alcohol's inhibitory effect on bone remodelling, which has been demonstrated in men. Several recent large studies have suggested that moderate alcohol consumption may lead to increased bone mineral density in postmenopausal women.[51] Whether increased bone mineral density leads to a reduced fracture risk has yet to be determined.

Psychiatric disorders

All psychiatric diagnoses are more prevalent in alcohol-abusing women than in either non-alcohol-abusing women or alcohol-abusing men. Only antisocial personality disorder is more prevalent in male alcoholics. Studies indicate that the prevalence of depression is 30 to 40% in alcohol-abusing women. Interestingly, women with alcohol problems seem to have a much higher rate of 'dual' diagnoses, in which a primary affective disorder predated their chemical dependence, than men with alcohol problems.

In the Epidemiologic Catchment Area Study,[52] depression was primary and alcoholism was secondary in 66% of alcohol-abusing women. In contrast, alcoholism was primary and depression was secondary in 78% of alcohol-abusing men. Many women cite worsening depressive symptoms as their main reason for entering an alcohol treatment programme. This information may help primary care physicians target their preventive efforts and tailor their treatment recommendations.

Alcohol-abusing women attempt suicide four times more often than women who do not have alcoholic problems.[53] Among adults with alcohol use disorders, the suicide rate in women equals that in men, but women attempt suicide more often than men. Anorexia and bulimia are also more prevalent in alcohol-abusing women (15–32%), significantly higher than the prevalence in the general population (anorexia, 1.5%; bulimia, 7%).[54]

Psychosocial consequences

Women experience significant psychosocial consequences from their alcohol use disorder. Family and marital problems are more common among women, whereas job and legal problems occur more often in men. Women are more likely to be divorced after entering treatment; they often report a fear of losing custody of their children as an important motivating factor for treatment. Women with alcohol problems are more likely to be victims of alcohol-related aggression, such as domestic violence and rape. Women who misuse alcohol often have a male partner with alcohol problems, and alcohol use in men is highly linked with partner abuse.

The elderly and drinking

Although the prevalence of alcohol dependence and problem drinking in the elderly is lower than in the young, it is nevertheless common and associated with considerable morbidity and mortality. Problem drinking in this age group often goes undetected. One primary care study identified 10% of older patients as having current evidence of alcoholism, yet fewer than half had this documented in their medical records.[55]

Elderly people are less likely to disclose their problem and health professionals have a lower degree of suspicion when assessing them for medical, psychiatric, or social problems. The presentation of older people differs from that of their younger counterparts. They may for example present with falls, confusion, or depression.[56] Sensible drinking limits do not apply to the elderly population, who, like adolescents, have lower tolerance to alcohol and suffer increased sensitivity to the effects at lower blood alcohol levels.[57]

Elderly people have been shown to be as likely to benefit from treatment as younger people although pharmacological interventions can be more hazardous because of coexisting medical problems. It is probably wise for elderly patients to be admitted to hospital for detoxification because of the increased risk of confusion and fluid and electrolyte problems. Benzodiazepine associated detoxification should be undertaken with care owing to increased sensitivity to adverse effects and altered pharmacokinetics.

Alcohol and the young is discussed in Chapter 17.

Further reading

Ritson B. ABC of Alcohol: Treatment of alcohol related problems. *BMJ* 2005; **330**: 139–74

Drug Misuse and Dependence – Guidelines on Clinical Management Annex 8: Alcohol and Drug Misuse. www:doh.gov.uk/drugs.

Alcohol Concern. Brief Interventions FactSheet 15 1997. www:alcoholconcern.org.uk.

Edwards G, Marshall J, Cook C. *The Treatment of Drinking Problems, A Guide for the Helping Professionals*, 3rd ed. Cambridge: Cambridge University Press, 1997.

Drug and Therapeutic Bulletin, see: DTB 1997: 35:73–4. www.which.net/dtb.

RCGP Assessment and Brief interventions in Alcohol Misuse. Training for Primary Care Professionals 2002/3.

www.smmgp.demon.co.uk

Royal College of Physicians. Alcohol – can the NHS afford it. Recommendations for a coherent alcohol strategy for hospitals. A report of a Working Party of the Royal College of Physicians. London: RCP, 2001

References

1. Cabinet Office: Prime Minister's Strategy Unit. *Alcohol Harm Reduction Strategy for England*. London: HMSO, 2004
   (available at: www.strategy.gov.uk/su/alcohol/ pdf/CabOffce%20AlcoholHar.pdf).

2. Wallace P, Brennan PJ, Haines A. Drinking patterns in general practice patients. *J R Coll Gen Pract* 1987; **37**: 35–7.

3. Gossop M. *NTORS, The National Treatment Outcome Research Studies: Improvements in Substance Use Problems at 6 Months Follow-up*. 2nd Bulletin, London: DoH, 1997.

4. Office for National Statistics. *Substance Misuse among Prisoners in England and Wales*. London: HMSO, 1999.

5. Greenfield T K. Individual risk of alcohol related disease and problems. In: Heather N, Peters T J, Stockwell T. (Eds). *International Handbook Alcohol Dependence and Problems*. London: Wiley, 2001.

6. Fiellin D A, Reid M C, O' Connor P G. Screening for alcohol problems in primary care: a systematic review. *Arch Int Med* 2000; **160(13)**: 1977–89.

7. National Institute on Alcohol Abuse and Alcoholism. *Screening for Alcoholism*. Alcohol Alert No. 8. Rockville, MD: The Institute, 1990.

8. Babor T F, De La Fuente J R, Saunders J, Babor M. *AUDIT: The Alcohol Use Disorders Identification Test, Guidelines for Use in Primary Health Care*. Geneva: World Health Organization, 1989.

9. Ewing J A. Detecting alcoholism: The CAGE questionnaire. *JAMA* 1984; **252**(14): 1905–7.

10. Selzer M L. The Michigan Alcoholism Screening Test: The quest for a new diagnostic instrument. *Am J Psychiatry* 1971; **127**(12): 89–94.

11. Pokorny A D, Miller B, Kaplan H B. The brief M A S T: A shortened version of the Michigan Alcoholism Screening Test. *Am J Psychiatry* 1972; **129**(3): 118–21.

12. Allen J P, Maisto S A, Connors G J. Self-report screening tests for alcohol problems in primary care. *Arc Int Med* 1995; **16**: 1726–30.

13. O'Connor P G, Schottenfeld R S. Patients with alcohol problems. *N Engl J Med* 1998; **338**(9): 592–602.

14. Holbrook AM, Crowther R, Lotter A, *et al*. Meta-analysis of benzodiazepine use in the treatment of acute alcohol withdrawal. *Canadian Med Assoc J* 1999; **160**(5): 649–55.

15. Lingford-Hughes A R, Welch S, Nutt D J. Evidence-based guidelines for the pharmacological management of substance misuse, addiction and comorbidity: recommendations from the British Association for Psychopharmacology. *J Psychopharmacol* 2004; **18**: 293–335.

16. Williams D, McBride A J. The drug treatment of alcohol withdrawal symptoms: a systematic review. *Alcohol and Alcoholism* 1998; **33**(2): 103–15.

17. Victor M, Adams R D. The effect of alcohol on the nervous system. *Res Publ Assoc Nerv Ment Dis* 1953; **32**: 526.

18. McMicken D B. Alcohol withdrawal syndromes. *Emerg Med Clin North Am* 1990; **8**: 805–16.

19. Earlywine M. Personality risk for alcoholism covaries with hangover symptoms. *Addict Behav* 1993; **18**: 415–20.

20. Victor M, Brausch C. The role of abstinence in the genesis of alcoholic epilepsy. *Epilepsy* 1967; **8**: 1–20.

21. Gill J S, Shipley M J, Tsementzis S A, *et al*. Alcohol consumption: a risk factor for hemorrhagic and non-hemorrhagic stroke. *Am J Med* 1991; **90**: 489–97.

22. Hillbom M, Kaste M. Alcohol intoxication: a risk factor for primary subarachnoid hemorrhage. *Neurology* 1982; **32**: 706.

23. Browne M, Anton R, Malcolm R, *et al*. Alcohol detoxification and withdrawal seizures: Clinical support for a kindling hypothesis. *Biol Psychiatry* 1988; **23**: 507–14.

24. Lechtenberg R, Worner TM. Relative kindling effect of detoxification and non-detoxification admissions in alcoholics. *Alcohol* 1991; **26**: 221–5.

25. Royal College of Physicians. *Alcohol – can the NHS Afford it? Recommendations for a Coherent Alcohol Strategy for Hospitals*. Report of a Working Party of the Royal College of Physicians. London: RCP, 2001.

26. Drummond C. Pharmacological approaches to the treatment of excessive drinking and alcohol dependence. Expert Rev. *Neurotherapeutics* 2002; **2**(1): 119–25 (available at: www.future-drugs.com).

27. Agency for Healthcare Research, Quality. *Pharmacotherapy for Alcohol Dependence*. Rockville, MD: AHRQ, 1999.

28. O'Farrell T J, Fals-Stewart W. Family-involved alcoholism treatment: an update. *Recent Dev Alcohol* 2001; **15**: 329–56.

29. Maxwell S, Shinderman M S. Use of naltrexone in the treatment of alcohol use disorders in patients with concomitant major mental illness. *J Addict Dis* 2000; **19**: 61–9.

30. Srisuraponont M, Jarusuraisin N. Opioid antagonists for alcohol dependence. Cochrane Database Syst Rev CD001867. Chichester: John Wiley, 2000.

31. Moncreieff J, Drummond D C. New drug treatments for alcohol problems: a critical appraisal. *Addiction* 1997; **92**: 939–47.

32. Chick J, Howless H, Morgan M Y. Ritson B. United Kingdom Multicentre Acamprosate Study (UKMAS): a 6-month prospective study of Acamprosate versus placebo in preventing relapse after withdrawal from alcohol. *Alcohol Alcoholism* 2000; **35**: 176–87.

33. Fox G C, Loughlin P, Cook C C H. Acamprosate for alcohol dependence (Protocol for a Cochrane Review). In: *Cochrane Library*. Issue 3. Chichester: John Wiley, 2004.

34. World Health Organization. Brief Intervention Study Group. A cross-national trial of brief interventions with heavy drinkers. *Am J Public Health* 1996; **86(7)**: 948–55.

35. Wallace P. Cutler S, Haines A. Randomised controlled trial of general practitioner intervention in patients with excessive alcohol consumption. *BMJ* 1988; **297(6649)**: 663–8.

36. Kristenson H, Öhlin H, Hultén-Nosslin M B, *et al.* Identification and intervention of heavy drinking in middle-aged men: results and follow-up of 24-60 months of long-term study with randomized controls. *Alcoholism: Clinical and Experimental Research* 1983; **7(2)**: 203–9.

37. Fleming M F, Barry K L, Manwell L B, *et al.* Brief physician advice for problem alcohol drinkers: A randomized trial in community-based primary care practices. *JAMA* 1997; **277(13)**: 1039–45.

38. Edwards G, Orford J, Egert S, *et al.* Alcoholism: A controlled trial of 'treatment' and 'advice.' *Journal of Studies on Alcohol* 1977; **38(5)**: 1004–31.

39. Bien T H, Miller W R, Tonigan J S. Brief interventions for alcohol problems: A review. *Addiction* 1993; **88(3)**: 315–36.

40. Graham A W, Fleming M S. Brief interventions. In: Graham A W, Schultz T K, Wilford B B. (Eds). *Principles of Addiction Medicine*. 2nd ed. Chevy Chase, MD: American Society of Addiction Medicine, Inc., 1998; 615–30.

41. O'Connor P G, Schottenfeld R S. Patients with alcohol problems. *New Engl J Med* 1998; **338(9)**: 592–602.

42. Heather N, Rollnick S, Bell A. Predictive validity of the Readiness to Change Questionnaire. *Addiction* 1993; **88(12)**: 1667–77.

43. Miller W. Motivational interviewing with problem drinkers. *Behavioural Psychotherapy* 1983; **11**: 147–72.

44. Chang G, Goetz M A, Wilkins-Haug L, Berman S. A brief intervention for prenatal alcohol use: an in-depth look. *Journal of Substance Abuse Treatment* 2000; **18**: 365–9.

45. Abel E L, Hannigan J H. Maternal risk factors in fetal alcohol syndrome: provocative and permissive influences. *Neurotoxicology and Teratology* 1995; **17**: 445–62.

46. Frezza M, di Padova C, Pozzato G, *et al.* High blood alcohol levels in women: the role of decreased gastric alcohol dehydrogenase activity and first-pass metabolism. *New Engl J Med* 1990; **322(2)**: 95–9

47. Randall C L, Roberts J S, Del Boca F K, *et al.* Telescoping of landmark events associated with drinking: a gender comparison. *J Stud Alcohol* 1999; **60(2)**: 252–60.

48. Becker U, Deis A, Sørensen T I, *et al.* Prediction of risk of liver disease by alcohol intake, sex, and age: a prospective population study. *Hepatology* 1996; **23(5)**: 1025–9.

49. Smith-Warner S A, Spiegelman D, Yaun S S, *et al.* Alcohol and breast cancer in women: a pooled analysis of cohort studies. *JAMA* 1998; **279(7)**: 535–40.

50. Hernandez-Avila M, Colditz G A, Stampfer M J, *et al.* Caffeine, moderate alcohol intake, and risk of fractures of the hip and forearm in middle-aged women. *Am J Clin Nutr* 1991; **54(1)**: 157–63.

51. Ganry O, Baudoin C, Fardellone P. Effect of alcohol intake on bone mineral density in elderly women: the EPIDOS Study. Epidemiologie de l'Osteoporose. *Am J Epidemiol* 2000; **151(8)**: 773–80.

52. Regier D A, Farmer M E, Rae D S, *et al.* Comorbidity of mental disorders with alcohol and other drug abuse. Results from the Epidemiologic Catchment Area (ECA) Study. *JAMA* 1990; **264(19)**: 2511–8.

53. Gomberg E S. Suicide risk among women with alcohol problems. *Am J Public Health* 1989; **79(10)**: 1363–5.

54. Lilenfeld L R, Kaye W H. The link between alcoholism and eating disorders. *Alcohol Health Res World* 1996; **20(2)**: 94–9.

55. Callahan C M, Tierney W M, Health services use and mortality among older primary care patients with alcoholism. *J Am Geriatr Soc* 1995; **43**: 1378–83.

56. Reid M C, Anderson P A. Geriatric substance use disorders. *Med Clin North Am* 1997; **81**: 999–1016.

57. O'Connell H, Chin A V, Cunningham C, Lawlor B. Alcohol use disorders in elderly people – redefining an age old problem in old age. *BMJ* 2003; **327**: 664–7.

CHAPTER 13

Cannabis

Hans-Christian Raabe and Clare Gerada

IN THIS CHAPTER

Introduction

On 29 January 2004 the House of Commons voted to downgrade all preparations
of cannabis from Class B to Class C. Although this move was recommended by the
Home Affairs Select Committee,[1] the House of Lords,[2] and the Police Foundation
(though opposed by the Police Federation, drug prevention organisations, and
some mental health charities),[3] it still leaves some confusion as to how primary
care workers should address cannabis use. The drug remains illegal and harmful
and therefore every effort should be made to discourage or at least reduce its use.
The GP and primary care nurse, therefore, have an important role in emphasising
the risks and harms associated with use of the drug and in advising users on ways
they can reduce these.

Prevalence

Cannabis is easily the most used illicit drug in the United Kingdom. The 2002/03
British Crime Survey, published by the Home Office, showed that over 3 million
16–59-year-olds have used cannabis in the past year (almost 11% of the population). Around 2 million people have done so in the past month.[4] Over a quarter
of all 16–24-year-olds used cannabis in the past year – the highest prevalence rate
of any European country.[5] This high rate of prevalence is worrying, but perhaps
unsurprising, in the context of a country with a large youth drug problem and
little in prevention or treatment techniques for cannabis use.

Drug policy in the United Kingdom focuses increasingly on Class A drugs. The
government's new 'communications campaign' in 2003, for example, was aimed
at young people and their parents and devoted to emphasising the risks of Class A
drugs, ignoring any of the potential risks associated with cannabis use.

Supplying cannabis remains a serious offence, however, carrying a penalty of up to 14 years in jail. Yet the availability of the drug is extremely high, with 68% of young people stating it is 'very easy' or 'fairly easy' to get hold of the drug.[5] Realistically, with the wide-scale use of cannabis so established in the United Kingdom, cutting down supply is a near-impossible task. Britain's 'cannabis economy' is worth £5 billion a year with a further £6 billion of consumer expenditure linked to the cannabis market due to 'the munchies' (increased appetite).[6]

Constituents of cannabis

Studying the constituents of cannabis highlights its dangers and the unavoidable effects of long-term use, particularly reinforced when compared with tobacco. Cannabis contains over 400 chemicals, about 60 of which are cannabinoids (compounds with a chemical structure related to delta-9-tetrahydrocannabinol (THC) – the main active chemical). It is reported that cannabis has become markedly stronger over the past 20–30 years, with an increase from about 0.5% THC to 5% while specially grown varieties may contain up to 30% THC. A 'reefer' in the early 1980s contained about 10 mg of THC, whereas a modern 'joint' may contain around 300 mg.[7]

The contention that cannabis is stronger today has been disputed. It seems that home-grown cannabis has increased in strength significantly over the past decade. Hydroponic cannabis may have a THC content of 10–20% whereas before the 1990s it was of poorer quality. The average THC of cannabis resin and herbal cannabis has been in the range of 4–5% for many years.[8] A review by the European Centre for Drugs and Drug Addiction in 2004 has concluded that over the last three decades there have been modest changes in THC levels and these are largely confined to the relatively recent appearance on the market of intensively cultivated domestically produced cannabis. Cannabis of this type is typically potent.[9]

The nature of cannabinoids mean that they remain in the body for a long time; it takes up to one month to eliminate a single dose of THC obtained from one cannabis cigarette.[10] Ten per cent of THC, a fat-soluble substance, can persist for up to a month in the brain with 50% lasting for a week. The brain of a person who smokes cannabis only once a week is therefore never free of THC. This contrasts with alcohol, which is eliminated from the body much more quickly.

Cannabis can be baked into cakes or biscuits, but it is normally smoked. Compared with tobacco smoking, cannabis is associated with a nearly five-fold greater increment in the blood carboxyhaemoglobin level, an approximately threefold greater increase in the amount of tar inhaled, and retention in the respiratory tract of one-third more inhaled tar. The smoke from cannabis contains the same constituents (apart from nicotine) as tobacco smoke, including bronchial irritants, tumour initiators (mutagens), tumour promoters, and carcinogens. The tar from cannabis smoke also contains greater concentrations of benzanthracenes and benzpyrenes, both of which are carcinogens, than the tar in tobacco smoke. It is plain to see that any beliefs held by young people that cannabis is a harmless drug are worryingly uninformed.

Box 13.1 **From the cannabis plant three types of drug can be produced**

Marijuana (marihuana, grass, pot, draw, weed etc.) is the simplest cannabis product from the dried plant material – potencies range from 0.3–22%

Hashish (cannabis resin, soap bar, Afghan, etc.) is produced from the resin extracted from the plant, often kneaded into sticks or flat lumps or even powder – THC content varies between 2% and 25%, or higher. Can contain substances such as diesel fuel, plastics, henna, coffee and even heroin

Cannabis extract (hashish oil, liquid cannabis) is the most concentrated form of cannabis, produced through distillation of the cannabis plant. THC concentrations vary between 10% and 60%. This form is rare in the illegal market

Indoor cannabis (skunk, northern lights) grown typically using hydroponic systems, potencies vary from 2–22%

Routes of use

Marijuana is usually mixed with tobacco and rolled into special cigarettes called 'joints'. Hashish is often mixed with tobacco and smoked in cigarettes, pipes, or 'bongs'. Cannabis smoke is usually inhaled rapidly and kept in the lungs for a time to maximise its effect. Users can smoke cannabis through a variety of means – for example, rolled in a cigarette, through bongs (which can be made from glass, brass, aluminium, acrylic), plastic bread bags, or buckets (litre coke bottles placed in bucket of water). Cannabis can even be smoked through a coconut.

Hashish is swallowed in tea or mixed with sugar or other edible products.

The effects of cannabis use

Acute

Cannabis, like most drugs, can precipitate both temporary and permanent effects in the user. The acute toxicity of cannabis is very low, with no confirmed reports of human deaths attributed to cannabis poisoning in the medical literature, although there has been a single report in a national newspaper of a possible acute death following cannabis use (see Box 13.2).

Box 13.2   **Death attributed to cannabis poisoning**

A man of 36 is believed to have become the first person in Britain to die directly from cannabis poisoning. Lee smoked six cannabis cigarettes a day for 11 years, an inquest heard. His death, which was registered as having been caused by cannabis toxicity, led to new warnings about the drug, which is due to be reclassified this month as a less dangerous one. 'This type of death is extremely rare,' Prof John Henry, a toxicologist at Imperial College, London, said after the inquest. 'I have not seen anything like this before. It corrects the argument that cannabis cannot kill anybody.' Post-mortem tests showed a high level of cannabinoids in his blood, was free from disease and had not drunk any alcohol.

Source: Richard Savill, *Daily Telegraph*; 20 January 2004

Generally the harmful effects of cannabis are related to its ability to impair perceptual-motor coordination and to those of inhaling toxic smoke into the lungs and respiratory system.

One of the serious temporary effects of cannabis is that it impairs the user's ability to drive, sometimes for up to 24 hours. Many studies have shown that cannabis impairs balance, tracking ability, hand-eye coordination, reaction time, and physical strength.[11] These effects can occur with a dose as low as 20 mg of THC. Furthermore, the fat-soluble nature of cannabis means the effects are far more long-lasting than those of alcohol. In a simulation, airline pilots could not land their planes a full 24 hours after taking only 20 mg of THC. Worryingly, the pilots were unaware of any problem.[12]

An Australian study underlined the often unreported danger of cannabis use and driving. Of all the drivers under the age of 45 killed in traffic accidents over a four-year period, more than one-third of drivers were found to have evidence of recent cannabis use but either no alcohol or very low alcohol levels.[13]

Cannabis use also temporarily impairs learning ability, which for young people smoking the drug regularly, can be a serious problem. Skills related to attention, memory, learning, and organising are severely impaired in heavy cannabis users and can remain so for over a day after the last time the drug was taken. Studies have proved that students who smoke cannabis attain lower grades than those who do not.[14] See Box 13.4.

Long-term effects

The long-term effects of cannabis are potentially wide-ranging, and evidence is mounting that cannabis is linked to mental illness, as well as lung damage. The latter has long been accepted, but the extent of the lung damage caused by cannabis is worrying. In 2002 the British Lung Foundation published a report entitled *Cannabis – a Smoking Gun?*[15] By studying existing evidence the report found that smoking three to four cannabis cigarettes a day causes the same acute and chronic bronchitis and equivalent degree of damage to the bronchial mucosa as smoking 20 or more tobacco cigarettes a day. Common long-term effects of cannabis use include a significantly higher prevalence of chronic and acute respiratory symptoms such as chronic cough, chronic sputum production, wheeze, and acute bronchitis than are found in non-smokers. There have been several reports of severe lung damage including severe emphysema occurring in people under 30. This emphysema is different in nature and occurs at a significantly younger age than the equivalent symptoms that cigarette smokers are prone to develop.[16]

A definite relationship between cannabis and damage to other areas of the body cannot be established so easily, but there are a number of case studies reporting cancers of the pharynx, larynx, and mouth in young adults with a history of cannabis use. In normal circumstance these cancers rarely occur in anyone under the age of 60.[17]

Smoking cannabis is also associated with a weakened immune system as the drug adversely affects the functioning of T cells, natural killer cells, and macrophages that help protect the airways against micro-organisms. Macrophagal ability to produce a variety of chemicals that play a key role in the immune response to infection and malignancy has also shown to be impaired by cannabis smoking.[18]

Cannabis and mental illness

The adverse effects described above are easily comparable with tobacco smoking. A now widely accepted concern, which distinguishes cannabis from tobacco, is a potential link with mental illness. There is considerable clinical evidence linking cannabis to schizophrenia, psychosis, anxiety, and depression. Earlier and heavier cannabis use exacerbates the risk. A doubling in the prevalence of schizophrenia in London in the past three decades cannot be decisively linked to an increase in cannabis use, but equally this cannot be ruled out on current evidence. Patients with a recent onset of psychosis are twice as likely to have smoked cannabis (but not to have taken alcohol or other illicit drugs) than those without psychosis.[19] Dopamine mediates the psychotic symptoms in conditions such as schizophrenia and THC is shown to raise the level of cerebral dopamine in the body.

The link between cannabis and mental illness dates back to a study of Swedish conscripts in 1987,[20] but it is only studies in the past few years that have really aroused concern. A Dutch study of some 4000 people showed that those taking large amounts of cannabis at the initial interview were seven times more likely to have psychotic symptoms three years later.[21] Even a group of initially healthy individuals had an increased risk of psychosis, while an expansion of the original Swedish Army study showed that the trend described still held when people showing early signs of mental illness at the time of initial recruitment were discounted.

In combination with this evidence is the continuing suggestion that risk is increased with particularly early cannabis use. A New Zealand-based study showed a 4.5 times higher risk of developing psychosis among those who started using cannabis at 15 rather than 18. Again this trend held, if slightly diminished, when those displaying psychotic-like ideas at the age of 11 were excluded.[22]

A recent review examined nearly 50 longitudinal studies, of which only 16 were able to reveal reliable evidence supporting the association between cannabis use and later psychosocial problems, although the authors were careful to emphasise that it was not possible to conclude that there was a causal link – in other words there is no knowing if cannabis leads to harm or if harm leads to cannabis use. In the accompanying commentary, a contributor added, 'There is some reason to believe that cannabis contributes to psychosocial problems in adolescents and young adults ... though ... there is little reason to believe that criminalisation has had a strong effect on the extent of cannabis use by young people.'[23]

Cannabis and pregnancy

One final effect of cannabis, albeit in a special circumstance, is on an unborn child. In a study of 12,424 mothers, cannabis smoking during pregnancy has been associated with low birth-weight, short gestation, and malformations.[24] It may be, however, that these effects are more related to the effects of tobacco ingestion rather than a direct effect of cannabis.

Addiction

Cannabis has the potential for dependency and regular use can induce a withdrawal syndrome, tolerance, escalation of dosage, craving, increasing importance of drug taking over other activities, and difficulty in controlling use.[25] The risk of dependence occurring is around 10–15% – a similar figure to that associated with alcohol dependence.

Treatment options

Box 13.3   **Case history**

Charles, a 45-year-old successful IT consultant running his own business presents in morning surgery wanting something to help him sleep. He feels very tense most of the time and finds that he cannot relax. On questioning it emerges that he smokes up to six cannabis joints a day – starting first thing in the morning to help overcome the anxiety of opening his emails and finding 'hundreds of emails'. He is worried about this cannabis use and also the concomitant tobacco use. He does not drink alcohol, but is aware that he uses cannabis as an alternative. He has tried to stop smoking cannabis but finds it very difficult, and feels so irritable after a few hours that he has to restart. He uses no other drugs, though in his youth had tried cocaine.

✓ What can you do to help?

✓ Is there a place for nicotine replacement products?

✓ What should you tell the patient about the risks caused by his cannabis use?

Treatment options for dependence are scant, but opinion, especially in the United States, has tended towards motivational interviewing techniques, which have had some success in promoting abstinence. Major research undertakings across the Atlantic such as the 1996 Marijuana Treatment Project have promoted the use of these techniques, but in reality they are only a form of counselling marketed around cannabis use. No pharmacotherapy exists to help cannabis addicts achieve abstinence other than those used to combat tobacco addiction. HIT (a charity aimed at providing information and educational material to users and health professionals on different drugs) has produced a self-help website for people who want to reduce or stop their cannabis use. This can be found at www.cannabishelp.org.uk.

The degree of impairment from the combined use of alcohol and cannabis needs to be highlighted in discussions of cannabis use and driving.

Therapeutic uses of cannabis[26]

Cannabis has been widely used as a medicine for over 5,000 years in China, India, the Middle East, and other parts of the world. There is suggestive evidence that it is effective against nausea and vomiting and as an analgesic and that it is valuable for combating the loss of appetite and weight loss experienced by patients

Box 13.4 **Acute effects of cannabis**

✓ Unprovoked euphoria, laughter

✓ Talkativeness and animation

✓ Changes in perception of time, space, and distance

✓ Increased self-esteem

✓ Impaired learning ability and concentration

✓ Diminished short-term memory

✓ Sleep disturbance

✓ Increased appetite ('munchies')

✓ Conjunctivitis ('red-eyes')

with cancer and AIDS, for the relief of muscle spasms in patients with multiple sclerosis, and in the treatment of glaucoma. There should be no barrier to the conduct of random allocation trials designed to compare cannabis with existing treatment and if cannabis proves superior to these existing remedies there should be no bar to its being made available to appropriate patients in the appropriate formulation. Such trials are currently being conducted. Its increased medical use, however, might lead to some diversion and abuse of prescribed medication.

Conclusions following reclassification

The reclassification of cannabis as a Class C drug in 2004 in the United Kingdom fitted well with the government's focus on Class A drugs that are the foundations of the most serious crime, individual, and community problems. This chapter has shown how many health risks still apply to cannabis use regardless of its classification. It is too early to judge whether the downgrading of cannabis will prompt a marked increase in its use, but if young people conclude that cannabis is virtually harmless then it is likely to do so. It is extremely important, therefore, that GPs continue to emphasise that cannabis is not harmless.[27]

Although one cannot say that cannabis use leads inexorably to other more dangerous drugs, there is still a relationship between cannabis and other drugs. Almost all heroin users began their drug use with cannabis and therefore to 'focus on class A drugs' and neglect cannabis is shortsighted. Sweden, with a very strong focus on drug prevention in general and cannabis in particular, has the lowest usage rates of cannabis in Europe, but also the lowest rates of cocaine, amfetamines, and ecstasy use. When in Lambeth (London) the police turned a 'blind eye' to cannabis, all other drug use increased too.

Cannabis remains increasingly popular among young people and the steady increase in its use over the past 50 years shows no sign of reversing. As there is a distinct lack of strategy to tackle the growing prevalence of cannabis dependence, a GP's role will be confined to the education and counselling of users based on the mounting evidence of the effects of cannabis use.

Reducing the harm from cannabis use

The health professional's role should be to try to reduce the risks and harms associated with their patients' drug use. HIT (www.hit.org.uk) have produced excellent leaflets designed for drug users, and have recently reissued one on cannabis. Doctors, nurses, and pharmacists would do well to read this small publication so that they are as informed as their patients. See Box 13.6.

Box 13.5   Summary of adverse effects of cannabis[28]

Acute effects

✓ anxiety and panic, especially in naive users

✓ impaired attention, memory, and psychomotor performance while intoxicated

✓ possibly an increased risk of accident if a person drives a motor vehicle while intoxicated with cannabis, especially if used with alcohol and/or tranquilisers

✓ increased risk of psychotic symptoms

✓ increased risk of low-birth-weight babies if smoked in pregnancy

✓ increased risk of myocardial infarction

Chronic effects (probable)

✓ chronic bronchitis and histopathological changes that may be precursors of malignant disease

✓ cannabis dependence syndrome characterised by an inability to abstain from or to control cannabis use, craving, and tolerance to the physical and mental effects of the drug. The risk of dependence is estimated at less than 20% if the drug is taken more than five times and 10% for those who have ever used. 15–30% of users report difficulty in controlling their use and withdrawal symptoms are common in this group

✓ subtle impairments of attention and memory that persist while the user remains chronically intoxicated, and this may or may not be reversible after prolonged abstinence

✓ impaired educational attainment in adolescents and underachievement in adults in occupations that require high-level cognitive skills

Possible adverse effects (to be confirmed)

✓ increased risk of cancers of the oral cavity, pharynx, and oesophagus; leukaemia among the offspring exposed in utero

✓ emphysema

Groups that are at higher risk of experiencing these adverse effects

✓ adolescents with a history of poor school performance, or who initiate cannabis use in their early teens

✓ women who continue to smoke cannabis during pregnancy at increased risk of low-birth-weight babies

✓ people with schizophrenia, asthma, bronchitis, alcohol and other drug dependence

Summary of effects in non-vulnerable individuals

✓ panic attacks

✓ toxic psychosis

✓ functional psychosis

Summary of effects in vulnerable individuals

✓ individuals with mental disorder at increased risk of misusing cannabis

✓ 4–6 times increased risk of cannabis misuse in schizophrenia

✓ a probable risk factor for schizophrenia

✓ worsening some symptoms of schizophrenia and increasing rate of relapse

✓ in heavy use short-term reversible cognitive impairments in adolescents

Reprinted with permission from Elsevier (*Lancet* 1998; **352**: 1611–16).

Box 13.6   Techniques and tips for reducing the risk

Users should do the following:

✓ Not hold the smoke in their lungs – they don't get more stoned and they increase the amount of tar and other dangerous chemicals that stick to their lung tissue

✓ Not inhale too deeply – sucking on a bong or using a bucket may cool the smoke but it also forces it deeper into the lungs, increasing the amount breathed in

✓ Clean weed properly – the bulk of THC is in the sticky tops and flowers, so the stem, leaves and other bits should be taken out

✓ Not use a cigarette filter for a roach – cigarette filters increase the ratio of tar to THC by 30% and reduce the amount of THC that gets through by 60% (a piece of plain card is better)

✓ Not use many papers – three skinners are big enough and this will cut down the amount of burnt paper inhaled

✓ Avoid using plastic bottles, rubber hoses, PVC, aluminium or foil to smoke cannabis with – these all give of toxic fumes when hot (pipes from glass, or brass cause fewer risks)

✓ Clean bongs and pipes properly after use – germs can hang around long enough to infect users and their friends

✓ Avoid sharing joints – germs can be passed from one person to another on the wet roach

Reproduced from HIT with permission

Further reading

Hall W, Pacula R L. *Cannabis use and dependence: public health and public policy.* Cambridge: CUP, 2003.

References

1. Home Affairs Committee. *The Government's Drugs Policy: Is It Working?* Third report of session 2001–2002. London: HMSO, 2002.

2. House of Lords Select Committee on Science and Technology. *Cannabis: the Scientific and Medical Evidence.* London: HMSO, 1998.

3. Runciman R. *Drugs and the Law.* Report of the Independent Inquiry into the Misuse of Drugs Act 1971. London: The Police Foundation, 1999.

4. British Crime Survey. *Findings 229: Prevalence of Drug Use: Key Findings from the 2002/03 British Crime Survey.* London: Home Office, 2003.

5. Crime in England and Wales. 2001/02 British Crime Survey. London: Home Office, 2002.

6. *The Observer.* Cannabis economy brings in £11 billion. 02/02/03.

7. Gold M S. Marijuana. In: *Comprehensive Handbook of Alcohol and Drug Addiction.* New York: Marcel Dekker Inc., 1991; 353–76.

8. King L A, Drugs Intelligence Unit Manager Forensic Science Service, in a submission to the Lords Science and Technology Committee. 8 May, 1998; pp 218–19.

9. European Monitoring Centre for Drugs and Drug Addiction. EMCDDA insights. An overview of cannabis potency in Europe. Luxembourg: Office for Official Publications of the European Communities, 2004.

10. Maykut M O. *Health Consequences of Acute and Chronic Marijuana Use*. Oxford: Pergamon Press, 1984; 328.

11. Golding J F. Cannabis. In: *Handbook of Human Performance: Health and Performance*. Vol. 2. New York: Academic Press, 1992; 175.

12. Leirer V O, Yesavage J A, Morrow D G. Marijuana carry-over effects on aircraft pilot performance. *Aviation, Space and Environmental Medicine* 1991; **62(3)**: 221–7.

13. Tutt, D BauerL, Arms J, *et al*. Cannabis and Road Death: An Emerging Injury Prevention Concern. *Health Promotion Journal of Australia* August 2001; **12(2)**.

14. Lynskey M, Hall W. The effects of adolescent cannabis use on educational attainment. *Addiction* 2000; **95(11)**: 1621–30.

15. British Lung Foundation. *A smoking gun? The impact of cannabis smoking on respiratory health*. London: British Lung Foundation, 2003.

16. Johnson M K, Smith R P, Morrison D, *et al*. Large lung bullae in marijuana smokers. *Thorax* 2000; **55**: 340–2.

17. Donald P J. Marijuana and upper aerodigestive tract malignancy in young patients. In: Nahas G G, Latour C, Hardy N and Dingea P. (Eds). *Physiopathology of Illicit Drugs: Cannabis, Cocaine and Opiates*. Oxford: Pergamon Press, 1991.

18. Baldwin G C, Tashkin D P, Buckley D M, *et al*. Alveolar macrophages derived from the lungs of tobacco, marijuana and cocaine users are functionally compromised. In: *Problems of Drug Dependence*. Proceedings of the 57th Annual Scientific Meeting of the College on Problems of Drug Dependence, NIDA Research Monograph Series 162, 1996.

19. Zammit S, Allebeck P, Andreasson S, *et al*. Self-reported cannabis use as a risk factor for schizophrenia in Swedish conscripts of 1969: historical cohort study. *BMJ* 2002; **325**: 1199–201.

20. Andréasson S, Allebeck P, Engström A, Rydberg U. Cannabis and schizophrenia: a longitudinal study of Swedish conscripts. *Lancet* 1987; **ii**: 1483–1485.

21. Van Os J, Bak M, Hanssen M, *et al*. Cannabis use and psychosis: a longitudinal population-based study. *Am J Epidemiology* 2002; **156(4)**: 319–27.

22. Arseneault L, Cannon M, Poulton R, *et al*. Cannabis use in adolescence and risk for adult psychosis: longitudinal prospective study. *BMJ* 2002; **325**: 1212–3.

23. Macleod J, Oakes R, Copello A, *et al*. Psychological and social sequelae of cannabis and other illicit drug use by young people: a systematic review of longitudinal, general populations studies. *Lancet* 2004; **363(9421)**: 1579–88.

24. Linn S, Schoenbaum S C, Monson R R. The association of marijuana use with outcome of pregnancy. *Am J Public Health* 1983; **73**: 1161–4.

25. Johns A. Psychiatric effects of cannabis. *Br J Psychiatry* 2001; **178**: 116–22.

26. Robson P. Therapeutic aspects of cannabis and cannabinoids. *Br J Psychiatry* 2001; **178**: 107–15.

27. Gerada C. Cannabis and the general practitioner – going to pot. *Br J Gen Pract* 2003; **493**: 598–99.

28. Hall W, Solowij N. Adverse effects of cannabis. *Lancet* 1998; **352**: 1611–16.

| # Tobacco use

Deborah Arnott and Clare Gerada

Introduction

This chapter draws heavily on Action on Smoking and Health (ASH) response to the Department of Health's consultation papers on public health, *Choosing Health? A Consultation on Action to Improve People's Health* (accessible at: www.dh.gov.uk)[2] which has led to the publication of a white paper on public health for England.

It is inconceivable that today's health professionals are not well aware of the risks of smoking. The original studies defining many of these risks were conducted on British general practitioners and as the initial results began to be disclosed doctors were amongst the first to give up smoking. In 2004, the 50-year follow up of smokers in this study found that smokers died on average about 10 years younger than lifetime non-smokers, and stopping smoking at age 60, 50, 40 or 30 years, gained, respectively, about 3, 6, 9, or 10 years of life expectancy.[1]

Today, the debate on the risks of smoking has moved on, the debate now is around whether smoking should be banned in the workplace and how we can prevent secondary damage from smoking. In the Choosing Health White Paper the UK government has announced that it will be legislating to stop smoking in almost all workplaces, with exemptions only for pubs and bars that don't serve food and clubs. Scotland plans to go even further with a complete ban on smoking. Doctors play an important part in this debate and indeed the British Medical Association conference in 2004 overwhelmingly passed a motion to urge the government to ban smoking in public places and is continuing to lobby for a complete ban on smoking in the workplace throughout the UK.

Policy context

Smoking is the biggest single cause of preventable illness and premature death killing around 106,000 people in the United Kingdom each year.[3] It is also the biggest single cause of inequalities in health. Improving the nation's health requires a significant reduction in the number of people who smoke. The health professional's role is not an easy one. Although 70% of smokers want to give up, less than 5% succeed each year. Tobacco in smokable form is the most highly addictive drug legally and illegally available (even when compared with heroin or cocaine) with 90% of regular smokers starting smoking before they are 18 and most having a life long addiction.[4]

Epidemiology

Between 1970 and 1990, the United Kingdom showed the fastest reduction in cigarette smoking in the world although this decline seems to have reached a plateau over the past decade, with around 27% smoking in 1994 and 25% in 2002 (16+). Young people are most likely to smoke; the highest prevalence is amongst men and women aged 20–24 (40% and 35% respectively compared with around 17% in the over 60s). In 2001, 10% of children aged 11–15 smoked at least one cigarette each week. Girls continue to smoke more than boys, with 11% of girls and 8% of boys saying that they smoked at least one cigarette a week.[5] Although the most recent data suggest that smoking is again in decline, it is only by about 0.4% per annum. If current rates of decline in smoking prevalence continue, smoking prevalence will still be at 22% by 2011, and it would take until 2024 to reach 17%, the level now seen in California, with one of the lowest prevalence rates in the developed world.[6] See Figure 14.1.

Nicotine dependence

Nicotine dependence is recognised in ICD-10 and DSM-IV as a psychiatric disorder. The defining features include failed attempts to abstain, powerful urges to use nicotine, and withdrawal symptoms on cessation. An estimated 80% of cigarette smokers are classifiable as dependent by DSM-IV criteria.

Smoking and social class

Smoking follows a social class gradient with smoking prevalence decreasing as one moves up the social scale. The social class gradient has increased as the

Figure 14.1 **Prevalence of smoking of manufactured cigarettes in Great Britain 1974–2022**

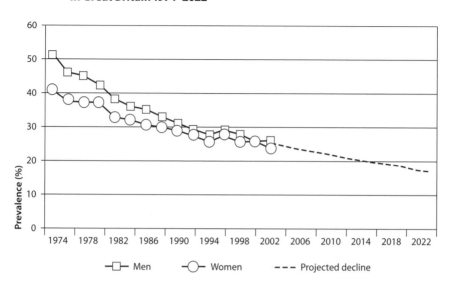

Data source: 1974–88 General Household Survey; 200-02 ONS; 2002–projected; source of graphic – ASH [7]

number of smokers has decreased, because the decline in smoking prevalence has been far higher in social Class I than in other social classes. Smoking remains highest amongst those from manual as opposed to non-manual socioeconomic groups (32% compared to 21%). Smoking is more than any other identifiable factor the cause of the variance in healthy life expectancy between those in need and those that are most advantaged.[8]

The impact of smoking on health inequalities is carried down from generation to generation. Children whose parents smoke are three times as likely to smoke themselves and are also more heavily exposed to the harmful effects of tobacco smoke pollution. As a result, children from more deprived families have a higher risk of cot death, the onset of asthma as well as asthma attacks, respiratory diseases, and ear infections. Children in social class V may be doubly disadvantaged because they are also more likely to go on to become smokers themselves and suffer the effects of smoking, in particular lung cancer, heart disease, and lung disease.

Prevention

As most smokers begin in their late teens it might seem a sensible policy to commence prevention strategies with preteens. Research shows, however, that unless this is part of a comprehensive programme of personal health and social education, youth smoking prevention policies are largely ineffectual. At best they may delay the onset of smoking but they have little impact on overall smoking prevalence.[9]

So what does work? The best evidence on this comes from California where a comprehensive tobacco control strategy has led to significant falls in smoking both amongst adults and amongst young people. Smoking prevalence is now around 17% for the population as a whole. The evidence shows that the most effective policies in helping to protect children from second-hand smoke, by reducing adult smoking, are also likely to be most effective in preventing children from starting smoking themselves.

The United Kingdom has put in place the foundation of a comprehensive tobacco control strategy, as set out in its white paper on tobacco *Smoking Kills*, published in 1998.[6] These include 'stop-smoking' services many of which involve general practitioners and include smoking cessation products available on the NHS; an advertising ban; public education and mass media campaigns; and a policy of maintaining high prices aimed at ensuring that tobacco does not become more affordable over time. Although laudable in their aims, this strategy may not go far enough until a ban on public smoking is introduced.

Smoking in prisons

Smoking rates amongst prisoners are very high, perhaps not surprising considering the dual impact of high numbers of prisoners coming from socially excluded sections of society and the boredom produced by incarceration. Over three-quarters of all prisoners smoke and half are moderate or heavy smokers.[10]

Smoking in the workplace

Legislation to require all employers to ensure that their workplaces are smoke-free is a key public health measure for a number of reasons. First, second-hand smoke is dangerous to the health of non-smokers and in particular is a workplace health and safety risk. Secondly, ending smoking in the workplace would probably be the single simplest and most effective means of cutting smoking prevalence rates. Thirdly, this intervention would most benefit poorer and socially excluded communities. Evidence suggests that when a workplace becomes smoke-free it can reduce smoking rates amongst workers by up to 4%, as well as reducing consumption levels,[11] and as workers in lower paid jobs are far more likely to work in places where smoking is allowed, smoke-free workplaces would also help reduce health inequalities.

Smoke-free environments are likely to impact on the young and help reduce their levels of smoking. For young people smoking is a social activity and spreads 'like an infectious disease which spreads from one person to another'. Smoke-free legislation that prevents young people from smoking in coffee bars, pubs, bars, clubs, and other places where they congregate, therefore, is an effective means of reducing the numbers starting to smoke. For example, research has shown that young people in colleges with a no-smoking policy for staff and students were half as likely to smoke as those in colleges that allowed smoking. And those who did smoke consumed fewer cigarettes.[12]

There is also evidence from Australia that smoke-free workplaces can be effective in reducing smoking in the home. In 1989 only 17% of workers were protected by a ban on smoking in the workplace. By 1995 this had risen to 66%. It is reported that the proportion of adults not smoking in front of children rose from 14% in 1989 to 33% in 1996. Those who worked in places where smoking was totally banned were more likely to ask their visitors not to smoke than those who worked where smoking was allowed.[13]

Media, advertising, and publicity

Advertising can both promote and prevent tobacco use. Long gone are the days when doctors and nurses were used to persuade people of 'health benefits' of the product though in more modern times there is concern about marketing and the role model effect of smoking in films and on TV. Smoking depicted in films has returned to levels observed in 1950 when smoking was nearly twice as prevalent as it is today. Research shows that children and young people in particular are influenced to try cigarettes by viewing role models smoking.[14]

Advertising can also reduce smoking among young people.[15] Public education campaigns can provide excellent value for money, costing under £1,000/life year saved.[16,17]

Total advertising bans can reduce smoking consumption by between 4% and 16%.[18] Tobacco advertising is a known risk factor for youth smoking.[19] Children are more likely to smoke brands that are heavily promoted and advertising reinforces the habit.

Graphic health warnings on cigarette packs are effective.[20]

Smoking in public places – Ireland's smoking ban

Ireland introduced the first natiowide ban on smoking in enclosed workplaces in the European Union on 29 March 2004. To date, 96% of pubs and restaurants have complied, with the majority displaying the required no smoking signs. Anyone caught smoking illegally by health inspectors enforcing the ban can be fined up to 3,000 euros (around £2,400). Psychiatric hospitals, hotel bedrooms, prison cells, and nursing homes are exempt from the ban.

A report on the workplace ban by the Office of Tobacco Control found that there was overwhelming support for the legislation and the ban has been hailed by many as a success.

Other countries are following suit. For example, in Australia smoking is prohibited in all airports, government offices, health clinics, and workplaces.

Pricing and taxation

Tobacco tax is an important component of health, as well as fiscal policy. As with most consumer products, price affects use, hence the greater the price, the less the use. Increasing the real price of cigarettes decreases cigarette consumption *and* the prevalence of smoking. Overall in the United Kingdom, smoking prevalence currently falls by around 0.3% per 1% real increase in price, although this ratio may fall as prices rise further and smoking is reduced to a 'hard core', whose demand for cigarettes is less price sensitive. Real increases in price through taxation can also be achieved only if smuggling is controlled.[21] The late 1990s saw the market share of smuggled cigarettes increase considerably although it has fallen in recent years since HM Customs and Excise introduced its smuggling strategy in 2000. The volume of cigarettes successfully smuggled into the United Kingdom was estimated to have fallen by 1.5 billion in 2001–2, the first time this had happened for a decade. Over the past two years it has fallen by a further 4 billion, a drop of nearly 30%.

Tobacco tax evasion still accounts for over £3 billion in tax losses (see Table 14.1), 41% of the total collected. This is many times more than fuel (4%) or alcohol (9%). Smuggling grew because of the willingness of tobacco manufacturers to export brands popular in the United Kingdom to end markets, such as Andorra and Cyprus, where there was little domestic demand for these cigarettes and from where they were re-exported as smuggled products back to the United Kingdom. With greater control put on the smuggling of legally produced cigarettes the well-established distribution chains for smuggled products are now turning to counterfeit. Counterfeit cigarettes as a proportion of smuggled cigarettes seized by customs have risen from 15% in 2001 to over 50% by 2003–4, and the proportion is believed to be continuing to increase. Contraband cigarettes can be bought at around half the price of premium brands, £2.50 for a packet of 20, compared with nearly £5 for a packet of a leading UK brand.

The lesson is that if the cost of a drug is low, use will increase, if tax is increased to drive down use then smuggling needs to be tightly controlled or it will create an illicit market, which can potentially decrease the price and increase use, particularly amongst the most vulnerable and the young.

Table 14.1 **Revenue collection and evasion estimates in major excise regimes for 2001–2**

	Revenue collected (£m)	Revenue evaded (£m)
Fuel (GB)	21,900	850
Tobacco	7,800	3,180
Alcohol	6,900	650

Source: Customs Annual Report and Accounts 2002–3, Customs Pre-Budget Report on Measuring and Tackling Indirect Tax Losses December 2003

Supporting quitters, cutting prevalence

'Stop smoking' interventions that provide behavioural support, counselling, and pharmacotherapy are all effective, with primary care being an important point of initiation for this treatment. Systematic reviews have demonstrated that simple advice from a physician has a positive effect in triggering quit attempts.[22] Best practice (regular counselling support and pharmacotherapy) increases the chance of sustained long-term cessation in any quit attempt by a factor of four.[23-25]

All smoking cessation interventions provide excellent value for money, costing less than £1,000 per life year saved, which is better than most other interventions in medicine[15,26] and far better than most interventions recommended to date by the National Institute for Clinical Excellence.[27] Currently the stop smoking services are reaching just over 2% of smokers a year. Their reported 4-week success rate of 50% is likely to translate into approximately an additional 0.2% of smokers quitting over the long term who would otherwise not have done so. Although there is variation across the country nationally, the services have achieved success in line with what was predicted from the research literature and should continue to receive funding at the current level.

Stop smoking interventions, however, although they are much more effective in reducing disease risk than most other current routine medical practices, are still not routine and systematic.

Stopping smoking halves the risk of recurrence of myocardial infarction, a much greater and more cost-effective impact than that achieved by other routine interventions such as therapy with aspirin, beta blockers, ACE inhibitors, or statins, but in clinical practice is the least likely intervention to be applied.

Smoking cessation is the only intervention that halts the development of chronic obstructive airways disease or reduces the risk of lung cancer, but only half of all UK chest specialists have direct access to a smoking cessation counsellor.[28]

Smoking rates are similar for diabetics and non-diabetics, but smoking increases the risk of serious disease and death in diabetics from 4 to 11 times.

Stopping smoking before surgery can have a dramatic impact on outcome. In hip and knee operations it reduces postoperative complications by two-thirds and duration of stay in hospital by 15%.

Smoking and primary care

The new general medical service contract (nGMS) offers quality points (and therefore income) for targets relating to smoking. For example, within the section concerned with secondary prevention in coronary heart disease, seven points are awarded for achieving 90% in recording patients' smoking habits and a further four points if this same percentage has a record that smoking cessation advice has been offered in the past 15 months. Similarly, points are awarded in the sections for stroke and transient ischaemic attack, hypertension, diabetes, and chronic obstructive pulmonary disease.

Smoking cessation products

Nicotine replacement products can be prescribed to patients on FP10s.

No single delivery method is more effective than others.

Nicotine replacement treatment (NRT) is currently produced as:

▸ transdermal patch (varying doses, 16-hour and 24-hour duration)

▸ gum (2 mg and 4 mg)

▸ inhalator

▸ nasal spray (0.5 mg per dose)

▸ sublingual tablet (2 mg)

▸ lozenge (1 mg, 2 mg and 4 mg).

Nicotine replacement therapy increases the chance of achieving abstinence for at least six months. These figures arise from many high quality randomised controlled trials with biochemical verification of smoking status at follow up (usually from expired air carbon monoxide). There is some evidence to suggest that combinations of NRT products are more effective overall than single products, and that combinations are safe. NRT delivers pure nicotine which is only one of the components smokers already obtain from cigarettes. Long-term NRT use does not pose a cancer risk, or a risk of COPD or other respiratory disease. NRT use is safe in patients with stable coronary heart disease. NRT may have a harmful effect on the fetus, but it is believed that it does so to a lesser extent than smoking. A minority of smokers transfer dependence from cigarettes to NRT. Such patients would probably resume smoking if they could not continue NRT use.

In highly dependent smokers 4 mg gum is more effective than 2 mg gum and higher dose patches are more effective than lower dose patches. There is no clear evidence that the 24-hour patch is more effective than the 16-hour patch and no evidence that tapering patch dose after eight weeks improves effectiveness.[29]

Other smoking cessation products

The atypical antidepressant bupropion is also marketed for smoking cessation. It is contraindicated in people with a past history of seizures and its safety has not been well established in pregnancy and young people under 18 years old. Its adverse effect profile may make it less suitable than NRT, which can be purchased over the counter.

Randomised controlled trials comparing NRT with bupropion have had conflicting results. Simon *et al.* carried out a randomised placebo-controlled study where all recipients received additional cognitive behavioural counselling. The results showed that the addition of brief seven-week bupropion did not significantly affect quit rate.[30]

An earlier study by Hughes *et al.* found that whereas concomitant behavioural or supportive therapy increases quit rates, which should be encouraged, they are not essential. However, combining patch or patch with gum with bupropion increases the quit rate compared with placebo.[31]

Brief intervention

Even simple, one-off advice from a doctor during a routine consultation is associated with 2% of smokers quitting smoking without relapse for one year. Advice from trained counsellors who are neither doctors nor nurses also increases cessation rates compared with minimal intervention. Brief advice from health professionals, as with alcohol treatment, is a proven cost effective method of promoting smoking cessation.[26] Yet the proportion of smokers recalling receipt of advice on smoking from any health professional in the past five years has fallen between 1996 and 2002 from 46% to 42%.[32]

Smoking cessation is now an integral part of the new primary care contract with points given to recording smoking and for referring or providing smoking cessation interventions. It may be that including smoking cessation as an enhanced service may add to the number of doctors delivering this service.

Summary of treatment for smoking

Nicotine replacement therapy

▶ All NRT products are effective in assisting smoking cessation.

▶ Combinations of NRT products can safely be used (e.g. patch plus inhalor) and may be more effective. If a single product is ineffective, it is worth trying a combination.

▶ Higher dose products are more effective for heavily dependent smokers (4 mg gum, or standard rather than low dose patches).

▶ Additional behavioural support (as provided in specialist smokers' clinics) is not essential but improves overall success rate.

▶ NRT can be used in patients with chronic disease, including cardiac disease.

▶ Although effectiveness is not established, NRT can be considered on an individual basis for pregnant women and for young people (under 18).

Bupropion

▶ Bupropion is an effective intervention for assisting smoking cessation.

▶ Bupropion should be stopped when a quit attempt has failed.

▶ Bupropion is unsuitable for adolescents, pregnant women, and people with a history of seizures.

Nicotine with other substance misuse

Compared with the general population, smoking prevalence is increased about threefold in those who are also dependent on alcohol and/or illicit drugs. Approximately 80% of alcohol-dependent patients are reported to smoke cigarettes and alcohol dependence is ten times more common in smokers than non-smokers. In illicit drug users, estimates of cigarette smoking are also around 80%.

It appears that a history of alcoholism does not reduce the effectiveness of nicotine substitution in smoking cessation, though higher doses of nicotine patches may be required in patients with active or past alcohol problems. Importantly, addressing their smoking does not have an adverse effect on recovery from alcohol or illicit drug misuse.

Tobacco and nicotine regulation

The public health goal in relation to smoking tobacco must be to reduce the death and disease it causes. Reducing tobacco or nicotine consumption is not an end in itself. It should not be forgotten that it is the tobacco smoke that kills people not the nicotine, but it is the nicotine that people are addicted to and not the tobacco smoke. There is now substantial experience with medicinal nicotine taken in the form of smoking cessation products. Although addictive, the main harm from nicotine is related to the method of use: inhaling hot smoke. Taken by any route other than smoking reduces the risk by up to 100 times. Where smokers cannot give up their nicotine habit, converting to forms of nicotine other than smoked tobacco will reduce their risks of morbidity and premature mortality to levels similar to non-smokers.

Certain groups are particularly at risk, for example there are significantly higher smoking rates and levels of tobacco consumption amongst those with mental health problems than amongst the general population. Studies have shown smoking rates to be as high as 80% amongst people with a diagnosis of schizophrenia and people with depression are more likely to smoke and have more difficulty giving up. Nicotine in safer, non-smoked forms is produced, licensed, and marketed, however, only as an aid to stopping smoking, not as a harm reduction substitute to smoking. As pointed out by the Royal College of Physicians and others, there is enormous potential to narrow health inequalities and dramatically cut the numbers dying from smoking by substituting safer forms of nicotine for smoked tobacco for longer-term use, not just to help cessation in the very short-term.

Conclusion

Smoking amongst professional groups is seen as an embarrassment and becoming less and less common (even in private). The same cannot be said for other socio-economic groups. It is worrying that young people are continuing to take up the habit, many of them to become lifelong smokers. Targeting our interventions at young people seems a sensible way forward but if smoking is to be the exception rather than the norm it can be achieved only through government policies, such as: raising the price of tobacco, ongoing media and education campaigns to discourage smoking, and by banning smoking in all workplaces, including enclosed public places. The health professional's role is perhaps to keep informing political leaders of the risks that the population of tomorrow face if smoking cigarettes continues at its present rate.

Further reading

Britton J. (Ed). *ABC of Smoking Cessation*. Oxford: Blackwell BMJ Books, 2004.

References

1. Doll R, Peto R, Boreham J, Sutherland I. Mortality in relation to smoking: 50 years' observations on male British doctors. *BMJ* 2004; **328**: 1529.

2. Department of Health. *Choosing Health? A consultation on action to improve people's health*. London: HMSO, 2004 (available at: www.dh.gov.uk).

3. Health Development Agency. *The Smoking Epidemic in England*. London: HDA, 2004.

4. US Public Health Service. *Preventing Tobacco use among Young People: A report of the Surgeon General*. USA: Office of the Surgeon General, 1994.

5. Office of National Statistics. *Smoking Related Behaviour and Attitudes*, 2002. London: HMSO, 2003.

6. Jarvis MJ. Monitoring cigarette smoking prevalence in Britain in a timely fashion. *Addiction* 2003; **98**: 1569–74.

7. Action on Smoking and Health. ASH response to *Securing good health for the whole population*. London: ASH, 2003.

8. Department of Health. *Smoking Kills: a White Paper on Tobacco*. London: HMSO, 1998.

9. Reid D, McNeill A D, Glynn T J. Reducing the prevalence of smoking in youth in Western countries: an international review. *Tobacco Control* 1995; **4(3)**: 266–77.

10. Marshall T, Simpson S, Stevens A. Use of health services by prison inmates: comparisons with the community. *Journal of Epidemiology Community Health* 2001; **55(5)**: 364–5.

11. Fichtenberg C M, Glantz S A. Effect of smoke-free workplaces on smoking behaviour: systematic review. *BMJ* 2002; **325**: 188–91.

12. Charlton A, While D. Smoking Prevalence among 16–19 year olds in sixth form colleges and further education. *Health Education Journal* 1994; **53**: 28–39.

13. Borland R, Mullins R, Trotter L, White V. Trends in environmental tobacco smoke restrictions in the home in Victoria, Australia. *Tobacco Control* 1999; **8**: 266–71.

14. Dalton M A, Sargent J D, Beach M L, *et al.* Effect of viewing smoking in movies on adolescent smoking initiation: a cohort study. *Lancet* 2003; **362**: 281–5.

15. Siegel M, Biener L. The impact of an antismoking media campaign on progression to established smoking: results of a longitudinal youth study. *Am J Public Health* 2000; **90**: 380–6.

16. Parrott S, Godfrey C, Raw M, *et al.* Guidance for commissioners on the cost-effectiveness of smoking cessation interventions. *Thorax* 1998; **53** (S5, Part 2): S1–S38.

17. Tengs T O, Adams M E, Pliskin J S, *et al.* Five hundred life-saving interventions and their cost-effectiveness. *Risk Analysis* 1995; **15**: 369–90.

18. Smee C, Parsonage M, Anderson R, Duckworth S. Effect of tobacco advertising on tobacco consumption: a discussion document reviewing the evidence. London: DoH, 1992.

19. Preventing tobacco use among young people: A report of the Surgeon General. Washington: US Public Health Service, Office of the Surgeon General, 1994.

20. Hammond D, Fong G T, McDonald P W, *et al.* Impact of the graphic Canadian warning labels on adult smoking behaviour. *Tobacco Control* 2003; **12**: 391–5.

21. Wanless D. *Securing Good Health for the Whole Population*. Final Report. London: HMSO, 2004.

22. Silagy C, Stead L F. Physician advice for smoking cessation (Cochrane Review). In: *The Cochrane Library*, 4. Chichester: John Wiley, 2002.

23. Fiore M C, Bailey W C, Cohen S J, *et al. Treating Tobacco Use and Dependence*. Rockville, Maryland: Department of Public Health and Human Services; 2000 (available at: www.surgeongeneral.gov/tobacco/treating_tobacco_use.pdf).

24. Raw M, McNeill A, West R J. Smoking cessation guidelines for health care professionals. *Thorax* 1998; **53** (Suppl 5, Part 1): S1–S19.

25. West R, McNeill A, Raw M. Smoking cessation guidelines for health professionals: an update. *Thorax* 2000; **55**: 987–99.

26. Parrott S, Godfrey C, Raw M, *et al.* Guidance for commissioners on the cost-effectiveness of smoking cessation interventions. *Thorax* 1998; **53**(S5, Part 2): S1–S38.

27. Raftery J. NICE: faster access to modern treatments? Analysis of guidance on health technologies. *BMJ* 2001; **323**: 1300–3.

28. Campbell I A, Lewis K E, Preston L A. Surveys and assessment of secondary care smoking cessation services in the UK, 2001–2003. *Thorax* 2003; **53** (Suppl III): iii42–iii43 (Abstract).

29. Silagy C, Ketteridge S. The effectiveness of physician advice to aid smoking cessation. In: Cochrane Collaboration. *Cochrane Library*. Chichester: John Wiley, 1998.

30. Simon J A, Duncan C, Carmody T, Hudes E S. Bupropion for smoking cessation. *Arch Int Med* 2004; **164**: 1797–803.

31. Hughes J R, Goldstein M G, Hurt R D, Shiffman S. Recent advances in the pharmacotherapy of smoking. *JAMA* 1999; **6(281)**: 72–6.

32. Lader D, Meltzer H. *Smoking Related Behaviour and Attitudes*, 2002. London: Office for National Statistics, 2003.

CHAPTER 15

Injecting drug use and harm reduction

Emer Coffey, David Young, and Clare Gerada

IN THIS CHAPTER

Injecting drug use || *Prevalence* || *Injecting* || *Injecting sites* || *Problems associated with injecting* || *Death* || *Needle sharing and different drugs* || *Overdose* || *Infection* || *Hepatitis B* || *Hepatitis A* || *Hepatitis C* || *AIDS/HIV* || *Harm reduction*

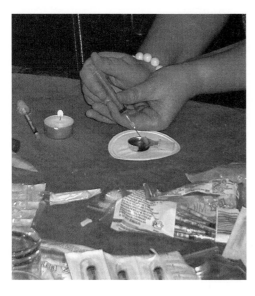

Injecting drug use

It is important for doctors, nurses and pharmacists to engage effectively with injecting drug users and to have some knowledge of the drugs injected, the injecting equipment used and the potential risks associated with each stage of the process. Injecting drug use has been a popular form of administration ever since the hypodermic syringe was invented in the 19th century. Ironically, injecting was thought to reduce the risk of morphine addiction as it bypassed the stomach.

Prevalence

Using a capture–recapture method the prevalence of intravenous drug use, for 2000/01, was calculated for three large UK cities (Brighton, Liverpool and London). Between 1.2 and 3.3% of those between 15–44 were found to be intravenous drug users with less than one in four in treatment.[1] The estimated rate of injecting drug use using Regional Drug Misuse Database data across England varied from zero to 1% of the population confirming that a large number of injecting drug users are not currently in treatment.[2]

Injecting

Most injecting drug users inject their drugs intravenously, but subcutaneous injection ('skin-popping') is also common. Intramuscular injection may occur intentionally or when the individual misses the vein or the subcutaneous space.

The most commonly injected drugs are heroin, cocaine, and anabolic steroids. Amfetamines, buprenorphine, methadone,[3] benzodiazepines,[4,5] and barbiturates are also injected; in fact any water-soluble drug may be injected. Heroin, cocaine and amfetamine are bought from the black market in powdered form and then combined with water and mixed into a solution in a spoon or a foil prior to injecting. The solutions are then injected directly into a vein, a muscle, or subcutaneous tissue. Drugs are often 'cut' with all kinds of substances to make them go further: glucose powder, flour, talcum powder, or even chalk. Injecting these under the skin can cause abscesses and other infections.

When injecting a drug the onset of drug effects are about 15–30 seconds for the intravenous route, and 3–5 minutes for the intramuscular or subcutaneous route. Drug effects from inhaling a drug begin in 7–10 seconds, and drug effects from intranasal use begin in 3–5 minutes.

Injecting sites

Drug users often have 'favourite' injecting sites. These depend on the ease of finding a viable vein and therefore these preferred sites are subject to frequent change. The results from a sample of 200 injecting drug users interviewed about their bodily injection sites found that the mean number of injection sites ever used by subjects was 3.1, with a mean of 2.0 sites used in the previous six months. Sixteen per cent of subjects had injected in five or more sites. Almost all (99%) had injected in the cubital fossa. The next most popular site was the forearm (71%). Other sites included the hand (53%), foot (19%), leg (18%), neck (10%), and groin (6%). There was a clear progression in sites used, from the cubital fossa at initial injection to the use of sites such as the groin after ten years of injecting. Female intravenous drug users used significantly more injection sites than men and reported more injection-related problems. The use of more injection sites was independently associated with a greater number of injection-related problems and a greater number of drug classes ever injected.[6]

Problems associated with injecting

The main problems associated with injecting drug use are overdose (either deliberate or accidental) and local or systemic infections (due to needle sharing, injecting technique, and unsafe sexual behaviour).

Death

Drug users are at substantially greater risk of premature death than their non-drug using peers. Longitudinal studies indicate yearly mortality rates of between 1% and 3% among heroin users. The excessive mortality rates among heroin users have been variously estimated to be between 6 and 20 times those experienced among others of the same age and gender. The causes of death are many, including HIV/AIDS, hepatitis, violence, overdose.[7]

An Australian study showed that the mortality rate for people regularly using illicit opiates was more than 13 times greater than that observed for the general community. It is estimated that 9.4% of total mortality in Australians aged 15–39 years of age can be attributed to regular use of illicit opiates.[8] Death from the direct toxic effects of a heroin overdose is usually associated with respiratory depression, coma, and pulmonary oedema. Death from direct effects of cocaine is often associated with cardiac dysrhythmias and conduction disturbances, leading to myocardial infarction and stroke. The 'typical' heroin overdose death is of an older, heroin-dependent male who is not currently in drug treatment, that is an experienced heroin user rather than a naive or recreational user. The circumstances of such a death are likely to involve the use of other central nervous system drugs, such as benzodiazepines and alcohol, in conjunction with heroin. A 'true' heroin overdose, involving only heroin, appears to be in the minority of deaths attributed to overdose.[7] (See also Chapter 2.)

Needle sharing and different drugs

Needle and equipment sharing is not uniformly found. Methamfetamine and cocaine users are more likely to share injecting equipment than users of other drugs and women are more likely to share than men.[9-11] The risk of blood-borne virus transmission amongst steroid injectors is low, probably because of hygienic use of injecting equipment and low levels of sharing.[12]

Overdose

Overdose of heroin following injection is a common experience, with 38% of a south London sample of injecting drug users self-reporting that they had experienced an overdose. The majority (54%) had witnessed someone else overdose. Overdosing is not a solitary experience; over 80% of subjects who had overdosed had done so in the presence of someone else, but only 27% reported ambulances having been called. Factors found to be associated with overdose were: age at which injecting began; sex (women being more likely to experience overdose); use of alcohol; and polydrug injection.[13] Different batches can have different strengths and overwhelm regular users; users therefore should be advised that if buying from a new source, always to try a bit first to check the strength.

Infection

Injecting drug use causes medical problems by introducing pathogens and other contaminants into the body via shared needles and a lack of sterile preparation and injection techniques. Damage to veins occurs for a number of reasons including repeated injections over the same site, using blunt and/or dirty needles, and severe chemical irritation caused by adulterants.

Injecting cocaine is often associated with more skin damage than other substances, probably because of its local anaesthetic effects: the user is unaware of any local injury or infection. Between the beginning of 2000 and the end of December 2002, there were 33 clinically diagnosed cases of wound botulism in the United Kingdom and Ireland. All cases had injected heroin into muscle or by 'skin popping'. The clinical diagnosis was confirmed by laboratory tests in 20 of these cases.[14]

Hepatitis B

It is estimated that 21% of injecting drug users in England and Wales have evidence of past or current hepatitis B (HBV) infection.[15] Since 1988 injecting drug users have been targeted for vaccination, despite this, both availability of vaccination and uptake are recognised to be poor in the United Kingdom.[16] Proactive provision of HBV vaccination through widely available services is critical for protecting this difficult to reach target group and should be delivered in, and form an important part of, primary care.

The presence in the blood of antibodies to a virus indicates that one has at one time been infected with or vaccinated against the virus. In contrast to other blood-borne viruses that commonly affect intravenous injecting drug users (HIV, hepatitis C) there is an effective vaccine against HBV. Thus, in the case of HBV, the proportion of injecting drug users who do not have antibodies (anti-HBs or anti-HBc) against the virus constitutes the potential vaccination population and is an important indicator of the need for a vaccination programme. Current HBV infection is indicated by the presence in the blood of HBsAg, and can be an indication of either recent or chronic infection. High levels of current infection suggest a high future level of severe, long-term complications and a widespread transmission to others through high-risk injecting behaviour or unsafe sex.

Immunisation

Hepatitis B vaccination should be considered an essential component of the care offered to drug users in primary care.

Practices who opt to provide a National Enhanced Service to patients suffering from drug misuse under the nGMS contract will be expected to undertake six-monthly audits of hepatitis B screening and immunisation data of this patient population (www.doh.gov.uk/gmscontract/nesdrug.pdf).

Poor patient attendance is often reported as a major barrier. To address this issue, vaccination needs to be carried out opportunistically at the time when the drug user makes contact with the practice, for example at the time of methadone prescribing. Practices should keep a stock of HBV vaccine.

Pre-vaccination testing

It has been standard practice to advise that clinicians wait for hepatitis B test results before giving the first dose of vaccine to prevent vaccination of those who have already been infected or who have already been vaccinated. For practical reasons the current expert advice has been to shift the emphasis away from testing and towards protection of the drug user by vaccination. Pre-testing should never act as a barrier or delay to vaccination. Drug users should have access to vaccination without testing. If a drug user wishes to be tested, the first dose of vaccine should be offered at the same time.[17] Delaying vaccination can do harm because a drug user may become infected before the next visit or may not return.

Primary vaccination schedule

A pragmatic approach to vaccination schedule is recommended. Emphasis needs to be placed on giving as many doses as possible. Even incomplete vaccination schedules offer some protection.[18] Accelerated schedules (0, 1, and 2 months or 0, 7, and 21 days) are now widely recognised as the most appropriate for people at high risk including drug users. A study of homeless drug users at an inner city primary care centre found a sevenfold higher completion rate with the 0, 7, and 21 day schedule compared with the conventional six-month schedule.[19] The 0, 7, and 21 day schedule is being promoted by the Department of Health for prisons and is the most strongly recommended regimen.[20] In addition, services need to ensure that there is a robust system for recall.

Booster doses and post-vaccination testing

Current best practice is to give a booster at 12 months if an accelerated schedule is used. Follow up of injecting drug users for booster doses can be difficult. It seems sensible to recommend that resources would be better invested in improving uptake and completion of three-dose schedules than in seroconversion testing or boosters.

Post-vaccination testing for seroconversion is not generally recommended unless the drug user is known to be immunodeficient, for example because of HIV infection.

Promotion of vaccination

Prominent display of posters and use of leaflets promoting HBV vaccination may be helpful. Promotion of vaccination is dependent on motivated, knowledgeable staff. In drugs services, uptake rates have been found to be higher where staff training and confidence were better.[21] GPs and practice nurses may also need training and awareness sessions to ensure greater uptake of vaccination.

Vaccination of partners and children of drug users

Hepatitis B can be transmitted through sexual contact and non-sexual intimate contact. Children infected with HBV have a higher risk of chronic infection than adults. Drug users should be advised about the risk of transmission of HBV to their partners and children. Partners and children should be routinely offered vaccination.

Organising the vaccination of families may not be straightforward. Families may not be registered with the same practice as the drug user. Some drug users may be reluctant to disclose the risk to their partners. Healthcare workers need to work with drug users to advise them of the risks and promote the routine offering of vaccination to partners and children.

Monitoring of vaccination

Local information on vaccine uptake and completion is crucial in order to judge the quality of the service and plan achievable improvements. The minimum standard for monitoring recommended by the National Treatment Agency is the number of vaccinations received by a drug user.[22] An easy recording system is needed.

Treatment

The impact of treatment for infection is developing rapidly. In recent years, increasingly effective treatments for chronic HBV have become available. In January 2004, NICE recommended combination therapy with pegylated interferon and ribavirin for six months to one year (www.nice.org.uk/Docref. asp?d=10224). Treatment is successful in clearing the infection, with no detectable virus in the blood six months after treatment has ceased in up to 55% of patients. This needs expert referral and assessment at a tertiary referral centre. The NICE guideline envisaged that patients with current injecting drug use and those with alcohol problems could still receive this treatment.

Hepatitis A

Injecting drug users are at high risk of hepatitis A (HAV) infection owing to poor living conditions. The virus is probably spread through faecal contamination of drugs or injecting paraphernalia. Blood-to-blood spread through needle sharing during viraemia is also possible.

Hepatitis A vaccination of injecting drug users infected with HCV and/or with chronic liver disease has been recommended for many years because of the risk of more serious illness if they became infected.[23] The Public Health Laboratory Service Advisory Committee on Vaccination and Immunisation expanded this recommendation in 2001 to include all injecting drug users.[24] As for HBV it is better to immunise first rather than pretest and risk losing the opportunity because of non-attendance at follow up.

Hepatitis A vaccine is available as a single component vaccine or combined with HBV vaccine (Table 15.1). The likelihood of a drug user returning for a subsequent dose needs to be taken into account when selecting the single vaccine or the combined vaccine. One dose of HAV vaccine confers greater protection against HAV than one dose of the combined vaccine because the combined vaccine has only half the amount of HAV antigen than the single component vaccine has.

Table 15.1 **Licensed schedules of hepatitis A and B vaccines**

Hepatitis vaccines	Schedule
Single A	Two doses with second dose after 6–12 months. Second dose may be delayed for up to 3 years
Combined A and B	Routine: 0, 1, 6 months
	Accelerated: 0, 7, 21 days with booster ideally at 12 months

Suggested criteria for audit

Criteria for audit should be kept simple. The minimum criteria should be:

▸ the number and percentage of drug users who have received one dose of HBV vaccine

▸ the number and percentage of drug users who have received two doses of HBV

▸ the number and percentage of drug users who have received three doses of HBV.

Other criteria to consider include:

▸ the number and percentage of drug users who have been offered HBV vaccination

▸ the percentage of drug users who have received one and two doses of HAV vaccine.

Hepatitis C

Prevalence

Around 0.4% of the general population and equating to 200,000 people are infected by hepatitis C (HCV). Overall prevalence of HCV infection amongst injecting drug users in England and Wales was 34% in 1998/99 and 33% 2000/01. There are major differences between regions, with prevalence being much higher in London and the north-west of England than elsewhere.[26] Prevalence of anti-HCV is lower among more recent initiates to injecting. Prevalence in England and Wales in users who began injecting in the past three years was 8% in 1998, 9% in 1999, and 8% in 2000. These data suggest that there may be a window of opportunity for prevention early in an injecting career. The prevalence for this group was 16% in 2001, and the increase was observed for both and males and females, within and outside London.[27] The Department of Health's *Strategy for Hepatitis C in*

England has estimated that 0.4% of the general population of England, equating to around 200,000 people, are chronically infected with HCV, of whom the majority are unaware of their infection.[28] These figures are partly based on a large study of antenatal women.[29] HCV is more infectious than HIV and can be transmitted more easily through injecting materials other than syringes, such as cotton, spoons, and water (but is far less readily transmitted sexually).

Routes of transmission

The major route of HCV transmission in the United Kingdom is by sharing injecting equipment, usually by blood-contaminated needles and syringes, though if contaminated with infected blood other equipment can also spread the infection. Mother-to-baby transmission is very uncommon, with upper estimates of around 6%. This rate is increased to around 14–17% where there is co-infection with HIV. Hepatitis C does not spread through breast milk. Sexual transmission is very rare, with studies suggesting that less than 5% of the regular sexual partners of people with HCV infection becoming infected.

Natural history

The majority of people infected with HCV suffer no symptoms when they become infected; some may feel slightly unwell and in rare cases become jaundiced. About 60–80% of people who acquire the infection become chronically infected; the remainder clear the infection spontaneously. Chronic infection may be asymptomatic for many years and the majority of these live a normal life expectancy. Around one in five to one in twenty of those chronically infected may develop serious liver disease after 20 years. A small proportion may develop liver cancers. Certain factors are associated with more rapid progression to severe liver disease, these are:

▸ over 40 years old at the time of infection

▸ alcohol consumption

▸ male

▸ co-infected with hepatitis B or HIV

▸ on immunosuppressive therapy.

Who should be tested?[30] Antibody testing should be considered for:

▸ anyone who has ever injected drugs

▸ current injecting drug users

▶ recipients of blood (before Sept 1991), or blood products (before 1986 in the UK) – if not already tested

▶ regular sexual partners of those with HCV (risk of sexual transmission low approx 5%)

▶ children born to mothers with HCV (risk of transmission 6%; may be higher if co-infected with HIV; N.B. test result may be difficult to interpret in children under 18 months old, owing to the presence of maternal antibodies)

▶ people who may have had unsterile medical treatment abroad

▶ people who may have had ear piercing, body piercing, tattooing, or acupuncture with unsterile equipment.

Reasons to be tested

▶ allaying anxiety even if result is positive

▶ positive test allowing early monitoring and intervention by a specialist if required

▶ opportunity to immunise against hepatitis B and A (co-infection significantly worsens prognosis)

▶ encouraging the patient to change patterns of behaviour such as injecting drug use or excessive drinking whether the result is positive or negative.

Life insurance and mortgage issues

A negative HCV test has no impact on ability to get life insurance or a mortgage. A positive test may make it more difficult to get life insurance policy or a mortgage linked to a life policy.

AIDS/HIV

An estimated 41,000 HIV infected people are alive in the United Kingdom; about a third of these have undiagnosed infections.[31] Men who have sex with men remain the group at greatest risk of HIV though the number of new cases infected through heterosexual sex has risen in recent years, most probably acquired outside the United Kingdom, mainly in sub-Saharan Africa.

Although the potential still exists for HIV transmission through injecting drug use there is no evidence of significant current HIV spread amongst intravenous drug users in the United Kingdom. It was the threat of HIV/AIDS amongst drug users that spurred the current move away from abstinence-based treatment into one of reduction. The ACMD reported in *AIDS and Drug Misuse Update*:[32]

> *Awareness of the HIV-related risks of injecting drug use has grown significantly and has provided a focus for harm reduction activities. Greater efforts are now needed to reduce the extent of drug use itself, and particularly of drug injecting, together with a wider recognition that* all *interventions to discourage drug misuse will contribute to HIV prevention.*

The ACMD recommended a series of actions directed towards:

▸ encouraging cessation of drug use

▸ discouraging new recruitment into experimentation with drugs

▸ discouraging regular drug use among experimental drug users

▸ discouraging drug injecting among potential injectors

▸ discouraging sharing of injecting equipment

▸ encouraging current injectors to switch to safer practices, or oral use

▸ ensuring all drug users have access to advice on safer sexual and injecting practices as well as access to clean injecting equipment.

Through the foresight of the ACMD and the implementation of its recommendations, HIV-spread needle sharing was largely prevented through the establishment of needle exchange schemes, which helped the United Kingdom to have a lower HIV prevalence rate than other countries. We cannot be complacent, however, and must be forever reinforcing harm reduction messages to our patients.

Harm reduction

Safer injecting

The 'safest' injecting sites are found in the antecubital fossa and in the superficial veins in the forearm. Users should be encouraged to rotate these safe sites and to avoid more harmful ones such as the groin and neck. Watching a patient run through their injecting technique can be very informative. If patients do insist on injecting into the groin then showing them the simple technique of how to avoid the femoral artery, by placing their fingers protectively on top of it, can be life saving.

Commercial sterile disposable spoons 'stericups' can be purchased for small amounts of money; these reduce the risks of dirty equipment and needle sharing.

Self-help information can be useful. For example, one US source issues a series of postcards, each aimed at providing information and harm reduction advice about each stage of injecting, from caring for veins to dealing with overdose (www.any positivechange.org/bvcsi.html).

Other advice about safer injecting can be obtained from Addaction, a leading UK charity working solely in the field of drug and alcohol treatment (www. addaction.org.uk/Drugsafeinject.htm). Amongst other things, this site explains to the user details which needles are best for different sites, why it is unsafe to inject tablets or oral methadone, and what to do if the user inadvertently hits an artery. HIT, a Liverpool based organisation, produces information for the health professional and the user on ways to reduce the risks of injecting, as well as publications on methadone treatment, opiate detoxification, and rehabilitation (www. hit.org.uk/publicationsBySubject.asp?subject=Safer-Injecting&sub=32).

Safer injecting rooms (drug consumption rooms)

Safer injection rooms, or drug consumption rooms, are legally sanctioned, low threshold, supervised facilities designed to reduce the risks of injecting and allow the hygienic consumption of pre-obtained drugs under professional supervision in a non-judgmental environment.[33,34] They usually provide access to sterile injection equipment, information about drugs and health care, treatment referrals, and access to medical staff.[35] Some offer counselling and hygienic and other services of use to itinerant and impoverished individuals.[36] Most prohibit the sale or purchase of illegal drugs.

Safer injecting rooms are not available in the United Kingdom though this situation may change in light of the UK Home Affairs Select Committee recommendation 'that an evaluated pilot programme of safe injecting houses for heroin users is established without delay and that if this is successful, the programme is extended across the country'.[37] At the present time there are a number of drug consumption rooms in Europe (Germany,[38] Switzerland, Spain,[39] and the Netherlands) and in Sydney, Australia. Evaluation is still in the early stages though the main successes reported are that they:[40]

▸ help providers contact a hard-to-reach population

▸ alleviate health problems related to injecting drugs

▸ reduce the risk of overdose[41]

▸ lessen nuisances and risks of public drug use.[42]

Although drug consumption rooms are broadly welcomed as a public health measure there are many difficulties that need to be addressed before they become part of mainstream treatment services, not least of which is the sanctioning of

Safer injecting

www.clas-sharedcare.org/Patient_Handouts/Safer_Injecting/safer_injecting.html

Remember, injecting drugs is very dangerous. You are at risk from blood-borne viruses, physical health complications such as abscesses, thrombosis and septicaemia. You also run a higher risk of overdosing.

What are you injecting? • You may be able to get help with safe and legal medication. Discuss this with your local drug agency.

What do you use when preparing your drug for injection? • It's better to use Vitamin C powder or citric acid. Most needle exchanges in street agencies will supply citric acid. This is much safer than lemon juice as some research suggests that using this can lead to eye infections. Vinegar is a safer option than lemon juice, but this can cause burning and pain.

What size works do you use? • It's always better to use the smallest size needles and syringes such as 1ml insulin syringes. Your local needle exchange will be able to offer you advice on sizes available. The more volume you inject, the more damage you are causing to your veins.

Filter • Always use a filter when preparing for a fix. When you've finished throw it away. Reusing filters can be dangerous as you can never be sure how much gear is left in it, and people have been known to OD.

Tourniquets • Try not to use something which is rigid such as a leather belt. It's better to use something with a bit of 'give' such as a tie or elasticated material. Only keep it on for 1 minute. If you can't find a vein, try another site.

Finding a vein • If you're a regular injector, change your injecting site each time. This allows your veins a rest. Know the difference between an artery and a vein. If you accidentally hit an artery you'll notice bright red blood, which may spurt. Remove the needle and apply firm pressure for at least 10 minutes. If in doubt, get medical help immediately.

   Injecting in the groin and neck is very dangerous – get help from your local drug agency.

Use the needle exchange • Many chemists provide a needle exchange service. Try the local drug agency or outreach bus. Always use new needles and syringes and dispose of them safely in a sharps container, returning it to the exchange.

Get vaccinated • Ask your GP for hepatitis B vaccination. Think about being tested for hepatitis B and C.

Get more information about local drug services and hepatitis.

unregulated and unsupervised illicitly obtained drugs. Workers within the facility may seek to influence their choice of drugs, dose, and technique, but it would be counterproductive to have rules that drive injecting drug users out of the facility by insisting on too many rules of engagement. Supervised injecting centres are are not intended for treating individual addictions, although they can have within them services that can address the individual's psychological, social, and physical health.

Strang et al.[43] argue for the development of supervised injectable maintenance clinics as a useful addition to current treatment services and something that would provide a missing link in current treatment services. The attendee would be a known patient, receiving treatment from a doctor, and self-administering the prescribed injectable maintenance (for example, injectable heroin or injectable methadone) supervised by a nurse or other worker within the clinic. Only drugs prescribed by a doctor, in the dose and route prescribed, would be sanctioned. Such treatment for the most severe heroin addicts would be a tertiary service, although GPs may be in the position to offer primary care advice and support to the clinic attendees.

The European Monitoring Centre for Drugs and Drug Addiction (EMCDDA) have recently reported on drug consumption rooms.[44] The main results of this report are that attendees welcome the service, in particular the availability of hygienic, medically supervised spaces in which to inject. The typical 'clients' were in their mid 30s with a long history of injecting and polydrug use – just the group identified by many researchers as being at highest risk of death from overdose. Most of the attendees were male (70%) and of the women attending a large number were engaged in the sex industry. Not surprisingly, many of those attending were homeless or living in unstable accommodation. Of those attending the German drug consumption rooms, 5% lived on the streets, and of those attending near Madrid the rate of homelessness was 42%, and in the Can Tunis of Barcelona it was 60%. Staff at drug consumption rooms reported that clients needed information about basic hygiene risks; when this was provided the majority went on to inject in a safe hygienic manner.

Further reading

Department of Health. *Hepatitis C Guidance for those Working with Drug Users*. London: DoH, 2001 (available at: www.dh.gov.uk/assetRoot/04/01/96/49/04019649.pdf).

Royal College of General Practitioners. Guidance for hepatitis A and B vaccination of drug users in primary care and criteria for audit. London: RCGP, 2005.

References

1. Hickman M, Higgins V, Hope V, *et al*. Injecting drug use in Brighton, Liverpool, and London: best estimates of prevalence and coverage of public health indicators. *J Epidemiol Community Health* 2004; **58(9)**: 766–71.

2. Frischer M, Heatlie H, Hickman M. Estimating the prevalence of problematic and injecting drug use for Dug Action Team areas in England: a feasibility study using the Multiple Indicator Methadone. Home Office Online Report, 34/04. 2004.

3. Lintzeris N, Lenne M, Ritter A. Methadone injecting in Australia: a tale of two cities. *Addiction* 1999; **94(8)**: 1175–8.

4. Darke S, Topp L, Ross J. The injection of methadone and benzodiazepines among Sydney injecting drug users 1996–2000: 5-year monitoring of trends from the Illicit Drug Reporting System. *Drug Alcohol Rev* 2002; **21(1)**: 27–32.

5. Fry C L, Bruno R B. Recent trends in benzodiazepine use by injecting drug users in Victoria and Tasmania. *Drug Alcohol Rev* 2002; **21(4)**: 363–7.

6. Darke S, Ross J, Kaye S. Physical injecting sites among injecting drug users in Sydney, Australia. *Drug Alcohol Depend* 2001; **62(1)**: 77–82.

7. Darke S. Zador D. Fatal Heroin 'Overdose': A Review. *Addiction* 1996; **91(12)**: 1765–72.

8. Bennett G A, Velleman R D, Barter G, Bradbury C. Gender differences in sharing injecting equipment by drug users in England. *AIDS Care* 2000; **12(1)**: 77–87.

9. Tyndall M W, Currie S, Spittal P, *et al*. Intensive injection cocaine use as the primary risk factor in the Vancouver HIV-1 epidemic. *AIDS* 2003; **17(6)**: 887–93.

10. Molitor F, Ruiz J D, Flynn N, *et al*. Methamphetamine use and sexual and injection risk behaviors among out-of-treatment injection drug users. *Am J Drug Alcohol Abuse* 1999; **25(3)**: 475–93.

11. Bennett G A, Velleman R D, Barter G, Bradbury C. Gender differences in sharing injecting equipment by drug users in England. *AIDS Care* 2000; **12(1)**: 77–87.

12. Crampin A C, Lamagni T L, Hope V D, *et al*. The risk of infection with HIV and hepatitis B in individuals who inject steroids in England and Wales. *Epidemiol Infect* 1998; **121(2)**: 381–6.

13. Powis B, Strang J, Griffiths P, *et al*. Self-reported overdose among injecting drug users in London: extent and nature of the problem. *Addiction* 1999 Nov; **94(11)**: 1745–6.

14. Brett M M, Hallas G, Mpamugo O. Wound botulism in the UK and Ireland. *J Med Microbiol* 2004; **53** (Pt 6): 555–61.

15. Department of Health. Unlinked Anonymous Surveys Steering Group, Prevalence of HIV and hepatitis infections in the United Kingdom 2001. London: DoH, 2002.

16. Lamagni, T L, Davison K L, Hope V D *et al*. Poor Hepatitis B vaccine coverage in injecting drug users: England, 1995 and 1996. *Communicable Disease and Public Health* 1999; **2(3)**: 174–7.

17. Heptonstall J. Strategies to ensure delivery of hepatitis B vaccine to injecting drug users. *Communicable Disease and Public Health* 1999; **2(3)**: 154–6.

18. Lamden K H, Kennedy N, Beeching N J, *et al.* Hepatitis B and Hepatitis C virus infections: risk factors among drug users in Northwest England. *Journal of Infection* 1998; **37**: 260–9.

19. Wright N, Campbell T, Tompkins C. Comparison of conventional and accelerated hepatitis B immunisation schedules for homeless drug users. *Communicable Disease and Public Health* 2002; **5(4)**: 324–6.

20. Piper M. Senior Prison Health Advisor, Department of Health (personal communication), 2003.

21. Morrison D, Gilchrist G, Ahmed A. Potential of specialist drug services to deliver hepatitis B vaccination. *Communicable Disease and Public Health* 2002; **5(4)**: 321–3.

22. National Treatment Agency for Substance Misuse, *Models of Care for the Treatment of Drug Misusers. Part 2: Full reference report* 159. London: National Treatment Agency for Substance Misuse, 2002.

23. Salisbury D M, Begg N T. (Eds). *Immunisation Against Infectious Disease.* Edward Jenner (Ed.) bicentenary edition. London: HMSO, 1996.

24. Crowcroft N S, Walsh B, Davison K L, *et al.* Guidelines for the control of hepatitis A virus infection. *Communicable Disease and Public Health* 2001; **4**: 213–27.

25. National Treatment Agency for Substance Misuse, *Models of Care for the Treatment of Drug Misusers. Part 2: Full reference report* 159. London: National Treatment Agency for Substance Misuse, 2002.

26. Judd A, Hickman M, Jones S, McDonald T, *et al.* Incidence of hepatitis C virus and HIV among new injecting drug users in London: prospective cohort study. *BMJ* 2005; **330**: 24–5.

27. Unlinked anonymous surveys steering group. *Prevalence of HIV and Hepatitis Injections in the United Kingdom* 2001, London: DoH, 2002.

28. Department of Health. *Hepatitis C Strategy for England.* London: DoH, 2002.

29. Balogun M A, Ramsey M E, Parry J V, *et al.* The prevalence and genetic diversity of hepatitis C injection in antenatal clinical attenders in two regions in England. *Epidemiology and Infection* 2000; **125**: 705–12.

30. Department of Health. *Hepatitis C: Essential Information for Professionals and Guidance on Testing.* London: HMSO, 2004 (available at: www:doh.gov.uk/publications).

31. CDSC (Communicable Disease Surveillance Centre), ICH (Institute for Children's Health) (London), SCIEH (Scottish Centre for Infection and Environmental Health) (2002), HIV and AIDS in the United Kingdom; 2001: an update. London: SDS.

32. Advisory Council on the Misuse of Drugs. *AIDS and Drug Misuse Update.* Report by the Advisory Council on the Misuse of Drugs. London: ACMD, 1993.

33. Consumption Rooms as a Professional Service in Addictions Health: International Conference for the development of guidelines. *Guidelines for the operation and use of consumption rooms* 1999 (available at: www.adf.org.au/injectingrooms/guidelines.pdf) (Accessed 11 Nov 2003).

34. Van Beek I. The Sydney medically supervised injecting centre: a clinical model. *J Drug Issues* 2003; **22**: 625–38.

35. Kimber J, Dolan K, Van Beek I, *et al.* Drug consumption facilities. An update since 2000. *Drug and Alcohol Review* 2003; **22**: 227–33.

36. Wright N, Tompkins C. Supervised injecting centres. *BMJ* 2004; **328**: 100–02.

37. Government reply to the third report from the Home Affairs Committee: The Government's Drugs Policy: Is It Working? Session 2001–2002 HC 318. London: HMSO, 2002.

38. Stoever H. Consumption rooms – a middle ground between health and public order concerns. *J Drug Iss* 2002; **32**: 597–606.

39. European Monitoring Centre for Drugs and Drug Addiction. *Annual report on the state of the drugs problem in the European Union and Norway.* Luxembourg: EMCDDA, 2002.

40. Joint Select Committee into Safe Injection Rooms, Parliament of New South Wales. *Report on the establishment or trial of safe injection rooms.* Australia: Parliament of New South Wales. 1998; 284.

41. Medically Supervised Injecting Centre Evaluation Committee. *Final report on the evaluation report of the Sydney medically supervised centre.* Sydney: MSIC Evaluation Committee, 2003.

42. Jacob J, Rottman J, Stoever H. Entstehung und Praxis eines Gesundheitsraumangebotes für Drogenkonsmierende. Abschlußbericht der einjährigen Evaluation des ‚drop-in Fixpunkt,‘ Hanover. Oldenburg: Bibliotheks und Informationssystem der Universitat Oldenburg, 1999.

43. Strang J, Fortson R, Supervised fixing rooms, supervised injectable maintenance clinics – understanding the difference. *BMJ* 2004; **328**: 102–3.

44. European Monitoring Centre for Drugs and Drug Addiction. European report on drug consumption rooms, EMCDDA. Luxembourg: Office for Official Publication of the European Communities, 2004.

CHAPTER 16

Beyond pharmaceutical treatments

Gordon Morse

IN THIS CHAPTER

Introduction ‖ *'Talking' treatments* ‖
'Hands-on' treatments ‖ *Discussion*

Introduction

Because, in one narrow sense, drugs are the problem in substance misuse, non-pharmaceutical interventions have been seen as the answer to treat those with drug dependency problems. Pharmacological interventions are important and much of this book has been devoted to a discussion of the evidence for substitute treatment. Nevertheless there are good reasons to employ non-pharmaceutical strategies: substance misuse often stems from the desire and perceived need to self-medicate some sort of distress, be it anxiety, depression, social phobia, early life trauma, or other social or psychological damage. To introduce new pharma-cotherapies where there has also been autonomous drug misuse both reinforces the erroneous belief that some sort of drug treatment is necessary, and introduces new drugs into the soup, which may themselves be abused. It is rational therefore to look for non-pharmaceutical interventions, which can either palliate or more effectively deal with distress, or otherwise help to decrease reliance on psychoac-tive drugs.

Inevitably these interventions tend to be championed by abstinence-based services, frequently non-medical ones. In response, there has been a historic dis-respect of alternative or complementary therapies by the medical establishment for a number of reasons. Undoubtedly there is an issue of professional rivalry, but there is also the want of a well-researched scientific evidence base for many of these therapies, which frequently lead to the conclusion that therefore they must be ineffective. There is an arrogance in medicine that because our treatments are researched and trialled they are therefore the only treatments of value. The fact that our treatments are often disliked by patients, have adverse effects, and considerable failure rates of their own seems to be disregarded by technocracy in its endeavours to justify itself.

There are no good treatments for substance misuse. There are many treatments, some of which have some value at some times in some people, but the very fact that we have an epidemic of morbidity and mortality arising from substance misuse in this country and throughout the world is evidence, if we needed it, that we cannot afford the luxury of ruling out any treatment if it has value.

Some drug services, usually those in the non-statutory sector but also a number of specialist services, have started to look at some of these non-pharmaceutical therapies as a way of broadening their effectiveness and their appeal, and especially, of retaining patients in treatment.

The National Treatment Agency's *Models of Care*[1] cites 'large numbers' of both residential and community based services offering complementary therapies, although The Task Force to Review Services for Drug Misusers in 1996 concluded, 'Most of the reports [on the use of complementary therapies in drug treatment] are fairly positive, but there are almost no data to support the claims of effectiveness'.[2] These therapies are claimed to be useful, particularly in assisting the uncomfortable process of withdrawal from dependency ('detox') and supporting abstinence thereafter as a pragmatic response, no doubt partly because conventional medicine and pharmacology have little to offer. But some of these non-pharmaceutical strategies have, in recent years, gained some good data testifying to their usefulness and will be discussed in this chapter. These treatments tend to fall into two categories:

'Talking' treatments

▶ counselling (which may include psychological therapies such as cognitive behavioural therapy, cognitive analytic therapy, coping skills training, cue exposure treatments)

▶ group therapy

▶ '12 Step' or 'Minnesota method' programmes as in Alcoholics Anonymous and Narcotics Anonymous.

'Hands-on' treatments

There are many, but notably:

▶ acupuncture (including 'neuroelectric therapy')

▶ herbal remedies

▶ aromatherapy

▶ also shiatsu, reflexology, various relaxation techniques, meditation.

Most of these interventions sit outside conventional primary care, but where practitioners with special clinical interest are tasked with administering or commissioning a range of services for drug misusers, they should be aware of these strategies, and may want to commission some of them. There follows a brief appraisal of some of the evidence for some of these treatments:

'Talking' treatments

Counselling

Counselling has been used widely in helping people to deal with drug or alcohol misuse, or more specifically, to help people deal with negative emotions and behaviours that become cues to use drugs or alcohol. Counselling has been a mainstay of treatment services in the United States for more than 50 years, and in the past 20 years or so has been taken up with similar enthusiasm in the United Kingdom and throughout the world. This enthusiasm, it must be presumed, is because counselling is useful – it must work. And yet there is a distinct paucity of good, reproducible evidence that has scientific and statistical validity to substantiate that counselling does indeed work. Contrary to what some cynics might believe, this is not because counselling is ineffective – there is a vast body of anecdotal or observational evidence to refute that claim – but it is because it is so difficult to measure.

The reasons are not difficult to see: counselling is not like a course of tablets to be taken by a patient – it is not a series of quantifiable units with effects that can be measured or assayed. Counselling is a generic term given to verbally communicated interventions that employ many styles; most counsellors use an eclectic blend of techniques that combine many different influences, such as transactional analysis, cognitive approaches, motivational interviewing, psychoanalytic therapies (again of varying styles), and so forth.

The blend of styles used will depend upon the training of the individual counsellor and the approach that best suits the individual patient. Also the patients themselves vary enormously not only between each other but also in themselves, according to many life events that are beyond the influence of the counsellor. These sorts of variation are far wider than the relatively small differences between different people's physiologies, which is why measuring the effects of pharmacotherapies is so much easier.

The author's own prejudice is this: how can we even contemplate a substance misuse service without using the services of skilled counsellors? Harm reduction, essential as it is, is limited to a narrow physical agenda; if harm reduction goes well, it can help to bring stability into a person's life, but it offers little to the person who uses drugs and alcohol to self-medicate their distress. How can we begin to help a patient to deal with life's vicissitudes without addressing the person?

And that is what counselling is about: it is the process of helping people to understand themselves, how they relate with others, and why they feel the way they do. It is about using that understanding to avoid triggers to drug use, or to deal with those triggers in a healthier and more productive way. Quintessentially, it is about helping a person to think and behave healthily. A substance misuse service without counselling is like a ham sandwich without mustard.

In fact some of these counselling therapies have been well researched and have a certain amount of evidence to back them.

Cognitive behavioural therapy is well known and accepted in general medicine and can be useful, particularly in demonstrating self-destructive, sabotaging behaviours that patients may be unaware of.[3,4]

Cognitive analytic therapy,[5] less well known but very useful, aims to create with patients narrative and diagrammatic reformulations of their difficulties, and has the added benefit of being time limited and hence inexpensive.

Cue exposure and coping skills training or variations on that theme form the basis of the generic strategy known as 'relapse prevention'. Gossop *et al.* in the widely respected National Treatment Outcome Research study made mention of the need for relapse prevention strategies, particularly since a number of studies have testified to the effectiveness of these techniques.[6-10]

Group therapy may be nothing more than self-help groups of patients discussing common problems and common strategies. Shared experiences and treatment can be very powerful: they allow greater insights into a person's behaviour by using the perspectives of others in the group who may have identified similar problems in themselves. Groups act as a sort of resonance chamber within which individuals will have their reactions and behaviours amplified for all to see. And groups confer the additional benefit of increasing self-efficacy by using the observations of the patients themselves to be therapeutic.

'12 Step' or 'Minnesota method' groups have been an extraordinary phenomenon since their inception in the 1940s. The original groups set themselves up with no professional input to address their alcohol dependency and became known as Alcoholics Anonymous' (AA). As the years have passed, the same philosophy has been extended to all addictive drugs (Narcotics Anonymous), specific drugs such as cocaine (CA), and also sex (SA), gambling (GA), and other behaviours that are banded together as 'addictions'. AA groups are available in most cities in the world and many smaller country areas as well. They remain 'anonymous' in as much as they are open only to those who admit to their dependency and ask for help – there is no trained or professional input, and each group will behave in slightly different ways, reflecting the different personalities within it.

246

Contrary to the widely held belief, they are not faith-based: one does not have to hold a religious belief, but the 'Steps' (towards recovery) become a sort of faith in themselves – that if you admit your powerlessness over your addiction to the group and ask for help, and if you keep to the programme, you will achieve sustained abstinence. The language employed can be arcane and off-putting to some, but there are a number of studies showing a close correlation between 12 Step meeting attendances, and duration of abstinence.[11-13]

Much research has been devoted to identifying the key triggers for relapse, most of which can be boiled down to the two biggest pre-determinants – demoralisation and isolation. 12 Step groups address these by being made up of those already recovering from addictions, which lends first-hand real optimism for recovery to the newcomer, and by offering a new peer group of those with healthy behaviours they address the isolation. Within these groups new relationships are often formed and employment can be found. Many people believe that they would not be alive today were it not for their involvement in the 'Steps'.

'Hands-on' treatments

These 'treatments' do not address the person as much as his or her symptoms. They are in effect non-pharmaceutical drugs that may help to palliate some symptoms of pain, anxiety, sleeplessness, or withdrawals. Aromatherapy, massage, herbal teas, shiatsu, reflexology, and other so-called 'complementary' therapies continue to enjoy enthusiastic application in various drug services. Again there is much anecdotal evidence testifying to their effectiveness, but little science. A much-vaunted criticism is that they are nothing more than placebo – by simply giving a patient one-to-one attention, which anyone would enjoy, they will come back for more. There may be some truth in that, but whatever the reason, research evidence has shown on numerous occasions that retention in treatment services is closely correlated with measurably better outcomes. So, whether their effects are direct, placebo, or both, they are indeed useful for retaining patients in treatment, and hence better outcomes may be expected.

Acupuncture using needles, either systemically or just in the ear, is gaining some real evidence of effectiveness in treating chemical dependency,[14] particularly cocaine abuse.[15]

Neuro-electric therapy is a sort of electrically augmented acupuncture, which has had some positive research findings.[16, 17] Claims are made about 're-educating' endorphin release, which have been cynically received as being pseudo-scientific and largely spurious speculation; this is a pity, as these treatments are inexpensive, and are at the very least comforting and supportive. But there is some science in these claims that merits further research.[18, 19]

Discussion

Why do people use drugs? Why do people want to take manifestly dangerous risks with their health for what might seem to be nothing more than 'cheap thrills'? Why do some people become addicted, and others are apparently able to use or stop using with ease and impunity? Why do some treatments work for some people and not for others?

These questions need to be asked of ourselves with every person we treat because with substance misuse above all other 'conditions', understanding the person is of paramount importance. Simply treating drug misuse as a disease that needs a specific treatment is not only to oversimplify the problem, but also to fundamentally misunderstand it.

There is no doubt that using psychoactive drugs is, for at least some of the time, rewarding. Disease is not rewarding. Drug use can make people who feel unwell feel better. Diseases do not make people feel better. It is no wonder therefore that, despite our best endeavours to 'treat' drug misuse as a disease and hence spare users from harm, they will frequently sabotage our efforts and continue to harm themselves.

Some doctors working with substance misusers in the United States like to categorise two sets of addicts, type A (or 1) and type B (or 2). Type A addicts will have simply become addicted to a chemical that is addictive – they will usually drift slowly into addiction, perhaps after starting to use the drug as a sociable activity. For some years, or even indefinitely, they may continue to have a reasonably well-ordered life. They need nothing more to develop an addiction, although they may or may not have a genetic predisposition to addiction. Most tobacco addicts and many cocaine and alcohol users may be of this type.

Type B addicts may or may not also have a genetic tendency, but will usually fall into addiction at a much earlier age. They may often become chaotic and will invariably be self-medicating with pre-existing psychological or social morbidity. It is said that there is a greater preponderance of type B addicts in heroin users by the time they contact treatment services, and many practitioners have recognised that large numbers of their patients have suffered serious early life trauma, usually sexual abuse.

Whether these descriptions are really two distinct subtypes or not, it is clear that although some simply become addicted to something that is addictive, many perceive a powerful 'need' for a drug, simply to make a wretched life feel better.

Whether we attempt to treat through the harm reduction approach, or through abstinence, in taking away a person's drug of choice we may be taking away their comfort and defence. This mechanistic approach to treating drug misuse through the disease model is insensitive and it is unsurprising that relapse is so common.

Young doctors today are prevailed upon to consider all conditions presenting to them in three dimensions – the physical, the psychological, and the social.

Surely there can be no condition quite like drug misuse that is both deeply rooted in all three dimensions, and impacts so deeply on all three dimensions of a person's health? And by implication therefore, no condition which needs so much more than a narrow physical response?

Acknowledgements

I am most grateful to my colleague Dr Fergus Law of the Bristol Specialist Drug Service, for his help with research and referencing some of the papers mentioned in this chapter.

References

1. National Treatment Agency for Substance Misuse. Models of care for treatment of adult drug misusers. National Treatment Agency: London, October 2002.

2. Department of Health, The Task Force to review services for Drug Misusers. Report of an Independent Review of drug treatment services in England. London: HMSO, 1997.

3. Ouimette P C, Finney J W, Moos R H. Twelve-step and cognitive-behavioural treatment for substance abuse: a comparison of treatment effectiveness. *J Consult Clin Psychol* 1997; **65(2)**: 230–40.

4. Finney J W, Noyes C A, Coutts A I, Moos R H. Evaluating substance abuse treatment process models: I. Changes on proximal outcome variables during 12-step and cognitive-behavioral treatment. *J Stud Alcohol* 1998; **59(4)**: 371–80.

5. Ryle A, Kerr I. *Introducing Cognitive Analytic Therapy: Principles and Practice.* Chichester: John Wiley, 2002.

6. Gossop M, Stewart D, Browne N, Marsden J. Factors associated with abstinence, lapse or relapse to heroin use after residential treatment: protective effect of coping responses. *Addiction* 2002; **97(10)**: 1259–67.

7. Anderson J G, Gilbert F S. Communication skills training with alcoholics for improving performance of two of the alcoholic's anonymous recovery steps. *J Stud Alcohol* 1989; **50(4)**: 361–7.

8. Rohsenow D J, Monti P M, Rubonis A V, *et al.* Cue exposure with coping skills training and communication skills training for alcohol dependence: 6- and 12-month outcomes. *Addiction* 2001; **96(8)**: 1161–74.

9. Monti P M, Rohsenow D J. Coping-skills training and cue-exposure therapy in the treatment of alcoholism. *Alcohol Res Health* 1999; **23(2)**: 107–15.

10. Rohsenow D J, Monti P M, Martin R A, *et al.* Brief coping skills treatment for cocaine abuse: 12-month substance use outcomes. *J Consult Clin Psychol* 2000; **68(3)**: 515–20.

11. Lloyd G. One Hundred Alcoholic Doctors: A 21 year Follow Up. *Alcohol and Alcoholism* 2002; **37(4)**: 370–4.

12. Moos R H, Finney J W, Ouimette P C, Suchinsky R T. A comparative evaluation of substance abuse treatment: I. Treatment orientation, amount of care, and 1-year outcomes. *Alcohol Clin Exp Res* 1999; **23(3)**: 529–36.

13. Brown T G, Seraganian P, Tremblay J, Annis H. Process and outcome changes with relapse prevention versus 12-Step aftercare programs for substance abusers. *Addiction* 2002; **97(6)**: 677–89.

14. Avants S K, Margolin A, Holford T R. Kosten T R. A Randomised Controlled Trial of Auricular Acupuncture for Cocaine Dependence. *Arch. Int Med* 2000; **160(15)**: 2305–12.

15. Lipton D S, Brewington V, Smith M. Acupuncture for Crack-Cocaine Detoxification: Experimental Evaluation of Efficacy. *Journal of Substance Abuse Treatment* 1994; **11(3)**: 205–15.

16. Patterson M A. Electro-acupuncture in alcohol and drug addictions. *Clin Med* 1974; **81**: 9–14.

17. Patterson M A. Treatment of drug, alcohol and nicotine addiction by NeuroElectric Therapy: analysis of results over 7 years. *Journal of Bioelectricity* 1984; **3**: 193–221.

18. Ulett G A, Han S, Han J S. Electroacupuncture: mechanisms and clinical application. *Journal of The Society of Biological Psychiatry* 1998; **44(2)**: 129–38.

19. Patterson M A, Patterson L, Flood N V, Winston J R, Patterson S I. Electrostimulation in drug and alcohol detoxification: significance of stimulation criteria in clinical success. *Addiction Research* 1993; **1(2)**: 131–44.

CHAPTER 17

Young people and substance use

Clare Gerada, Daphne Rumball,
and Beate Becker

IN THIS CHAPTER

Introduction ‖ Prevalence ‖ Risks for problematic use ‖ Gateway theory ‖ Alcohol and young people ‖ Smoking and young people ‖ Prevention of substance misuse ‖ Role of primary care ‖ Children Act 1989 ‖ Specialist treatment services ‖ Conclusion

Introduction

This chapter considers the needs of young people who use substances problematically. Substance use in young people is often multiple and frequently involves alcohol and illicit substances. The age range considered in reference material varies greatly and for the purpose of this chapter we will mainly consider those of 18 years or under.

Drug misuse is described as drug taking that harms health or social functioning. It may be dependent use (physical or psychological) or drug taking that is part of a wider spectrum of problematic or harmful behaviour. Both require therapeutic intervention. Drug use of a non-dependent type can cause harm (intoxication, illegality, health problems) but usually a lower level of medical intervention is required. General practitioners and other health and allied professionals employed in primary health care should have knowledge of the use and misuse of substances by children and adolescents. Their health promotion role is of particular importance regarding the initiation of help for this patient group and in primary and secondary prevention of drug related harm.

Prevalence

Substance misuse by young people has been a matter of concern amongst health professionals and others for a number of years.[1] This concern is justified as the

Box 17.1   **Case study**

Wayne, aged 14 years, attends the surgery with his mother. She is concerned that he has started to drink alcohol with his friends after school and that he has started smoking cigarettes. She is also worried that he may be using cannabis as she has seen cigarette papers in his bedroom. Wayne, she says, 'is a good boy'; he is doing well at school and up to now she has not had any problems with him. His dad left when he was six years old and does not have any contact with the family. He used to be violent to her and she thinks he had an alcohol problem. She really wants some advice from you about what to do and how to handle Wayne.

The practitioner needs to consider:

✓ Is Wayne using drugs and if so how engrained is this? Is he dependent?

✓ Is Wayne's use of alcohol risky or is he dependent?

✓ What do he and his mother understand of the risks that he may be taking?

✓ Who else needs to be involved at this stage (e.g. social services, specialist adolescent drug services, child and adolescent mental health services, school)?

✓ What interventions can be made concerning his smoking?

use of drugs and alcohol by young people shows an increase year on year. Alcohol, nicotine, and cannabis are the drugs most commonly used by young people, with more than half of 16-year-olds reporting having used an illegal drug, mostly cannabis. Thirteen per cent of drug users reported to the Drug Misuse Database are under 20 years. It does seem, however, from the results of recent surveys that drug use by the young is levelling off and may actually be dropping amongst 14–15-year-olds.[2] This finding is consistent with findings of other researchers where the use of any drug in the previous year by 16–19-year-olds fell from around one third in 1994 to just over one quarter in 2000.[3,4]

Risks for problematic use

Polysubstance use in adolescence, including alcohol, is usually problematic.

Drug use by the young must be viewed in context. Most illicit use in adolescence is transient and does not lead to lifelong addiction although there is a small group who continue to use and a significant number of these develop problems. There are a number of reasons why a young person exposed to a drug might continue beyond the experimental stage. When growing up, children and young adults are exposed to a wide range of risk factors that either alone or combined may lead to persistent drug use. Their genes, family influences, and early experiences will shape their psychological development. The incentives to try illicit drugs if offered will be dependent on the balance of incentives to use against the disincentives to use, which in turn are determined by factors such as parental influences, educational and employment opportunities, and societal norms and normative expectations, for example fear of arrest or school expulsion. The relative availably of drugs will be influenced by geographical issues (inner city, rural pockets of use), which in turn will influence the risk of the young person being exposed to a drug taking peer group. See Table 17.1.

The risks for illicit drug use overlap with those that lead to teenage pregnancy, conduct disorder, truancy, and scholastic failure, hence the UK government's desire in 1999 to combat these through the creation of a social exclusion unit. This led to the programme Positive Futures, fostering social inclusion.[5] Measures that combat poverty, poor housing, truancy, school failure, exclusion, and general measures to support vulnerable families will help reduce the risks of entering lifelong addiction. Less is known about protective factors against drug use, although the benefits of a stable family background, good education, and job opportunities enhance the likelihood of drug use forming a small and mainly harmless part of an individual's life. It is important to add that it is the quality of the parent–child relationship rather than family structure (for example single parent households) that appears to be the most important influence.[6]

Table 17.1 **Risk factors for persistent and problematic drug use**

Risk factors	Examples
Drug factors	Ability to produce mind altering, pleasurable effects
	Dependence potential (tolerance and withdrawal syndrome)
	Price
	Availability
Environmental factors	Social deprivation
	Poor housing
	Neighbourhood crime
	Lack of community supports
	Acceptance of drug use

continued over

Risk factors	Examples
Individual and interpersonal factors	Sex (men more than women)
	Age (adolescence and young adult)
	Scholastic failure
	Conduct disorder
	Unemployment
	Friends who use
	Attention deficit disorder
	Family attitudes to substance misuse, e.g. tolerance of drug use, approval of smoking and drinking behaviour

Resilient children have a repertoire of problem-solving skills and a belief in their own self-efficacy.[7] Primary and secondary prevention strategies need to address and focus on reducing multiple risks and on enhancing protective factors.

Protective factors include positive temperament and intellectual prowess.

Gateway theory

Much has been written about the so-called gateway theory of drug use. This theory postulates that the use of less harmful drugs, such as cannabis, introduces people to a criminal subculture where they meet other drug users and dealers who encourage them to experiment with other, often more harmful, drugs.

It is difficult to untangle the evidence and it is often presented to serve the purpose of the arguer. Certainly most heroin users have used cannabis, but very few cannabis users progress to heroin use. In one study, 96% of opioid users had used cannabis in the previous year but only 7% of cannabis users had ever taken heroin. There is a strong link between cigarette smoking and later drug use as young dependent smokers are 22 times more likely to have tried a drug than non-smokers.

An alternative to the gateway theory and one that intuitively seems more accurate is that progression from cannabis to more harmful drugs is more about individual vulnerability and risk than about exposure to these drugs. Frequent or regular cannabis users are more likely to have a history of antisocial behaviour and non-conformity, to perform poorly at school, and to use drugs to deal with emotional problems, suggesting that cannabis use is a consequence not a casual factor in predicting future drug use.

Alcohol and young people

Many parents, not to mention doctors, are more concerned with young people experimenting with cannabis than drinking heavily, despite binge drinking and the problems caused by this pattern of use being on the increase. The dangers of heavy and binge alcohol use far outweigh those of occasional cannabis use. Worldwide, 5% of all deaths of young people between the ages of 15 and 29 are attributable to alcohol use.[8,9] In the United Kingdom, consumption of alcohol beginning at some stage of adolescence is part of normal expected behaviour, except in relatively small cultural and religious communities. As children grow, so too will their intake of alcohol; most children by the age of 15 years have drunk alcohol, with a small but growing proportion drinking more per week then the recommended *adult* limits.

Results from the National Longitudinal Alcohol Epidemiologic Survey (a US study) (N = 27,616) suggested that early initiation to alcohol use is related to more frequent and higher quantity of alcohol use in later life and may even predict later cannabis use.[10] The study also shows that the lifetime alcohol dependence rate of those who initiate alcohol use by the age of 14 is four times as high as those who start at the age of 20. Adjusting for potentially confounding variables, the odds of dependence decreased by 14% with each additional year of delayed initiation.

Alcohol has been identified as a direct cause of school exclusions with 20% of school suspensions being for dinking alcohol at school. An indirect link is also apparent, with 16% of excluded pupils drinking alcohol every day compared with 3% of non-excluded pupils, and 20% of excluded pupils drinking three to four times a week more compared with non-excluded pupils. In many cases, the fact that a child is not at school can lead to increased drinking.

The Annual Report of the Chief Medical Officer of the Department of Health (England and Wales) highlights a worrying trend for teenagers who drink alcohol to consume larger quantities.[11] In 1998, average consumption among 11–15-year-old drinkers was 9.9 units of alcohol a week (1 unit contains 8 g of pure alcohol), compared with 6.0 units a week in 1992.

A major European study has recently provided comparative international data. The European School Survey Project on Alcohol and other Drugs (ESPAD) focusing on 15–16-year-olds showed that in the United Kingdom nearly 40% of young people had been drunk by the time they reached 13 years, over one-fifth of students had been intoxicated three times or more during the previous 30 days, and nearly one-third of students reported having five or more drinks in a row (binge drinking).[12] In each case the rates in the United Kingdom were among the worst of the 30 countries studied.

The Chief Medical Officer also raised a concern about the increasing number of deaths from chronic liver disease in young people. In the last 30 years of the 20th century this death rate amongst people aged 35 to 44 years increased eightfold in men and sevenfold in women; and amongst 25–34-year-olds a fourfold increase was seen over the 30-year period.

Media reports have indicated that in the United Kingdom up to 1,000 people a week suffer serious facial injuries as a result of drunken assaults, and 18,000 young people are scarred for life each year. In scientific studies alcohol use has been associated with delinquent and violent behaviours in young people, even after adjusting for personality and behavioural risk.[13,14] There was only a small direct effect of alcohol intoxication on violent behaviour after controlling for various relevant confounders (e.g. criminal activities) in a large national sample study of Norwegian adolescents aged 12 to 20 years; although in cross-sectional studies the size and strength of relationships need to be interpreted cautiously.

The range of harms related to alcohol use in young people make a straightforward classification and definition of alcohol misuse difficult, but include immediate harm to self through alcohol overdose and alcohol-related injury, immediate harm to others through drinking and driving and alcohol related injury, and longer-term harm to self through the development of inappropriate drinking behaviour and patterns.

Young children's and adolescents' metabolism of alcohol and response to intoxication differs from those of adults. Young people more often exhibit hypoglycaemia. At higher blood levels, both children and adolescents can suffer from hypothermia and respiratory depression. They are more likely to have seizures. Children and adolescents suffer coma at lower blood levels than adults.

The setting for acute intoxication amongst schoolchildren is largely experimental drinking, with peer pressure leading to binge drinking and then to intoxication. In later adolescence, drinking competitions are incentives to the young to binge drink and can lead to toxic overdose. Adolescents are susceptible to the 'happy hour' and cheap drink offers prominent in many clubs and public houses. These offers are implicated in the explosion of binge drinking and reckless behaviour found in many city centres at pub closing time.

Smoking and young people

This topic is dealt with in more detail in Chapter 14. Targets for reducing young people's smoking, from 13% in 1996 to 11% by 2005, and to 9% or less by 2010, were set in the government document *Smoking Kills, a White Paper on Tobacco* and are unlikely to be met.[15] Smoking prevalence is strongly related to age. Only 1% of 11-year-olds are regular smokers compared with 23% of 15-year-olds. Interestingly, young girls smoke more than boys. In 2002, 11% of girls were regular smokers, compared with 9% of boys.[2]

Prevention of substance misuse

Reducing the demand for drugs is a key component of the UK Drug Strategy,[16] with primary prevention activities focused on preventing the young from using, and secondary prevention on treating those who are already involved in drug taking. This strategy aims 'to enable people with drug problems to overcome them and live healthy crime-free lives' and 'to help young people resist drug misuse in order to achieve their potential in society'.

The effectiveness of drug and alcohol education programmes has always been difficult to assess.[17] Long-term randomised controlled studies are methodologically difficult and expensive to carry out. Compounding factors such as socioeconomic status, IQ, educational achievement, parental influences (including removing their children from schools where drug use is prevalent), and the skills of the educator are difficult to control for. External influences such as trends in drug use may change from year to year and from one small community to another. It would seem logical, given the time and influence of school on a young person, and that most children attend school, that school based prevention programmes could be effective in at least imparting information to young people about the risks associated with alcohol and drug taking. The evidence suggests that short-term reduction in both drug use and progression to frequent drug use may be achievable through school and community based programmes, but there is limited evidence of success in the United Kingdom.

The longer-term effects are less clear. Delivery of drug education programmes is now commonplace and incorporated into the curriculum of Personal, Social and Health Education (PSHE). Those that target personal development rather than drug based messages are more effective. General practitioners can and should be involved wherever possible in both primary care and secondary prevention. For example, an innovative project in south London uses primary care professionals to deliver aspects of PSHE to primary school children in the borough. Each practice is linked to a local school and aims to foster the close relationship that many of these children (and their parents) have with their family doctor and health visitor.

Box 17.2 **Project**

The Lambeth Education Link Project has been running for six years and at present serves 40 Lambeth schools; primary, secondary, special, and pupil referral units. The team takes health professionals into schools to deliver sessions on a range of health topics, such as Sex and Relationships, Drugs, Mental Health, and Healthy Lifestyles, with the aim of building community links and nurturing healthier, happier citizens (www.healthykids.org.uk).

With respect to drug prevention education in schools the Home Office Drug Prevention Advisory Service has laid out guidance as follows:[18]

National guidance: model for drugs prevention

Drug prevention programmes should:

▶ be evidence-based

▶ be clearly targeted

▶ have clear objectives

▶ reduce risk factors

▶ increase protective factors

▶ be consistent and/or linked to other programmes

▶ be sustainable.

Table 17.2   **Examples of drug prevention activity** [19]

Type of intervention	Comments
Social influence model	This aims to engage young people through a range of activities designed to increase personal and social skills
Brief interventions	These help to reduce and manage the number of problem users
Peer approaches	When peers are adequately trained and supported, they can be successful in school-based initiatives to engage vulnerable and 'difficult to reach' groups and provide credibility. Peer approaches appear to be beneficial to the peers themselves, providing positive experience and a potential path to career or personal development
Community programmes	Programmes such as Positive Futures are said to have helped young people raise their aspirations, relate better to others, increase their skills and competencies, and change their attitudes. Antisocial behaviour in the community can also be reduced
Diversionary activities	Young people excluded from mainstream education may be engaged through activities designed to interest them, such as driving lessons
Criminal justice intervention	These interventions, such as court diversion schemes and drug treatment and testing orders can be cost effective in terms of savings to health, welfare, and criminal justice systems

Drug prevention programmes as outlined by the Health Development Agency span primary and secondary prevention, that is prevention of initiation and prevention of further harmful use.[19] See Table 17.2.

The UK government spent £7.5m in 2004 trying to find the best method for implementing drugs education in schools.

Engaging and treating young people

A four-tier range of services has been described for local implementation:

Tier 1 Primary and direct access services should provide direct accessibility for the general public. This includes education, preventive work, and generic treatment and comprises primary care workers, for example GPs and health visitors, staff of non-statutory organisations, social workers, police officers, and school medical officers. Information and advice is offered as well as initial assessment of personal needs.

Tier 2 This service is provided by individual practitioners who have some specialist knowledge of drugs and alcohol misuse. They offer all of Tier 1 intervention plus drug-related prevention and targeted education, advice, and general counselling services.

Tier 3 Specialist agencies provide young people's specialist drug services and other specialised services including work with complex cases requiring multidisciplinary team-based work.

Tier 4 Very specialised care interventions are designed for specialised and intensive forms of intervention for young drug misusers with complex care needs. Services may include specialist residential services, specialist community based treatment teams, and mental health co-morbidity treatment teams.

General practitioners could be involved at various levels of this intervention system.

Role of primary care

Even where general practitioners feel unskilled in substance use or reluctant to offer care, they must, at least, be confident in recognising needs and be aware of the constitution of services that are appropriate to younger people, of their availability locally, and of the mechanisms for referring vulnerable children and adolescents to them. Services include those in the statutory and non-statutory sector, generic and specialist counselling, sexual health, psychiatric and specialist substance misuse services.

Depending on the local prevalence of drug use in young people, general practitioners and their teams may need to consider how to review the needs of young people in their practice, by, for example, promoting routine enquiry into the use of substances by young people. They should be able to give appropriate and accurate initial advice. If confident, GPs may counsel and support parents and families of young people who use/misuse drugs. Advice on safe sex and on harm minimisation, including hepatitis B immunisation, is particularly relevant.

The close association of mental health problems and substance use should be actively considered during consultations, especially depression, anxiety, and the early onset of psychotic illness.[20–23] The risk of self-harm should be considered. Family involvement through acknowledgement and support is not only good practice but increases the likelihood of treatment being effective.[20] Care should be taken to encourage constructive activities, educational goals, and the maintenance or development of supportive relationships.

Treatment is a difficult area for the non-specialist. On the one hand is the need to engage the young person, by providing ample opportunity for disclosure of use in a non-judgmental and confidential environment, and on the other hand is the need to respond to the legal requirement of involving parents and/or social services if the practitioner feels that the young person is suffering or at risk of suffering (Children Act 1989).[24]

If 'treatment' is considered there is the issue of consent. The provision of treatment, especially pharmacological interventions, requires informed consent and for those aged under 16 years parental consent is usually required. Some people under 16 years may be able to consent to their treatment, but only if they are assessed as competent, with a sufficient understanding of the nature and purpose of the proposed treatment, its risks and side effects, alterations and consequences. They must be assessed as having freedom from pressure and sufficient maturity to make the decision.[25] When a young person presents in a primary care setting with significant substance misuse problems the general practitioner has to weigh up the balance of maturity, circumstances, age, support systems, and drug use (amount, risk behaviour, etc.) before a decision is made to provide treatment. Any intervention provided should be age (and maturity) appropriate, rapidly accessible, and built on trustful relationships and confidentiality.[26]

It is important to exercise great caution in prescribing for adolescents. The Department of Health's guidelines on clinical management recommend that the GP seek advice of a specialist consultant in the case of a young person (under 18 years).[27] Specialists in adolescent substance misuse, however, are few and far between and it is not unknown for the GP to have greater specialist prescribing knowledge than the local child psychiatrist and greater skills in responding to adolescents than the adult service substance misuse specialist. Nevertheless, it is important to remember that prescribing should not be considered in isolation from the treatment of the rest of the young person's needs; in general these are best provided through the care of a specialist practitioner.

Children Act 1989

This act[24] is the legislative framework governing all young people in England. The major principles of the act are as follows:

▶ The welfare of the child is paramount.

▶ The child's wishes and views must be considered.

▶ There should be minimum statutory intervention.

▶ There is a duty to safeguard and promote the welfare of the child.

▶ Agencies working with children should cooperate and work together in the best interests of the child.

Specialist treatment services

The Health Advisory Service, in 1996 and again in 2001,[28-29] advised that services for young people should range across education, preventive work, and treatment in the community and comprise GPs and other primary care workers and specialist services requiring multidisciplinary team-based work. Identifying and supporting young people with drug problems is best achieved by complementing mainstream children's services with specialist prevention and treatment services. Guiding principles have been defined to promote specific qualities required for services for young people:[26] See Box 17.3.

Conclusion

Young people who use or misuse drugs do not fall into a homogeneous group. Each young person has to be carefully assessed, and treated on an individual, well-informed basis. The results can be rewarding and effective.

Box 17.3   **Principles to be applied for services working with young people[26]**

Accessible

1. **Appropriate:** a child or young person is not an adult

2. **Lawful:** services should aim to operate, in all cases, according to the principles of good practice

3. **Competent:** services must be competent to respond to the need of the young person

4. **Respecting and protecting:** the overall welfare of the individual child or young person is of paramount importance; the views of the young person are of central importance, and should always be sought and considered

5. **Collaborative:** services need to respect parental responsibility when working with a young person; a holistic approach is vital at all levels, as young people's problems tend to cross professional boundaries

6. **Coordinated:** services should recognise the role of, and cooperate with, the local authority in carrying out its responsibilities towards children and young people

7. **Effective:** a comprehensive range of services should be provided

8. **Targeted:** services must be child-centred

9. **Evaluated**

Further reading

Crome I, *et al.* (Eds). *Young People and Substance Misuse*. London: Gaskell, 2004.

References

1. British Paediatric Association, Royal College of Physicians. *Alcohol and the Young*. Report of a joint working party of the Royal College of Physicians and the British Paediatric Association. London: RCP and BPA, 1995.

2. Boreham R, McManus S. (Eds). *Smoking, Drinking and Drug Use among Young People in England in 2002*. London: HMSO, 2003.

3. Miller P, Plant M. Drinking, smoking and illicit drug use among 15–16 year olds in the United Kingdom. *BMJ* 1996; **313**: 394–7.

4. Ramsey M, Baker P, Goulden C, *et al*. Drug misuse declared in 2000: results from the British Crime Survey. London: Home Office Research Development and Statistics Directorate, 2001.

5. Home Office. *Positive Futures impact report*. London: HMSO, 2004
    (available at: www.drugs.gov.uk/NationalStrategy/YoungPeople/PositiveFutures).

6. McArdle P, Wiegersma A, Gilvarry E, *et al*. European adolescent substance use: the roles of family
    structure, function and gender. *Addiction* 2002; **97(3)**: 329–36.

7. Rutter M. Resilience in the face of adversity: protective factors and resistance to psychiatric
    disorder. *Br J Psy* 1985; **147**: 598–611.

8. Murray C J, Lopez A D. *The global burden of disease: A comprehensive assessment of mortality
    and disability from diseases, injuries and risk factors in 1990 and projected to 2020*. Cambridge,
    MA: Harvard School of Public Health on behalf of the World Health Organization and the World
    Bank, 1996.

9. Jernigan D H. *Global Status Report: Alcohol and Young People*. Geneva: World Health
    Organization, 2001.

10. Grant B F. Prevalence and correlates of alcohol use and DSM-IV alcohol dependence in the United
    States: Results of the National Longitudinal Alcohol Epidemiologic Survey. *J Studies on Alcohol*
    1997; **58(5)**: 464–73.

11. Donaldson L. *Annual Report of the Chief Medical Officer of the Department of Health*. London:
    Department of Health, 2001.

12. Hibbell B, Andersson B, Ahlstrom S, *et al*. *The 1999 ESPAD report: alcohol and other drug use
    among students in 30 European countries*. Stockholm: The Swedish Council for Information on
    Alcohol and Other Drugs (CAN), The Pompidou Group of the Council of Europe, 2000.

13. Rossow I, Pape H, Wichstrom L. Young, wet and wild? Associations between alcohol intoxication
    and violent behaviour in adolescence. *Addiction* 1999; **94(7)**: 1017–31.

14. Komro K A, Williams C L, Forster J L, *et al*. The relationship between adolescent alcohol use and
    delinquent and violent behaviors. *Journal of Child and Adolescent Substance Abuse* 1999; **9(2)**:
    13–28.

15. Department of Health. *Smoking Kills, A White Paper on Tobacco* (Cm4177). London: HMSO, 1998.

16. Home Office. *Tackling Drugs to Build a Better Britain: The government's 10-year strategy for tackling
    drug misuse*. London: HMSO, 1998.

17. Aggleton P. *Health Promotion and Young People*. London: Health Education Authority, 1996.

18. Drugs Prevention Advisory Service. *The DPAS Drug Prevention Compendium: A Prevention Guide
    for Drug Action Teams*. London: Home Office, 2003.

19. Millward L, Warm D, Coomber R, *et al*. *Evidence for Effective Drug Prevention in Young People*. A
    summary of findings arising from research activity to date. London: Health Development Agency,
    2004.

20. Zeitlin H. Psychiatric comorbidity with substance misuse in children and teenagers. *Drug and
    Alcohol Dependence* 1999; **55(3)**: 225–23.

21. Crome I B, Christian J. The development of a unique designated community drug service for
    adolescents: policy, prevention and education implications. *Drugs: Education, Prevention and
    Policy* 2000; **7(1)**: 87–108.

22. Wittchen H U, Nelson C B, Lachner G. Prevalence of mental disorders and psychosocial
    impairments in adolescents and young adults. *Psychological Medicine* 1998; **28**: 109–26.

23. Kandel D B, Johnson J G, Bird H R, *et al*. Psychiatric disorders associated with substance use among
    children and adolescents: Findings from Methods for the Epidemiology of Child and Adolescent
    Mental Disorders (MECA) Study. *J Abnorm Child Psychol* 1999; **25(2)**: 121–32.

24. Children Act, 1989 (available at: www.ntas.org.uk/childrenact.htm#CP).

25. British Medical Association and the Law Society. Assessment of mental capacity: Guidance for doctors and lawyers. London: BMA, 1995.

26. Standing Conference on Drug Abuse. *Young People and Drugs*. Policy guidance for drug interventions: London: SCODA, 1999.

27. Department of Health. *Drug Misuse and Dependence: Guidelines on Clinical Management*. London: HMSO, 1999.

28. Health Advisory Service. *Children and Young People: Substance Misuse Service Needs, The Substance of Young Need*. London: HMSO, 1996.

29. Health Advisory Service. *The Substance Young Needs Review 2001*. London: HMSO, 2001.

CHAPTER 18

Women and drug use

Clare Gerada and Sharon Dawe

IN THIS CHAPTER

*Introduction || Prevalence and sex differences || Crack cocaine ||
Injecting drug users || Antecedents of drug use || Special problems for
women who use drugs || Health needs of women drug users || Sexual
health || Family planning || Treatment for women || Identification
and screening || Referral to other agencies || Conclusion*

Introduction

Over the 20th century, in most Western countries, women made many great
strides in social equality, including winning the right to vote and to equal wages.
A by-product of this emancipation means that women are engaging in 'traditional' male activities, including the use of high levels of alcohol and illicit drugs,
resulting in a narrowing of the gap between sexes in terms of rates of substance
use disorders.

Primary care practitioners are well positioned to discuss the health effects of
alcohol and other drugs with women, to identify and counsel those with alcohol
use disorders, and to make appropriate referrals for treatment. This chapter dis-
cusses the causes and consequences of substance use in women.

Prevalence and sex differences

Although historically there have been significant sex differences in the rates of
substance use, with men using more illicit drugs and drinking larger amounts
of alcohol than women, in many countries the ratio is narrowing, especially in
the younger age groups. Whereas men are twice as likely to have taken drugs
than women, this pattern is not found in younger age groups.[1] There is a trend
among boys and girls aged from 12–17 years towards comparable rates of use and
initiation for alcohol, cocaine, heroin, and tobacco. The rates of illicit drug use are

also similar in young men and women (under the age of 26) with approximately 44% of women and 56% of men reporting use of an illicit drug in 2001.[2] If this age range is narrowed further to those under the age of 18 years, there are almost equal numbers of young men and women who report the use of illicit drugs in the previous year.

These trends are found elsewhere. For example, in Australia approximately 26% of young people aged between 14 and 19 years report recent use (past twelve months) of illicit drugs, with no reported difference between women and men,[3] and of 12–17-year-olds in the United States,[4] 16.2% of males and 16.5% of females reported alcohol use in the month prior.

Amongst drug users notified by treatment services to the Regional Drug Misuse Databases in England, heroin accounts for more than two-thirds of all the 11,000 new agency presentations, followed by methadone, cocaine, and then cannabis. Where injecting status was known, the proportion of women injecting in the past four weeks (38%) was lower than that for men (45%), but the level of sharing injecting equipment was higher (24% compared with 18%) with some evidence that women are more likely to share injecting equipment than men.[5,6]

Women are almost certainly under-represented in treatment settings with a reported ratio of 13:1.[7]

Although it is unclear what proportion of substance use reported in national surveys is problematic use, it seems unlikely that the proportion of young men whose substance use requires treatment is 13 times greater than that of young women. Of those women who do present for treatment, almost a third are in their early twenties (the proportion ranging from 27 to 30%).

Barriers to treatment have been investigated extensively in women drug users and there is a broad consensus that impediments to treatment are associated with women's difficulties in managing childcare responsibilities and their own substance use treatment needs. In an evaluation of an enhanced drug service for women that provided transport, child care, and outreach, participating women were more engaged in treatment and had a greater reduction in drug use compared with those women who received the standard care option.[8]

Crack cocaine

Women have been using crack cocaine since its introduction to the United Kingdom in the mid-1980s. US data for women show that, in the year 2000, smoked cocaine was the primary substance of abuse for 14% of all adult women admitted for treatment. The average age of these women was 35 and half of them had been using for more than 10 years. The majority of these women also use other drugs and almost half were dependent on alcohol.[9]

Injecting drug users

Women who inject drugs constitute a continuously increasing proportion of people infected with HIV.[10] Many factors serve to increase the already significant risks of HIV infection for women who inject drugs. These women are often unable to negotiate safer sex because of personal histories of sexual abuse. Relationships involving violence are common with heavier users of heroin and cocaine; heavy users are more likely to be hit, slapped, or shoved by their partners than light users or nonusers of these drugs.[11]

The drug injecting practices of women are also more likely to be affected by close personal relationships. In an analysis of the psychosocial risk factors for HIV transmission among injecting drug users, Brook and colleagues found that a woman's relationship with her significant other and family members was strongly associated with needle sharing. Women were less likely than men to inject alone and more likely to be influenced by others who inject.[12] Women reported sharing needles with their regular sexual partner more often than men did, being the second on the needle after their partner and being injected by their partner.[13]

Even when women are engaged in treatment services there is less reduction in risky injection and sexual practices than men.[14] As with needle sharing behaviour, unsafe sexual practice is also more common among women who report a history of childhood sexual abuse.[15] Women drug users often work in the sex trade to support both themselves and their male partners and this increases their risk for HIV infection; the more clients they report, the higher is their risk.[16]

Antecedents of drug use

There are many common risk factors for the development of substance misuse problems in men and women; these include chaotic family environments characterised by financial difficulties, parental substance abuse, and mental health problems. Early school failure and the development of behavioural problems have been widely reported and these, in turn, are associated with initial substance use and criminal activity.[17] For women, there are additional factors that contribute to their dependent and problematic use. Young women with substance abuse problems tend to be younger when they start using and have fewer years of formal education. High rates of childhood trauma, in particular childhood sexual abuse, are reported amongst women substance abusers and in later adult life they are exposed to high rates of domestic and sexual violence.[18]

Box 18.1   **Case study**

Kim is a 29-year-old woman. She was sexually abused by her stepfather as a child and began drinking heavily while still at school, aged 14. By 16 she was living with her heroin-using boyfriend and began heroin use herself around the age of 17. She had a habit of binge drinking and using heroin intravenously on a daily basis. She had a child taken into care when she was 22 and another at 26. She had never worked and funded her drinking and drug taking by a combination of benefit fraud, prostitution, and shoplifting. Kim's case illustrates several features found in substance using women:

✓ history of sexual abuse

✓ school failure

✓ no employment history

✓ drug-using partner who introduces her into drug taking

✓ polydrug use

✓ binge drinking

✓ parenting problems

✓ funding habit through prostitution

Special problems of women who use drugs

Table 18.1   **Risks associated with substance abuse in women**

Area of need	Risks
Physical health	Gynaecological problems and sexually transmitted diseases common
	Increased risk of reproductive complaints secondary to increased prevalence of pelvic inflammatory disorder and complications in pregnancy
	Increased vulnerability to HIV infection
	Same injection drug use-related problems as men for hepatitis and many other medical problems

Area of need	Risks
Psychological and social health	Increased risk of affective disorders (depression, anxiety, attempted suicide, low self-esteem)
	Low levels of coping skills
	High psychological distress
	Lack of confidence in communication skills
	Passivity in relationships
	Increased likelihood of being separated or divorced
	Smaller social networks
	More unresolved sexual issues
Economic and legal status	Poorer occupational functioning
	Often economically dependent on men through prostitution or exchanging sex for drugs, food, shelter etc
	Low levels of vocational training and job skills
	High rates of unemployment
	Majority have at least one legal conviction

Adapted from Jones *et al.*[19]

In women, heroin use is usually started through contact with a male drug-using partner and this use is also more likely to be funded through prostitution than it is in men.[20, 21] These factors lead to higher exposure to the risks of unsafe sex: sexually transmitted disease, unwanted pregnancies, and high rates of domestic and stranger violence, especially violence when exchanging sex for drugs or money. Women engaged in sex-for-money or sex-for-drugs exchanges are likely to be at greatest risk of both negative health and psychological and social consequences, particularly trauma associated with rape and physical violence with the result that many drug-using women meet diagnostic criteria for post-traumatic stress disorder.[22] Incarceration and arrest add substantially to a profile of enduring victimisation and perceived powerlessness.

The experience of multiple traumas both in early childhood and as adults has been proposed to have an enduring effect on personality style, in particular the ability to regulate, affect and inhibit impulsive behaviours.[23] As a consequence drug-using women have a range of personality or behavioural tendencies that are often referred to in a derogatory way as 'borderline traits' and dismissed as untreatable. This is unfortunate as such behaviours are understandable given the history of trauma. There are now several research studies that have focused on changing such behaviours with reasonable success.[24] It is not the role of the primary care team to undertake complex psychological treatment for such issues but sensitivity and understanding may help in the management of what often appears to be self-destructive behaviours. Liaison with appropriate mental health facilities where treatment may be provided is a critical role for the primary care team.

Women drug users are more likely than their male counterparts to have parental responsibility and all the responsibilities involved in providing adequate parenting whilst engaged in a drug-using lifestyle. Often mothers who are attempting to bring up their children in chaotic environments have the same set of difficulties and problems found in their own family of origin. Added to this is a lack of understanding or knowledge about how to be a 'good enough' parent to their children. Women substance misusers often perceive themselves as failed parents and, although drug use plays a role in parenting, contextual factors such as poverty and a mother's perception of the extent of her child's difficulties influence parenting style.[25] There is now growing evidence that an intergenerational pattern of substance abuse occurs with many young drug users reporting high rates of parental illicit drug abuse.[26]

Health needs of female drug users

The needs of female drug users are likely to include those associated with serious health and psychiatric problems, for example:

▶ poor nutrition and low weight

▶ low self-esteem, depression, anxiety

▶ if pregnant, increased risk of complications

▶ blood-borne viruses

▶ sexually transmitted diseases and pelvic inflammatory disease.

There is clinically important comorbidity between psychiatric illness and drug misuse, particularly in women. Women with affective disorders are more likely to present with alcohol and/or drug dependence. In turn, women who use drugs are more likely to experience significant depression and anxiety.[27]

Sexual health

Most female drug users are sexually active (84%) and, as a group, are reluctant to attend family planning or genitourinary medicine services. Drug services tend to concentrate their HIV prevention strategies on the reduction of injecting equipment sharing to the exclusion of strategies to change high-risk sexual activity. Although drug-using prostitutes usually report that they use safer sex techniques and condoms with their clients, fewer than a sixth will use condoms with their regular partner and only a quarter of all female drug users use any form of contraception.[28]

The misuse of opiates can suppress the production of luteinising hormone and follicle stimulating hormone from the pituitary gland. This disturbance affects menstruation but does not necessarily prevent ovulation. Heavy drug use can cause severe weight loss, which itself affects menstruation. Amenorrhoea is common amongst opiate users – related in part to poor health but also to low weight. There are unintended consequences of treatment. For example, when a woman first starts on methadone (or indeed any substitute medication) she may experience weight gain and return of menstruation. Ovulation may restart with drug treatment before menstruation returns. It is important therefore to discuss contraception with all female drug users. Conversely, those trying unsuccessfully to become pregnant may have restored fertility.

Pregnancy is discussed in Chapter 18.

Family planning

Providing family planning services to women who use drugs or alcohol is similar to providing these services to other women.

The clinician needs to take a history before deciding on the most appropriate treatment. The history should ask about current and past drug use, current alcohol use, and previous (or current) history of sexually transmitted diseases, including episodes of pelvic inflammatory disease, needle sharing, and infection with blood-borne viruses. Lifestyle issues, in particular the ease of taking regular medication, should also be looked into: there is little point giving a once a day oral contraception if the women is living in chaotic circumstances with frequent changes of address where she is likely to forget taking her medication.

The choice of contraception will depend on contraindications for the different options: a woman with high risk of sexually transmitted diseases should be discouraged from using an intrauterine device and one with liver disease or hepatitis C or B should avoid the oral combined contraceptive pill. The progesterone only pill may not be appropriate where there are concerns about stability.

A woman who is dependent on alcohol may need specialist assessment as her choices of family planning are likely to be predicated by the state of her liver and general physical state. It may be more appropriate in these women, where there are many physical problems, to take the safest option, which is the depot progesterone injection.

The new contraceptive devise, Implanon™ (Organon), could have a very useful place for drug-using women. Implanon is a progestogen only contraceptive implant. It consists of a small plastic rod about the size of a matchstick, which is inserted just under the skin on the inside of the upper arm. The rod is flexible and not likely to be visible. The hormone is released slowly from the device into the bloodstream over three years. Implanon is highly effective at preventing pregnancy. In clinical trials so far, no pregnancies have been reported by women using this implant. It is particularly useful for women who cannot tolerate oestrogen, which is contained in most oral contraceptives. Women who have difficulty remembering to take daily contraception may prefer this method. However, it should not be used in women who have severe liver disease.

Treatment for women

As this chapter has described, women drug users have complex needs, which are not always recognised or met by some existing drug services. For example, approaches to treatment need to be sensitive to the possible sexual and physical abuse histories of women, as well as the gender-specific potential consequences associated with substance abuse. Acknowledging and supporting both men and women who are primary carers of children is also a critical need for drug services and attending to issues that include parenting skills, and housing and schooling needs are as important as determining basic medical needs and drug stabilisation. These are as follows:

▶ food, clothing, and shelter

▶ transportation

▶ job counselling and training

▶ legal assistance

▶ literacy training and educational opportunities

▶ parenting management techniques

▶ couples counselling

▶ medical care

▶ child care

▶ social services

▶ social support

▶ psychological assessment and mental health care

▶ family planning services.

There are also other considerations in providing treatment for women, including the need for outreach efforts that involve community based workers and organisations; gender sensitive services to address self-esteem, anxiety, depression, sexuality, communication skills and personal health; screening for domestic violence; HIV intervention and skills development.

Identification and screening

The most important first goal is to engage women in treatment. Women are more likely than men to attend their general practitioner for general health, family planning and antenatal needs. Thus the general practitioner and practice nurse have the opportunity to identify drug and/or alcohol users and provide appropriate intervention. Primary care professionals are random in their questioning about drug use, with only 20% of general practitioners reporting that they 'occasionally' ask pregnant women about alcohol or drug use while 60% reported that they never asked.

Women are more likely to disclose their drug use to maternity staff than to their general practitioner, perhaps reflecting the concern for the adverse effects of their drug use on their infant. However, this may also reflect perceived indifference from primary care professionals to their drug use.[29]

The identification of women with a substance misuse problem can be done through the use of initial screening questions. Most screening instruments are sensitive to low-level misuse of a substance, but are less sensitive to determining a range of use and dependence (that is, they have a ceiling effect). Screening instruments have been developed to help clinicians identify women with substance misuse problems.

The AUDIT is a 10-item screening instrument developed by the World Health Organization designed to screen for a range of drinking problems and in particular for hazardous and harmful consumption. It is particularly suitable for primary health care settings and has been used in a number of different countries and with diverse cultural groups. Two instruments that were developed specifically to identify at-risk drinking in pregnant women are the T-ACE and the TWEAK.[30-32] Further research has suggested that both are also sensitive to the detection of alcohol problems in non-pregnant women. Both measures are easily administered and scored. A cut-off score of two or more on either measure is used to indicate that at-risk drinking may be present in pregnant and non-pregnant women.

Referral to other agencies

Women who access drug services often find that there are significant shortcomings in the care that is offered. A Home Office report has suggested a range of ways in which services can be improved to increase their accessibility. See Table 18.2. These include making stronger links, including shared guidelines/protocols and training, with staff and key partners, such as social workers, general practitioners, nurses, and midwives.

Primary care organisations can encourage women to access their services by addressing childcare issues, assisting in transport, and providing safe women only spaces. General practitioners can provide the opportunities for early intervention and signposting to appropriate treatment.

Table 18.2 **Factors influencing drug service provision for female drug users**

Lack of childcare and transport facilities	One of women's main areas of dissatisfaction with treatment services involves lack of childcare facilities. Childcare and other domestic responsibilities and lack of transport have been identified as key barriers to accessing services[33]
Stigmatisation and child protection issues	Fear that children will be removed from them prevents women from admitting to their drug-using problem
Lack of women only services	Some women feel intimidated talking in mixed counselling groups – usually dominated by men
Lack of provision for ethnic minority women	Accessing services may be more difficult for ethnic minority women than white women[34]
Poor social support networks	Support from significant others, especially partners, appears to be an important influence on whether women present and remain in treatment. Women, if they inject drugs, are more likely to have drug-using partner who also injects
Weakness in maternity services	Klee *et al.*, in 1995,[35] found that pregnant drug users received conflicting and confusing advice and information from maternity units. Findings from a survey of all the NHS maternity units in England and Wales showed that only 29% of units had formal links with local drug agencies and over 50% (57%) routinely admitted babies of drug-using women to high dependency units[36]
Negative attitudes of health professionals	Research has identified that health professionals have negative views of drug-taking women

Source: Becker *et al.*[30]

Conclusion

Primary care practitioners have a unique opportunity to educate women about their substance use and to identify those with problems. Early identification and intervention can significantly limit the adverse consequences of all substance abuse and clinicians need to recognise the differences in risk factors, presentation, and treatment relevant to women.

References

1. Ramsey M, Baker P, Goulden C, *et al. Drug misuse declared in 2000: results from the British Crime Survey*. Home Office Research Study 224. London: Home Office, 2001.

2. National Statistics Office. *Living in Britain 2001, Results of 2001 British Household Survey*. London: HMSO, 2001 (available at: www.statistics.gov.uk).

3. Goddard E. Higgins V. *Drug Use, Smoking and Drinking among Teenagers in 1999*. London: HMSO, 2000.

4. Substance Abuse and Mental Health Services Administration, Office of Applied Studies. *National Household Survey on Drug Abuse: Population Estimates 1993*. Rockville, MD: the Administration, 1994.

5. Hopwood M, Southgate E, Kippax S, *et al.* The injection of methadone syrup in New South Wales: patterns of use and increased harm after partial banning of injecting equipment. *Aust N Z J Public Health* 2003; **27**(5): 551–5.

6. Bennett G A, Velleman R D, Barter G, Bradbury C. Gender differences in sharing injecting equipment by drug users in England. *AIDS Care* 2000; **12**(1): 77–87.

7. Department of Health. *Statistics from the Regional Drug Misuse Databases on Drug Misusers in Treatment in England, 2000/01*. Bulletin 2001/03. London: DoH, 2001.

8. Marsh J, D'Aunno Smith B. Increasing access and providing social services to improve drug abuse treatment for women with children. *Addiction* 2000; **95**: 1237–48.

9. Drug and Alcohol Services Information System (DASIS) report: women in treatment for smoked cocaine. USA: DASIS, 2003 (available at: www.oas.samhsa.gov/2k3/FemCrack/FemCrack.cfm).

10. Canadian Centre on Substance Abuse and Canadian Public Health Association. *HIV, AIDS and Injection Drug Use: a National Action Plan*. Ottawa: CCSA, CPHA, 1997.

11. Brewer D D, Fleming C B, Haggerty K P, Catalano R F. Drug use predictors of partner violence in opiate-dependent women. *Violence Vict* 1998; **13**(2): 107–15.

12. Brook D W, Brook J S, Whiteman M, *et al.* Psychosocial risk factors for HIV transmission in female drug users. *Am J Addict* 1997; **6**(2): 129–57.

13. Freeman R C, Rodriguez G M, French J F. A comparison of male and female intravenous drug users' risk behaviours for HIV infection. *Am J Drug Alcohol Abuse* 1994; **2**(2): 129–57.

14. Camacho L M, Bartholomew N G, Joe G W, *et al.* Gender, cocaine and during treatment HIV risk reduction amount injection opioid users in methadone maintenance. *Drug Alcohol Depend* 1996; **41**: 1–7.

15. Whynot E. Women who use injection drugs: the social context of risk. *CMAJ* 1998; **159**: 355–8.

16. Strathdee S A, Patrick D M, Currie S L, *et al.* Needle exchange is not enough: lessons from the Vancouver Injection Drug Use Study. *AIDS* 1997; **11**: F59–F65.

17. Dawe S, Harnett P H, Staiger P, Dadds M. Parent training skills and methadone maintenance: clinical opportunities and challenges. *Drug and Alcohol Dependence* 2000; **60**: 1–13.

18. Wechsberg W M, Craddock S G, Hubbard R L. How are women who enter substance abuse treatment different than men? A gender comparison from the Drug Abuse Treatment Outcome Study (DATOS). *Drugs & Society* 1998; **13(1/2)**: 97–115.

19. Jones H E, Velex M L, McCaul M E, Svikis D S. Special treatment issues for women. In: Strain E C, Stitzer M L. (Eds). *Methadone Treatment for Opioid Dependence.* Baltimore: Johns Hopkins University Press, 1999; 251–80.

20. Powis B, Griffiths P, Gossop M, Strang J. The differences between male and female drug users: community samples of heroin and cocaine users compared. *Substance Use and Misuse* 1996; **31(5)**: 529–43.

21. Gossop M, Powis B, Griffiths P, Strang J. Sexual behaviour and its relationship to drug taking amongst prostitutes in south London. *Addiction* 1994; **89**: 961–70.

22. Falk R S, Wang J, Siegal H A, Carlson R G. The prevalence of psychiatric disorder among a community sample of crack cocaine users: an exploratory study with practical implications. *Journal Nervous Mental Disorders* 2004; **192**: 503–7.

23. Linehan M M. *Cognitive-Behavioural Treatment of Borderline Personality Disorder.* New York: Guilford Press, 1993.

24. Linehan M M, Dimeff L A, Reynolds S K. Dialectal behaviour therapy versus comprehensive validation therapy plus 12-step for the treatment of opioid dependent women meeting criteria for borderline personality disorder. *Drug and Alcohol Dependence* 2002; **67(1)**: 13–26.

25. Suchman N, Luthar S S. Maternal addiction, child maladjustment and socio-demographic risks: Implications for parenting behaviours. *Addiction* 2000; **95(9)**: 1417–28.

26. Brook J, Whiteman M, Zheng L. Intergenerational transmission of risks for problem behaviours. *Journal of Abnormal Child Psychology* 2002; **30**: 65–76.

27. Chander G, McCaul M E, Co-occurring psychiatric disorder in women with addictions. *Obset Gynecol Clin North Am* 2003; **30(3)**; 469–81.

28. Morrison C L, Ruben R M, Beeching N J. Female sexual health problems in a drug dependence clinic. *International Journal of STD and AIDS* 1995; **6**: 201–3.

29. White C, Best D, Farrell S, Gerada C, *et al. Services Providing for Substance Misusing Women who are Pregnant or Parenting.* A needs analysis in North Lambeth, 2001. National Addiction Centre, London (unpublished report).

30. Becker J. Duffy C. *Women Drug Users and Drugs Service Provision: Service-level Responses to Engagement and Retention.* DPAS 17. London: Home Office, 2002.

31. Sokol R J, Martier S S, Ager J W. The T-ACE questions: Practical prenatal detection of risk-drinking. *American Journal of Obstetrics and Gynecology* 1989; **160**: 863–8.

32. Russell M. New assessment tools for risk drinking during pregnancy: T-ACE, TWEAK, and others. *Alcohol Health and Research World* 1994; **18**: 55–61.

33. Marsh J C, D'Anino T A, Smith D B. Increasing access and providing social services to improve drug abuse treatment for women and children. *Addiction* 2000; **95(8)**: 1237–48.

34. Oyefeso A, Ghodse II, Keating A, *et al. Drug Treatment Needs of Black and Minority Ethnic Residents of the London Borough of Merton.* London: Addictions Resource Agency for Commissioners, 2000.

35. Klee II, Lewis S, Jackson M. *Illicit Drug Use, Pregnancy and Early Motherhood: an Analysis of the Impediments to Effective Service Delivery.* An interim report to the Department of Health Task Force to review services for drug misusers. London: DoH, 1995.

36. Morrison C. Siney C. Maternity services for drug misusers in England and Wales: a national survey. *Health Trends* 1995; **27(1)**: 15–17.

CHAPTER 19

Drug use by parents

Sharon Dawe and Clare Gerada

IN THIS CHAPTER

Introduction ‖ Pregnancy and drug use ‖ The impact of drug use on in utero *development and neonatal outcome ‖ Specific drug effects ‖ Treatment services for drug-using pregnant women ‖ Buprenorphine in pregnancy ‖ Treatment of neonatal abstinence syndrome – hospital or community? ‖ Impact of parental drug use on child outcome ‖ Treatment options for drug-using mothers in the postpartum period ‖ Treatment options that improve outcome for children ‖ Responsibilities of the primary care team ‖ Pre-birth planning meeting ‖ After the birth and beyond ‖*

Introduction

Box 19.1 **Case study**

Jane, aged 35 years, is a well-known patient of the practice. She was a rather chaotic heroin user in the past – injecting at least 1 g/day for a number of years. For the past two years she has been receiving a maintenance buprenorphine prescription from her general practitioner but has recently met up with an ex-boyfriend who had led her to start using crack cocaine.

She has a son aged eight years and there have been concerns about his erratic school attendance. In recent months, things seem to have deteriorated. She has begun to use crack cocaine on almost a daily basis, she has had to leave her flat and squat with friends through nonpayment of rent, and her son has been living occasionally with her and occasionally with his maternal grandmother.

Her relationship with her boyfriend is one marked by a great deal of domestic violence.

She presents to her general practitioner 13 weeks pregnant, desperate to try to 'make a go at becoming drug free'. Her drug use at this time is around 1 g heroin, crack cocaine, benzodiazepines, and cannabis. She also smokes 20 cigarettes per day and drinks around a bottle of strong cider per day.

Jane's case highlights many of the issues facing women who misuse drugs and/or alcohol, in particular issues around parenting and pregnancy.

As discussed in Chapter 18 many more women are developing problems with drug and alcohol use and as a consequence the number presenting who have parenting responsibilities is also increasing.

The outcome for children brought up in families in which either or both parents use drugs is often poor. However, drug use *per se* cannot be considered as the only, or even the critical, factor influencing this outcome. Outcome is the consequence of the particular balance of risk and protective factors present in each child's life.[1] For example, maternal drug use during pregnancy may have a direct impact on the development of the foetus, with the consequences of use a function of the nature and quantity of the substance(s) used. Maternal drug use in the early neonatal period may also impact on the quality of the mother–child relationship and this in turn will influence the nature of the relationship in later childhood.

The environmental and social factors associated with substance dependence can impact on multiple domains of family life. The use of illicit drugs brings with it additional lifestyle problems that arise from involvement in criminal activities including risk of arrest, imprisonment, and an association with drug dealers and users. Such risk factors may, in turn, be offset by protective factors such as a strong attachment to a significant carer, academic ability, consistent parenting practise with clear rules, and a socialised peer group in late childhood and early adolescence.

This chapter provides a brief review of the major effects of drug use during pregnancy, in the early postnatal period, and in later childhood. Treatments and strategies that have been demonstrated to reduce the risk factors and promote protective factors in children's lives where either or both parents misuse drugs are reviewed. Finally, suggestions are made regarding the adoption of empirically validated treatment strategies by the primary health care team that may increase protective factors.

Pregnancy and drug use

Exact prevalence rates of illicit drug use in pregnancy are difficult to obtain, as national surveys addressing the use of drugs by pregnant women are infrequent and the figures obtained are regarded as estimates.

There is, however, some consistency in the figures obtained across the United States, Australia, and the United Kingdom. The National Household Survey on Drug Abuse reported that approximately 3.4% of pregnant women had used an illicit drug in the past month.[2] Similar rates of drug use during pregnancy were reported by a national survey conducted in Australia.[3] There have been at least two surveys conducted on postpartum reports of prenatal substance use. The National Pregnancy and Health Survey conducted in the United States found approximately 1 in 1,000 pregnant women reported the use of heroin during their pregnancy.

Data from the United Kingdom, obtained by anonymous urine testing in 1,000 women (12 weeks gestation) found that a significant proportion tested positive for cannabis (8.5%) with fewer testing positive for opiates and cocaine (1.4% and 1.1% respectively).[4] A postal survey conducted in 1993 of maternity services in England and Wales estimated the incidence of babies born to drug-using women to be 0.81 per 1,000 deliveries.[5]

A survey conducted by the Home Office of all maternity units in the United Kingdom in 2000 found that 75% of responding agencies had contact with pregnant drug users. The maternity units estimated that 1% of deliveries were to problem drug users and a similar number to problem drinkers. The majority (82%) reported an increase in the number of pregnant drug users over the previous five-year period.[6] Many clinicians report that pregnancy appears to act as a catalyst for women with drug problems to seek treatment with the stated goal of minimising risk for their unborn child. Unfortunately there are a number of women who do not feel able to engage in treatment services, with concerns about the involvement of social services and previous adverse experiences with obstetric units being the reasons for their reluctance to make contact. It is not uncommon for women with such concerns to present late in pregnancy or even in labour,[7] thereby increasing the risk for both mother and child.

The impact of drug use on *in utero* development and neonatal outcome

Researchers and clinicians are still learning about the effects of drugs in pregnancy on the developing infant. (See Table 19.1 for summary.) Alcohol and drug use by pregnant women are harmful to the developing embryo and foetus, although teasing apart the specific contributions of each substance to adverse child outcome proves difficult in practice, not least because polydrug use (including routine use of cigarettes) occurs frequently in this population.

The risks to the neonate include intrauterine growth retardation, birth defects, altered neurological behaviour, and withdrawal syndromes. Subsequent behavioural, developmental, and neurological function may also be impaired.

Women who are using illegal drugs also have more infections such as hepatitis B and C, dental abscesses, chlamydia, gonorrhoea, herpes, HIV, and urinary tract infections. General ill health and poor diet are common. Thus, antenatal exposure to any drug should be seen as a possible marker for multiple medical and social risk factors all of which can adversely affect the developing foetus and pregnancy outcome.

Specific drug effects

Most adverse effects of antenatal drug exposure are short term, with catch-up growth and resolution of withdrawal and prior neurobehavioural abnormalities found over time. The exception to this is alcohol, which is linked to life-long impairments (i.e., growth retardation, nervous system anomalies including intellectual impairment and microcephaly) and possibly cigarette-related behavioural effects.[8] Bearing this in mind the sections below summarise the possible direct adverse effects of specific substances.

Opioids

The use of opioids during pregnancy is associated with low birth weight, premature delivery and small head circumference. Babies exposed to opiates in pregnancy are likely to experience neonatal addiction and withdrawal symptoms. The syndrome, characterised by irritability, hyperactivity, abnormal sleep, poor sucking, and high-pitched cry, can persist for two to three weeks after birth, longer in infants born to mothers who are heavy users of benzodiazepines.[9] There appears to be a significant relationship between maternal methadone dose at delivery and the severity of neonatal withdrawal,[10] the mean duration of hospital stay, the proportion of infants needing treatment and the mean duration of treatment; all increase markedly with increasing doses of methadone.

Severity of withdrawal tends to be more prolonged but more predicable with methadone than heroin and diminishes with maternal methadone doses of less than 30 mg by delivery.[11]

Other studies have failed to find a correlation between maternal dose at delivery and the risk of neonatal withdrawal.[12] Most importantly, with appropriate care and after controlling for socioeconomic status and cigarette smoking there are no long-term effects of *in utero* exposure and no differences between those exposed to opiates and those who are not in the short term.

Cocaine and amfetamines

In utero exposure to cocaine, with or without other drug exposure, is associated with significant increases in neonatal mortality from intrauterine growth retardation and prematurity.[13] The powerful vasoconstrictor effect of cocaine may be the factor in fetal growth retardation.

Spontaneous abortion and premature birth are also more frequent in women who use cocaine, with one study finding that the increased risk of spontaneous abortion was unrelated to cocaine dose.[14] The increased risk of abruptio placentae occurs only when cocaine is used close to delivery.[15]

There is a link between sudden infant death syndrome and *in utero* cocaine exposure and there have been reports of respiratory pattern abnormalities in cocaine-exposed infants as compared with methadone-exposed infants.[16]

Though 'crack babies' attracted considerable interest from the mid-1980s to mid-1990s there is no consistent evidence that intrauterine cocaine leads to long-term developmental problems in the children. Rather it is likely that the behavioural, developmental, and cognitive impairments found in the children of cocaine-using mothers are due to the constellation of environmental risks found in the households of severely cocaine-addicted mothers.[17,18]

Cannabis

There is some dispute whether cannabis causes direct teratogenic effects (as opposed to the effects caused by inhaling tobacco and its constituents). A recent study has found evidence that regular use of cannabis during pregnancy may result in a reduction of birth weight that is statistically independent of maternal and social background, maternal characteristics, or other substances used during pregnancy.[19]

Benzodiazepines

Benzodiazepines and their metabolites freely cross the placenta and newborn levels of benzodiazepines in the blood are about one to three times greater than maternal serum levels. An association between diazepam and an increased risk of cleft lip and/or palate and inguinal hernia has been suggested by several studies, although this is by no means conclusive.

Alcohol

Many pregnant women have drunk alcohol at some stage of their pregnancy and occasional consumption has not been linked to adverse child outcomes. The Royal College of Obstetricians and Gynaecologists in the United Kingdom recommends that although 'there is no conclusive evidence of adverse effects in either growth or IQ levels in moderate drinking ... women should be careful about alcohol consumption in pregnancy and limit this to no more than one standard drink per day'.[20]

The evidence that alcohol acts as a teratogen is extensive in both animal and human studies.[21] Heavy consumption of alcohol is associated with a range of abnormalities that are referred to as foetal alcohol syndrome and its less severe form, foetal alcohol effects.[22] The consequences of heavy alcohol use depend in part on timing of exposure with the primary teratogenic effects occurring during the first eight weeks of embryogenesis while exposure in later pregnancy affects growth, and behavioural and cognitive functioning. While there is a consensus amongst researchers that there is a relationship between high alcohol use and foetal alcohol effects, it is not clear at what dose such effects are likely to occur. Rates for foetal alcohol syndrome range from 0.05 to 0.3% of births and alcohol-related birth defects to as high as 0.5%.[23]

Maternal alcohol dependence can cause foetal alcohol syndrome characterised by:

▶ intrauterine growth retardation, with persistent postnatal poor growth in weight and height

▶ a pattern of specific minor physical anomalies that include a characteristic facial appearance

▶ central nervous system deficits, including microencephaly, delayed development, hyperactivity, attention deficit, learning difficulties.

These infants are reported to have a three and a half times elevated mortality rate.[24]

Table 19.1   **Summary of the effects of exposure to drugs on the foetus and infant**

Drug	Potential effects	Comments
Opioids	Small for dates Premature delivery Neonatal addiction Neonatal withdrawal syndrome	Small for dates effect persists even controlling for confounding variables. No differences in development by 2 years
Cocaine and amfetamines	Intrauterine death Premature delivery Intrauterine growth retardation (most consistent finding)	Conflicting evidence of the long-term sequela of long-term intrauterine expose to cocaine. Some report cognitive delay[1] although this is not consistently reported
Benzodiazepines	Opiate neonatal abstinence is prolonged if also exposed to benzodiazepines	No evidence of direct effect on foetal development
Tobacco	Spontaneous abortion Small for dates Stillbirth Premature delivery Sudden infant death	Maternal smoking is linked to increased risks of childhood asthma, sudden infant death, respiratory infections, and ear infections

Drug	Potential effects	Comments
Cannabis	If smoked similar effects to smoking tobacco cigarettes	It is unclear whether the effect is related to the route of use, i.e. smoking, rather than direct drug effect
Alcohol	Serious developmental problems, including delayed neurological development, growth impairments, and variety of physical abnormalities	Heavy drinking is common especially when on methadone maintenance

Treatment services for drug-using pregnant women

Pregnancy should be seen as a window of opportunity for recruiting women with a substance misuse problem into treatment. There is a strong consensus amongst clinicians that an encouraging and non-judgmental attitude towards the pregnant woman and her partner is important in enabling her to engage effectively with treatment services.[25]

Box 19.2   **Substitution treatment in pregnancy**

> ✓ Enables stabilisation of drug use and lifestyle
>
> ✓ Reduces need for additional illicit drug use
>
> ✓ Facilitates access to antenatal and other health care
>
> ✓ Reduces risks inherent in illicit drug use lifestyle

There have been many services established that aim to attract drug-using women into treatment in early stages of their pregnancy with some evidence that such services improve health and help the woman stabilise drug use which, in turn, is associated with better neonatal outcome.[26] (See Box 19.2 for principles and Table 19.2 for summary of management.)

The general practitioner is ideally placed to provide both antenatal treatment and assist in the stabilisation of drug use by careful prescribing practices. In order to encourage take-up of antenatal care, a pregnant drug-using woman needs to believe that the general practitioner adopts a non-judgmental and non-punitive attitude towards her drug use. This does not imply that such use should be condoned by those in the practice, but rather that a caring attitude is expressed with an emphasis on helping the woman achieve the best outcome for herself and her baby. Although drug use is clearly not in the best interest of the infant the detrimental effects of such use are compounded by erratic use and a lack of antenatal care. Providing an environment in which there is a strong and clear message that pregnant drug users will be fairly treated is an important first step in ensuring that women attend for care.

The general principles of best practice should underpin services for pregnant drug-using women. Stabilising drug use, in the case of opioid dependence, and helping to minimise other drug or alcohol use is essential. This can be done in conjunction with drug and alcohol treatment agencies. If the woman is reluctant to attend such agencies the general practitioner and the primary health care team may be in the best position to help her in her endeavour to reduce drug use.

For those women dependent on opioids, oral methadone substitution is strongly recommended. Methadone treatment for opiate addiction has been consistently associated with improvements in many domains of life including reduction in illicit drug use, illegal activities related to obtaining illicit drugs – including, for many women, prostitution – and an opportunity to address issues such as housing or parenting of other children. A stable dose of methadone ensures that the infant experiences minimal *in utero* withdrawal and is not exposed to drugs of unknown concentration and impurities. Given the above, the importance of providing adequate dosages of methadone is perhaps even more important than in the non-pregnant state. This can be as a steady dose or an initial maintenance dose that is then gradually reduced.

It is generally recommended that women are maintained on methadone rather than attempt detoxification during the pregnancy as this increases the chances that the woman remains in contact with her prescribing doctor and continues to receive antenatal care. Detoxification from opioids has also been associated with an increase in the risk of spontaneous abortion in the first trimester and adverse outcome, including neonatal death or preterm labour in the third trimester.[27,28]

It is important to realise that methadone doses may need to be increased as pregnancy progresses particularly in the last trimester as increased blood volume, metabolic changes, and drug metabolism of the foetal/placental unit may result in the onset of maternal withdrawal symptoms at what was previously an adequate dose.[29] It is critical that both doctor and patient are clear that this is not a consequence of the use of additional non-prescribed opioids, but rather a direct effect of pregnancy. Increasing the dose of methadone should in principle also increase the risk of neonatal withdrawal. Although there is some support for this, there are some surprising findings in which higher methadone doses have been related to higher birth weight and larger head circumference compared with lower doses.[30,31] The general conclusion drawn from these studies has been that the higher doses were more effective at minimising other non-prescribed drug use, in particular heroin, which has been associated with poorer outcome.

Buprenorphine in pregnancy

The safety of buprenorphine during pregnancy and breastfeeding remains uncertain at this stage owing to a lack of completed studies evaluating the safety of this medication in pregnancy. Research, however, is continuing and to date around thirty human studies have been reported with most being retrospective studies or single case reports.

Researchers have[32] reported on 15 cases of buprenorphine maintained pregnancies. Fourteen were transferred from either methadone or long-acting morphine and one inducted from street heroin onto buprenorphine. Induction on to buprenorphine occurred as a three-day inpatient admission without any report of foetal adverse effect. Birth outcome was unremarkable with no significant problems other than intrauterine growth retardation in one baby.

The most rigorous study to date compared outcomes of 93 pregnant women maintained on methadone with 153 women maintained on high dose buprenorphine.[33] The prevalence of neonate withdrawal was the same in both groups (65%). There were few differences in the two groups with the only neonatal difference being a slightly higher rate of prematurity in the methadone group (18% compared with 9%).

At the present time methadone maintenance remains the treatment of choice for pregnant and breastfeeding women because it is considered the safest option. Women who conceive whilst on buprenorphine treatment are currently advised to transfer to methadone maintenance.[34] Some pregnant women may decline to transfer to methadone treatment and the clinician will have to weigh up the balance of risks for pregnant women who may then resort to heroin use.

Table 19.2   **Summary of management of pregnant drug users**

Assessment	Pregnant drug users and their partners should be considered high priority and assessment undertaken as quickly as possible. Assessment in pregnancy is similar to that for any pregnant women – although there should be special emphasis on social factors and support networks
	Opioid antagonist (e.g. naloxone) challenge should not be undertaken in pregnant women owing to risk that acute withdrawal might precipitate miscarriage or premature labour
Substitution treatment	Methadone maintenance is the mainstay of management of opioid dependence in pregnancy

Continued over

Breastfeeding	As a general principal, breastfeeding should be encouraged for pregnant opiate dependent women maintained on methadone. The amounts of methadone secreted in breast milk are minimal and are unlikely to have any adverse effects on the neonates. Contraindications to breastfeeding include ongoing illicit substance use and HIV positive status. Hepatitis C positivity is generally not a contraindication to breastfeeding
Reduction	Withdrawal from methadone maintenance is not recommended owing to the high risk of relapse. If a patient does want to reduce it is probably best done in the second trimester. Reductions of between 5–10 mg per week are recommended

Treatment of neonatal abstinence syndrome – hospital or community?

Approximately half of infants suffering from neonatal abstinence syndrome require pharmacological treatment. A variety of agents, including morphine, methadone, chlorpromazine, phenobarbitone, and diazepam, have been administered with the aim of controlling withdrawal symptoms.[35] Despite the large numbers of infants requiring treatment for the syndrome, few agents have been examined in randomised trials with long-term outcome measures. Affected infants can require treatment for many months, leading to a prolonged stay on the neonatal unit. This has a major impact not only on maternal and infant bonding, but also on bed occupancy.

A hospital in Dublin reported that at any one time three neonatal beds were always occupied by infants with neonatal abstinence syndrome.[36] A proportion of such infants require neonatal care because of problems not directly related to their drug withdrawal, such as prematurity, but the duration of stay and associated hospital costs can be reduced for infants who are otherwise 'healthy' by discharging them home once they are stable on treatment. A concern regarding such an approach, however, is that parents who misuse drugs may not have sufficiently competent organisational skills to comply with the outpatient follow up schedule required by infants with medical needs.

In one survey only half of women who were misusing drugs kept their infants' outpatient appointments. It has been suggested that compliance with clinical attendance can be improved,[37] but this requires establishment of a hospital-based weekly follow up clinic with continuity of care provided by staff with whom the families have become familiar and that meets all the infants' needs, including vaccinations, sub-specialist appointments and prescriptions for the treatment of neonatal abstinence syndrome. In the United Kingdom, the general practitioner and the baby's health visitor are important in maintaining continuity of care and can be useful for monitoring treatment in the baby and mother. Whatever the follow up package adopted, community care for infants with neonatal abstinence syndrome and ongoing treatment needs must be adequately resourced. Whether such management, compared with prolonged hospital admission, is more cost effective in improving the long-term outcome of affected infants requires further research.

Impact of parental drug use on child outcome

There is now a substantial body of evidence indicating that parental drug and alcohol use is associated with a range of adverse child outcomes including behavioural, emotional,[38] financial, and social problems that taken together can impact adversely on child outcome.[39-42] The impact of parental substance misuse will vary according to the age and developmental stage of the child.

Parenting of a young infant, particularly one where there has been the need for special care and/or a protracted period in hospital after birth places considerable demands on parents. For young women especially, often single parents who are also attempting to remain on methadone programmes, this period of time is particularly fraught with difficulties. Women often report high levels of depressed mood on methadone and this may impact on maternal responsiveness to the child's needs. Maternal depression has been identified as one of the major risk factors for the development of emotional, behavioural, and somatic problems in children and may be influenced by a range of factors including marital relationship, lack of social support, and financial stress amongst others.[43]

As the children develop, behavioural difficulties emerge in the early toddler years, becoming established patterns of behavioural and emotional problems, in particular oppositional, defiant, and noncompliant behaviours in the preschool and early primary years.[43]

Poor outcomes are found across generations.[44] Specific problems found in substance abusing families include inconsistent parenting, poor limit setting, reversal of the parent–child care giving role, harsh discipline, violence, and neglect. The children are also at a greater risk of developing a substance misuse problem themselves.[45] Children of alcohol-dependent parents are at two to ten times greater risk of developing problematic alcohol use than other children and are at increased risk of other substance misuse and dependence, including nicotine.[46]

There are also high rates of child abuse and neglect in substance misusing families with the result that there is often intervention by social services. This was highlighted in a recent UK report that found that approximately 54% of drug-using parents had children living elsewhere (45% with other members of their family, and 9% in care). The proportion of parents not living with their children had increased since the previous survey in 1996. Figure 19.1 reproduces data derived from national surveys elucidating the number of drug-using parents in England and Wales. For more information, the reader is encouraged to read the full Advisory Council Drug Misuse Report, *Hidden Harm*.[6]

Figure 19.1 **Number of drug using parents (England, Wales)**

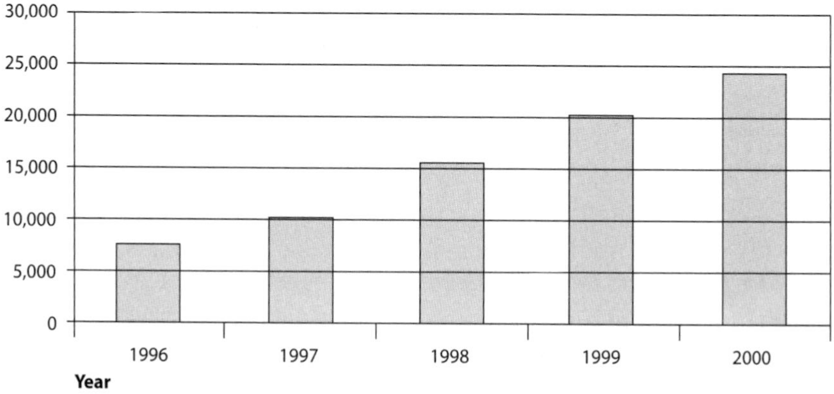

Data from Hidden Harm

There are a number of factors associated with the removal of a child from a family in which there is problematic drug use, with the primary reason being the high risk of child abuse and neglect.[47,48] Other factors associated with a more stable lifestyle, such as low risk sexual and injecting practices and minimal illicit drug and alcohol in the preceding six months, also increase the rates of mothers retaining primary care of their children.[49] Drug-using parents who had the care of their children had fewer risk factors than parents whose children lived elsewhere, with the former less likely to be sharing injecting equipment, having less regular use of stimulants, and having more stable accommodation.[50] See Table 19.3.

Children who have been taken into care also have poor developmental outcomes that include conduct problems and anxiety and depression and place greater demands on mental health services for treatment.[51,52] There is some evidence that the fostering experience can contribute uniquely to negative outcomes for children.[51] This highlights the importance of both improving the foster care system to ensure that problems are not compounded and developing interventions that decrease the potential for child abuse and neglect in substance using families.

Table 19.3 **Factors associated with greatest risk of a child not living with one or other parent**

Social risk factors	Health risk factors	Drug use risk factors
Homelessness or unstable accommodation	Depression	Heavy alcohol use
Poverty	High risk sexual behaviour	Drug use up to delivery
Living with another user	Two or more children	Heroin use (women)
Living alone or with strangers		Cocaine use (men)
Involvement with criminal justice system		High risk drug taking behaviour

Treatment options for drug-using mothers in the postpartum period

Intervention from the primary care team to support a drug-using mother with a young infant may well be associated with an improved outcome for both mother and infant. Interventions that focus on visiting high-risk mothers and their infants in their homes have been extensively evaluated, particularly in North America.

Since the early work of Olds and colleagues who demonstrated significant improvement at 15 years for those children whose high risk mothers had received intensive home visiting, there have been a number of systematic attempts to determine the qualities of home visiting programmes that are associated with the strongest effects. Based on the findings from a meta-analysis of 22 studies, MacLeod and Nelson concluded that home visiting of high risk families works to improve child outcome if the home visits cover a period longer than six months and consist of at least 12 visits.[53,54]

An ancillary issue relates to the professional background of the home visitor who in a number of home visiting models is a trained layperson with interest working with high risk families. Surestart in the United Kingdom uses these principles of targeting high risk families and aims to intervene early with problem families. It provides an intensive and flexible home visiting intervention which aims to reduce the level of maternal stressors impacting on child development whilst minimising the risk of child maltreatment and the potential harms of drug use on the child and the family. Mothers are encouraged to access services in the community to reduce levels of maternal stress and isolation.

A similar programme called the Parents Under Pressure (Babies) programme is also undergoing evaluation in Australia and engages drug-using women in the later stages of their pregnancy through the first 12 months of their infant's life. The focus of this programme is on either stabilisation or cessation of drug use (including tobacco), affect regulation, and establishment of social support networks.

General practitioners and health visitors can provide a critical role in helping women in the transition to parenthood by providing ongoing support through home visiting.

Treatment options that improve outcome for children

Although interventions with a focus on improving parenting skills have been shown to produce enduring change in children's behaviour,[55] there has been a growing consensus in the drug and alcohol field that families in which there is significant substance abuse require more intensive interventions that address a range of factors. Effective interventions in multi-problem families need to be flexible and highly individualised to address the particular issues of each presenting family. The somewhat simplistic model of parent training has been replaced by a more sophisticated model of parenting interventions in which the needs of the family are given greater emphasis, with programmes being specifically tailored to meet identified needs.

There have been encouraging findings from several research groups conducting intensive parenting interventions with multi-problem families. Henggeler and colleagues have developed an intensive, multisystemic intervention called multisystemic therapy. It has been evaluated in families in which there is either, or both, chronic juvenile offending and juveniles with substance use disorder.[56–58] This form of intensive intervention has been shown to produce better outcomes than 'usual services' provided to youth such as probation, individual counselling, and community-based eclectic treatment.[59] The major benefits found have been a reduction in delinquency and an improvement in family functioning.

Catalano et al. completed a large-scale randomised trial of an intensive behavioural family therapy programme, Focus on Families,[60] with parents on methadone maintenance with children aged between 3 and 14 years. The programme's intervention included relapse prevention for drug use and strategies for managing family conflict and parenting skills and was associated with lower rates of drug use and improvements in parental functioning compared with standard care.

Dawe and colleagues in Australia have developed the Parents Under Pressure programme, a multisystemic intervention that is designed to strengthen family relationships and teach effective child management techniques.[61] The programme emphasises the importance of the parents' management of their own emotional state using strategies outlined by Teasdale et al. and Linehan et al. as a precursor to effective parenting.[62, 63]

This focus is consistent with current research that highlights the negative impact of maternal psychopathology on the quality of parenting care provided to the child.[64,65] Compared with a brief intervention and standard care in the methadone clinic, those families receiving this intensive home based programme showed highly significant reductions in parental psychopathology including anxiety and depression, a reduction in child abuse potential, and an improvement in children's behaviour. These results were maintained to 12 months.

These studies demonstrate that intensive home based interventions can make significant changes in multiple-problem families. Although such interventions are time consuming, there is growing evidence that early interventions in multiple-problem families is cost effective and relatively inexpensive in terms of outcomes achieved.

There are now a number of studies in which the cost of conduct disorder, for example – a common outcome for children raised in families with substance abuse – has been estimated. In the United Kingdom, Scott and colleagues calculated that the average cost of children with conduct disorder was £15,382 (range £5,411 to as much as £40,896) over and above the normal expenditure by parents,[66] with the greatest cost falling on the families themselves, education authorities, health services, social services, and benefit agencies.[67] Follow up studies of antisocial children into adulthood show that by the age of 28 the mean individual cost was £70,019, a figure ten times higher than asymptomatic children.

Responsibilities of the primary care team

Parents with drug problems should be treated in the same way as other parents whose personal difficulties interfere with or lessen their ability to parent effectively. Engaging a pregnant drug-using women and her partner into treatment is probably the most effective intervention possible. Not only will it reduce her illicit drug use but it can also give her time to discuss and address other problematic areas.

The provision of adequate primary care for the children of problem drug users depends on both the child and the parent being registered with a GP and a parent who is willing to bring the child to the surgery.

The primary care team is an important aspect of care. Not only does a good practice ensure that the child has the basic child development tests, immunisations and so forth but they can also act as a focus of continuity and support for the parent. The primary care team can liaise with child and youth mental health services, where intensive parenting interventions are offered for multi-problem families. Although such services are currently few and far between in the United Kingdom, the need for such service development has been a major recommendation of the *Hidden Harm* report and in future years it is hoped that such services will become more accessible.

Prebirth planning meeting

Before birth, it is most likely that the GP and/or health visitor will be involved in a predelivery planning case conference in which potential risks are identified and strategies developed that may minimise these risks. An unborn child cannot be placed on an 'at risk' register and this planning meeting is merely to determine what, if any, anxieties there are amongst the professionals caring for the mother or father.

The GP and health visitor will often be well placed to provide information about the woman's previous history, her supports, and her housing or other difficulties. The GP may be asked to give some indication on how the woman has engaged in drug treatment and what the outcome of this treatment has been. The GP should give the information honestly and accurately – bearing in mind that they are not there to give expert advice but merely give an opinion based on their knowledge of the patient. Consent from the patient is required at this stage and it is good practice to discuss any report – written or verbal – with her beforehand and to encourage the patient and relevant family to be present at any meeting.

After the birth and beyond

A predischarge meeting may be called, especially if the baby has spent a length of time in a special care baby unit. In some cases, a child protection conference may be convened at any time after birth. These conferences are multiprofessional meetings, chaired by an independent person employed by a social services department who is not involved with the family. Depending on the age of the child, the participants include social workers, health visitors, doctors, teachers, police, psychologists, and nursery staff. Parents are invited to attend the conferences and if their age and understanding is sufficient, so will children.

It is important that any support offered by the primary care team is realistic and fits with current standard or normal primary care services. It is unlikely that in the long term a primary care team can provide intensive parenting interventions for example. Support in the immediate postnatal period may be possible and the importance of having a continuing relationship with a general practice – in which the medical needs of mother and child are met and regular, brief supportive counselling can be provided – should never be undervalued.

Further reading

Osborn D A, Cole M J, Jeffery H E. Opiate treatment for opiate withdrawal in newborn infants. In: Cochrane Collaboration. *Cochrane Library*. Issue 3. Chichester: John Wiley, 2004.

Standing Conference on Drug Abuse. *Drug-using Parents. Policy Guidelines for interagency working*. Local Government Drugs Forum, 1997.

References

1. Cicchetti D, Toth, S. Perspectives on research and practice in developmental psychopathology. In: Damon W. (Ed). *Handbook of Child Psychology*, 5th ed. Vol. 4. New York: John Wiley, 1998; 479–583.

2. Office of Applied Statistics, Substance Abuse and Mental Health Administration (SAMHSA). *National Household Survey on Drug Abuse* 1999 (available at: www.DrugAbuseStatistics.samhsa.gov).

3. Adhikari P, Summerill A. *National Drug Strategy Household Survey 1998*. Detailed findings. AIHW cat. no. PHE 27. Canberra: AIHW (Drug Statistics Series No. 6). NDSHS, 1998.

4. Farkas AG, Colbert DL, Erskine KJ. Anonymous testing for drug abuse in an antenatal population. *Br J Obstet Gynaecol* 1995; **102(7)**: 563–5.

5. Morrison C, Siney C. Maternity Services for drug misusers in England and Wales: a national survey. *Health Trends* 1995; **27(1)**: 15–17.

6. Advisory Council on the Misuse of Drugs. *Hidden Harm. Responding to the Needs of Children of Problem Drug Users*. London: Home Office, 2003.

7. Klee H, Lewis S, Jackson M. *Illicit Drug Use in Pregnancy and Early Motherhood: an Analysis of the Impediments to Effective Service Delivery*. London: DoH, 1995.

8. Chiriboga C A. Fetal Alcohol and Drug Effects. *Neurologist* 2003; **9(6)**: 267–79.

9. Coghlan D, Milner M, Clarke T, *et al.* Neonatal abstinence syndrome. *Irish Medical Journal* 1999; **92**: 123–5.

10. Dawe S, Gerada C, Strang J. Establishment of a liaison service for pregnant opiate-dependent women. *British Journal of Addiction* 1992; **87**: 867–71.

11. Osborn D A, Cole M J, Jeffery H E. Opiate treatment for opiate withdrawal in newborn infants. In: Cochrane Collaboration. *Cochrane Library*. Issue 3. Chichester: John Wiley, 2004.

12. Berghella V, Lim P J, Hill M K, *et al.* Maternal methadone dose and neonatal withdrawal. *Am J Obstet Gynecol* 2003; **189(2)**: 312–7.

13. Greene O, Varghese A, Tuamokumo F, *et al.* Perinatal outcome after cocaine + polydrug exposure. *Annals New York Academy of Sciences* 1998; **21(846)**: 396–8.

14. Ness R B, Grisso J A, Hirshinger N, *et al.* Cocaine and tobacco use and the risk of spontaneous abortion. *N Engl J Med* 1999; **340**: 333–9.

15. Ostrea E M, Brady M, Gause S. Drug screening of newborns by meconium analysis: A large scale, perspective, epidemiologic study. *Pediatrics* 1992; **89**: 107–13.

16. Bauer C R. Perinatal effects of prenatal drug exposure. *Clinics in Perinatology* 1999; **26**: 87–106.

17. Tronick E, Beeghly M. Prenatal cocaine exposure, child development, and the compromising effects of cumulative risks. *Clinics in Perinatology* 1999; **26**: 151–71.

18. Addis M, Ahmed S, *et al*. Fetal effects of cocaine: an updated meta-analysis. *Reprod Toxicol* 2001; **15**(4): 341–69.

19. Fergusson D M, Horwood J, Northstone K. Maternal use of cannabis and pregnancy outcome. *Br J Obstet Gynaecol* 2002; **109**: 21–7.

20. Wilkie S. Global overview of drinking recommendations and guidelines. *AIM Digest* (supplement) 1997; **4**: 2–4.

21. Clark C M, Li D, Conry J, *et al*. Structural and functional brain integrity of fetal alcohol syndrome in nonretarded cases. *Pediatrics* 2000; **105**(5): 1196–9.

22. Mattson S N, Schoenfield A M, Riley E P. Teratogenic effects of alcohol on brain and behaviour. *Alcohol Research and Health* 2001; **25**(3): 185–91.

23. O'Leary C. *Fetal Alcohol Syndrome: A Literature Review*. National Alcohol Strategy Occasional Paper. Canberra: Commonwealth Department of Health and Aging, Australia, 2002.

24. Habbick B F, Nawson J L, Synder R E, Casey R E. Mortality in foetal alcohol syndrome. *Canadian Journal of Public Health* 1997; **88**(3): 181–83.

25. Wilbourne P, Wallerstedt C, Dorato V, Curet L. Clinical management of methadone dependence during pregnancy. *Journal of Perinatal and Neonatal Nursing*, March 2001; **4**: 14.

26. Finnegan L P. Treatment issues for opioid–dependent women during the perinatal period. *Journal of Psychoactive Drugs* 1991; **23**: 191–201.

27. Kaltenback K, Berghella V, Finnegan L. Opioid dependence during pregnancy: Effects and management. *Obstet Gynecol Clin North Am* 1998; **(1)**: 139–51.

28. Zuspan F P, Gumper J A, Mejie-Zelay A, *et al*. Fetal stress from methadone withdrawal. *Am J Obstet Gynecol* 1977; **122**(1): 43–61.

29. Wilbourne P, Wallerstedt C, Dorata V, Curet L. Clinical management of methadone dependence during pregnancy. *Journal of Perinatal and Neonatal Nursing*, March 2001; **14**(4): 26–45.

30. Madden J D, Chappel J N, Zuspan F, *et al*. Observation and treatment of neonatal narcotic withdrawal. *Am J Obstet Gynecol* 1977; **127**(2): 199–201.

31. Kandall S R. Treatment strategies for drug exposed neonates. *Clin Perinatol* 1999; **26**(1): 231–243.

32. Schindler S D, Eder H, Ortner R, *et al*. Neonatal outcome following buprenorphine maintenance during conception and throughout pregnancy. *Addiction* 2003; **98**(1): 103–10(8).

33. Lejeune C S, Aubisson, Simmat-Durand London, *et al*. Withdrawal syndromes in neonates born to drug addictions on substitution treatment with methadone or high dose buprenorphine. *Ann Int Med* 2001; **152**(suppl 7): 21–7.

34. Dunlop AJ, Panjari M, O'Sullivan, H, et al. Clinical guidelines for the use of buprenorphine in pregnancy. Fitzroy, Turning Point Alcohol and Drug Centre 2003 (available at: www.turningpoint.org.au/library/CTG_Bup_Pregnancy_060104.pdf).

35. Johnson K, Gerada C, Greenough A. Treatment of neonatal abstinence syndrome. *Archives of Disease in Childhood* 2003; **88**: F 2–5.

36. Coghlan D, Milner M, Clarke T, *et al*. Neonatal abstinence syndrome. *Irish Medical Journal* 1999; **92**: 232–3.

37. Oei J, Feller J M, Lui K. Coordinated outpatient care of the narcotic-dependent infant. *Journal of Paediatrics and Child Health* 2001; **37**: 266–70.

38. Wilens T E, Biederman J, Kiely K, *et al*. Pilot study of behavioural and emotional disturbances in the high-risk children of parents with opioid dependence. *Journal of the American Academy of Child and Adolescent Psychiatrists* 1995; **34**: 779–85.

39. Zeitlin H. Children with alcohol misusing problems. *British Medical Bulletin* 1994; **50**: 139–51.

40. Rutter M, Rutter M. *Developing Minds: Challenge and Continuity across the Lifespan*. London: Penguin, 1992.

41. Barnard M. Forbidden questions: drug-dependent parents and the welfare of their children. *Addiction* 1999; **94**(8): 1109–11.

42. Hogan D M. Annotation: the psychological development and welfare of children of opiate and cocaine users: a review and research needs. *Journal of Child Psychology and Psychiatry* 1998; **39**: 609–19.

43. Cicchetti D, Rogosch F A, Toth S. Maternal depressive disorder and contextual risk. *Development and Psychopathology* 1998; **10**: 283–300.

44. Brook J, Whiteman M, Zheng L. Intergenerational transmission of risks for problem behaviours. *Journal of Abnormal Child Psychology* 2002; **30**: 65–76.

45. Nurco D, Blathcley R, Hanlon T, *et al*. Early deviance and related risk factors in the children of narcotic addicts. *American Journal of Drug and Alcohol Abuse* 1999; **25**: 25–45.

46. Sher K. Psychological characteristics of children of alcoholics. *Alcohol Health and Research World* 1997; **21**: 247–54.

47. Tracy E M. Maternal substance abuse: protecting the child, preserving the family. *Social Work* 1994; **39**: 534–40.

48. Chaffin M, Kelleher K, Hollenberg J. Onset of physical abuse and neglect: Psychiatric, substance abuse and social risk factors from prospective community data. *Child Abuse Neglect* 1996; **20**: 191–203.

49. Pilowski D, Lyles C M, Cross S I, *et al*. Characteristics of injection drug-using parents who retain their children. *Drug and Alcohol Dependence* 2001; **61**: 113–22.

50. Advisory Council on the Misuse of Drugs. Estimates of the scale of the problem. In: *Hidden Harm. Responding to the Needs of Children of Problem Drug Users*. London: Home Office, 2003: 20–8.

51. Dozier M, Albus K, Fisher P A, Sepulveda S. Interventions for foster parents: implications for developmental theory. *Development and Psychopathology* 2002; **14**(4): 843–60.

52. Leslie L K, Gordon J N, Ganger W, Gist K. Developmental delay in young children in child welfare by initial placement type. *Infant Mental Health Journal* 2002; **23**(5): 496–516.

53. Olds D, Henderson C R Jr, Cole R, *et al*. Long-term effects of nurse home visitation on children's criminal and antisocial behaviour. *JAMA* 1998; **280**(14): 1238–44.

54. Macleod J, Nelson G. Programs for the promotion of family wellness and the prevention of child maltreatment: A meta-analytic review. *Child Abuse and Neglect* 2000; **24**(9): 1127–49.

55. Dawe S, Harnett P H, Staiger P, Dadds M. Parent training skills and methadone maintenance: clinical opportunities and challenges. *Drug and Alcohol Dependence* 2000; **60**: 1–13.

56. Borduin C M, Henggeler S W, Blaske D M, Stein R J. Multisystemic treatment of adolescent sexual offenders. *International Journal of offender Therapy and Comparative Criminology* 1990; **35**: 105–14.

57. Henggeler S W, Melton G B, Smith L A, *et al*. Family preservation using multisystemic therapy: long term follow up to a clinical trial with serious juvenile offenders. *Journal of Child and Family Studies* 1993; **2**: 283–93.

58. Henggeler S W. Multisystemic therapy: an overview of clinical procedures, outcomes and policy implications. *Child Psychology and Psychiatry Review* 1999; **4**(1): 2–10.

59. Henggeler S W, Melton G B, Smith L A. Family preservation using multisystemic therapy: an effective alternative to incarcerating serious juvenile offenders. *Journal of Consulting and Clinical Psychology* 1992; **60**: 953–61.

60. Catalano R F, Gainey R R, Fleming C B, Haggerty K P, Johnson N O. An experimental intervention with families of substance abusers: One-year follow-up of the Focus on Families project. *Addiction* 1999; **94**: 241–54.

61. Dawe S, Harnett P H, Rendalls V, Staiger P. Improving family functioning and child outcome in methadone maintained families: The Parents Under Pressure Program. *Drug and Alcohol Review* 2003; **22**: 299–309.

62. Teasdale J D, Segal Z V, Williams J M, *et al.* (2000). Prevention of relapse/recurrence in major depression by mindfulness-based cognitive therapy. *Journal of Consulting and Clinical Psychology* 2000; **68**: 615–23.

63. Linehan M M, Dimeff L A, Reynolds S K. Dialectal behaviour therapy versus comprehensive validation therapy plus 12-step for the treatment of opioid dependent women meeting criteria for borderline personality disorder. *Drug and Alcohol Dependence* 2002; **67 (1)**: 13–26.

64. Beckwith L, Howard J, Espinosa M, Tyler R. Psychopathology, mother-child interaction, and infant development: Substance abusing mothers and their offspring. *Development and Psychopathology* 1999; **11**: 715–25.

65. Luthar S S, Cushing G, Merikangas K R, Rounsaville B J. Multiple jeopardy: risk and protective factors among addicted mother's offspring. *Development and Psychopathology* 1998; **10**: 117–36.

66. Scott S. Aggressive behaviour in childhood. *BMJ* 1998; **316**: 202–6.

67. Scott S, Knapp M, Henderson J, Maughan B. Financial cost of social exclusion: follow up study of antisocial children into adulthood. *BMJ* 2001; **323**: 1–5.

CHAPTER 20

Black and ethnic minorities

Alex Laffan and Clare Gerada

IN THIS CHAPTER

Introduction || Prevalence of use || Patterns of use || Causes of drug use ||
Barriers to treatment || Black and ethnic minority women || Good practice
and evidence of successful methods and models || Conclusion

Introduction

The term 'black and ethnic minority' (BEM) applies to all minority groups in the United Kingdom and the characteristics of these groups will vary enormously for each primary care practice. The patterns of drug use and the barriers or attractions to treatment can be very different for particular ethnic groups. The focus on treating opioid addiction in the United Kingdom in recent decades has simultaneously been a focus on the white working class, yet many of those from other BEM groups use other non-opioid drugs. This chapter will discuss ways that primary care practitioners and managers of services can ensure that BEM patients are given the treatment they require.

Prevalence of use[1]

Evidence from both quantitative and qualitative surveys strongly indicates that prevalence of drug use within BEM groups is increasing and that even where it is shown to be less than in the white population, it is still significant. The *Annual Report on the UK Drug Situation 2001* provides clear trends for drug use by ethnic minorities, reporting that lifetime drug use is currently lower among these groups than in the white population, with 28% of black people, 15% of Indians, and 10% of Pakistani/Bangladeshis having taken an illicit drug at some point in their lives.[2] This compared with 34% of the white population and white people also had higher rates for drug use across all classes of drug. The Indian population, although having lower overall drug use, had a lifetime use of Class A drugs equivalent to black people among 16–29-year-olds. It is the Indian 16–29-year-olds whose drug use is increasing at the most worrying rate.

The Thames Regional Drug Misuse Database 1999 shows a significant increase in South-Asian heroin users – mostly males and less than 20 years old – presenting for treatment.[3] Similarly, the 1997/98 Regional Drug Misuse Database for Anglia and Oxford records that over 30% of new cases presenting for treatment were from BEM communities, mostly South-Asian.[4] Across the United Kingdom, drug use is increasingly being reported amongst young BEM women.[5,6]

Patterns of use

A detailed literature review by the National Treatment Agency (NTA) gives a more in-depth guide into the use of individual drugs. Not surprisingly cannabis is the most widely used illicit drug among all groups mirroring non-BEM populations, but heroin use is becoming more common, especially in central and northern England.

There is also some evidence that cannabis users are moving steadily to more problematic drugs, particularly crack cocaine. So-called 'dance drugs' (ecstasy, LSD, amfetamines) appear to be used among ethnic minority groups although some evidence suggests that these drugs are regarded as 'white people's drugs' and use by minority groups is limited. Drugs that are used more by different populations are khat and methamfetamine.

Some groups around the country use khat, a stimulant consisting of the leaves and tender shoots of a plant, and its use amongst the Somali population in the United Kingdom has now been well documented.[7] Both these drugs are discussed in more detail in Chapter 11.

Causes of drug use

The causes of drug use amongst BEM people are likely to be more or less the same as for the general population, although as a group they are more exposed to the sociodemographic risk factors for drug misuse.[8] Since the early 1980s, there has been clear evidence that a concentration of the most serious drug related problems are in areas of high unemployment and social deprivation,[9,10] where the majority of young BEM people live. The vast majority of England's BEM groups are concentrated in some of the most deprived inner city areas,[11] where in some cases they are the majority, not the minority, population. Many of these communities are young and growing, with nearly half under the age of 25. BEM people figure disproportionately in statistics of those who are:

- ▶ unemployed[12]

- ▶ living in poverty[13]

▶ in the criminal justice arena[14]

▶ detained under the Mental Health Act 1983, especially some BEM groups in high and medium secure services[15]

▶ in ill health[16]

▶ excluded from school and in care[17]

▶ vulnerable to homelessness.[18]

Attempting to 'fit in' with white peers and to cope with the tension of being non-white amongst a predominately white community have also been cited as risk factors for use amongst young BEM groups.[19,20] For recently established BEM communities in the United Kingdom, there may be links between drug use and the experiences of war, torture, and trauma prior to coming to this country. Heroin use amongst Vietnamese people has been found to have begun in refugee camps in Hong Kong and is continuing amongst those now living in the United Kingdom.[21]

Barriers to treatment

An important element for health professionals is to understand and address the factors that entice minority communities into treatment and the barriers to care. Many examples of good practice are described later in this chapter, but primary care practitioners and health care managers will benefit from understanding what aspects of treatment can alienate BEM patients.

Unsurprisingly, there is a danger in the United Kingdom that treatment services can become too orientated towards the white population, especially in areas where local ethnic minorities are less apparent or more dispersed. This problem can emerge in drug services that are overly opiate-based, without addressing growing crack cocaine problems for example, among ethnic minority drug users. This bias is more likely to occur in agencies employing few or no BEM workers, who are more likely to appreciate local ethnic communities' particular problems.

Research shows that while primary care managers and black workers groups have broadly similar opinions of black drug use, there are noticeable contrasts when addressing the difference in patterns of drug use between white and black people.[22]

BEM groups are likely to be under-represented in surveys where fears about stigma within these communities may mean that drug use is not revealed to researchers or may be 'statistically' hidden if the proportion of BEM respondents is too small to conduct a meaningful analysis. The 2000 British Crime Survey

(BCS) included an ethnic booster sample and revealed higher proportions of BEM drug users than found by previous BCS surveys, although reported levels of drug use amongst BEM respondents remained lower than amongst white respondents.[23]

Black and ethnic minority women

A crucial point for primary care practitioners is the finding that BEM women are most likely to enter treatment later,[24] often missing out on harm minimisation interventions at an earlier stage. Regardless of the reasons for this, there is clearly a cultural barrier delaying these women's entrance into treatment. If such a trend is established locally, services must look at ways to target women in these communities.

Research from Australia shows that communication difficulties with ethnic minorities often result in reluctance among patients to return to treatment, a problem no doubt present in UK treatment services.[25] In Australia, ethnic minorities were more inclined to visit a GP than any other service, perhaps because of the less intimidating surroundings and the well-known guarantee of confidentiality, which is considered vital in ethnic communities where illicit drug use is completely unacceptable. There may also be factors such as differences in access, entitlement, and cost of health care in Australia.

With easily accessible, free, and excellent primary care services in the United Kingdom, it is hoped that primary care can be in the position to provide effective treatment to these women. The same study brought to light the scepticism among many ethnic communities that counselling by professionals can solve drug problems.[25] Such treatment methods are, even in Australia, based on Anglo-Saxon models and these can make ethnic minority patients feel uncomfortable and many drop out of treatment early. Outreach work, described below, should help bridge the cultural gap and inform communities of the benefits of counselling techniques.

Good practice and evidence of successful methods and models

The factors that dissuade black and ethnic minorities from entering treatment will vary from community to community, but a combination of good practice initiatives taken from below can be remarkably effective in combating them.

BEM people should not feel that they are subject to special treatment, some UK practices have shown ways of ensuring that these patients get a high quality level of care. The Black Drug Workers Forum North West (BDWF) cites several examples of good practice that should be of interest to primary care managers and practitioners.[22]

A common but effective example is the provision of leaflets in different languages. This is a good way of getting key messages across to ethnic communities and reducing the widely felt impression that some drug services are run by white people for white people. However, the BDWF reported that in many cases leaflets were left unused in cupboards and pointed out that providing leaflets in different languages can be of only limited use if staff do not have the language skills to back them up. Putting leaflets with clear messages on display, however, can serve a useful purpose.

As with many special groups, liaison between primary care workers and relevant agencies is an excellent way of promoting relations between ethnic communities and drug services. Such work can be extremely effective in overcoming the barriers mentioned earlier that put ethnic minority patients off entering treatment.

In 1991 the Social Services Inspectorate's study recommended the recruitment of black outreach workers. This is a promising way of reaching the black community, but as the BDWF found in Greater Manchester, levels of outreach work are low and form an ad hoc part of any attempt to attract ethnic communities into treatment. To be effective, outreach work should be used on a permanent basis, with the employment of ethnic outreach workers likely to further its good work.

The Department of Health has funded an initiative in which 47 projects, representing 25 ethnic groups, were recruited, trained, and supported to conduct drugs needs assessments in their own communities.[26]

Studies have found conclusively in favour of outreach work both as a way of raising awareness of drug services in the community and also as a method by which the drug services themselves can conduct a needs assessment within the community. The provision of outreach workers does not simply parachute them into communities to fulfil their project aims and disappear: a significant improvement in uptake of services can be expected.[27]

More detailed ideas for outreach work can be found in a study by Johnson and Carroll.[28]

A drug education project focused specifically on ethnic communities is a suitable way of engaging those who might otherwise miss out on drug education or be unaware of the drug services available. This should encompass working with families, young people, voluntary and religious groups, and professionals in the community.[29]

Finally, focusing a primary care drug service on the needs of BEM drug users – in Greater Manchester this might include a greater role for crack cocaine treatment – would ensure they received the best treatment, but this should not come at the expense of the needs of the population as a whole.

Overall the BDWF found most examples of good practice in Greater Manchester were isolated and even in the practices where efforts had been made there was a lack of permanency and commitment to initiatives. Sixty-five per cent of the drug services questioned did not evaluate their practices to see if intended outcomes were being met.[26] This is unacceptable and the sooner primary care practices realise that evaluation is as much a part of good practice as implementation the better. Several examples of good practice have been mentioned above, but not all of them will necessarily work in all situations; evaluation is therefore imperative.

There seems to be a telling lack of data within primary care practices regarding the ethnic backgrounds of patients. Despite a general unease about classifying people on racial grounds it is only by doing so that agencies can effectively target communities with the sort of initiatives described above. Without this information it is probable that agencies will miss important trends in the uptake of drug services among different ethnic groups, which can lead to alienated groups missing out on the education and encouragement they need before they seek help. The National Treatment Agencies *Models of Care* specifically recommends a better collection of data to avoid this.

The BDWF found two organisations in Greater Manchester currently attracting a sizeable number of black patients. Both were voluntary sector organisations and shared several common characteristics. These included a proactive approach to implementing equal opportunities policy and providing explicit organisation aimed at opposing all discrimination. They involved outreach work, liaised with external community agencies and employed a good mix of men, women, white, and ethnic minority employees providing a good variety of services that were not only opiate-based. It is real-life examples such as these that show that simple good practice measures do attract BEM patients who feel alienated by agencies that make no attempt to account for cultural differences.

An issue of importance is whether BEM people are best served by specialist or generic services. Specialist services have obvious benefits, such as a greater understanding of the culture of patients and a reduction in linguistic difficulties. Other studies have pointed to the disadvantages of this and that it may inadvertently impede mainstream services from developing appropriate ways of meeting the needs of this population. It is important that generic services continue to implement good practice in treating ethnic minorities so that specialist services are not a necessity. Where they do exist, close cooperation between generic and specialist services should be encouraged.

Conclusion

It is not practical, or indeed desirable, to focus a generic primary care practice entirely around the needs of BEM people. There is clear evidence that many agencies are failing to recognise that these communities will often need encouragement before using available drug services. Agencies that make no effort to overcome cultural barriers are failing in their duty to provide an effective service for all local communities.

This chapter has shown what aspects of drug services can lead to the alienation of ethnic minority patients and several simple good practice measures that can help reverse this. It does not take a radical overhaul of service provision to treat BEM people effectively, but simple measures such as a proactive equal opportunities policy, a good mix of workers, and long-term outreach work within the community are proven to work.

References

1. Sangster D, Shiner M, Sheikh N, Patel K. Delivering *Drug Services to Black and Minority Ethnic Communities*. DPAS/P16. London: Home Office Drug Prevention and Advisory Service (DPAS), 2002 (available at: www.drugs.gov.uk).

2. Home Office, *Annual Report on the UK Drug Situation 2001*. London: Home Office, 2001.

3. Centre for Research on Drugs and Health Behaviour. Thames Regional Drug Misuse Database. Short paper no. 3: *Trends in Reports of Asian Heroin Smoking*. London: CRDHB, Imperial College School of Medicine, 1999.

4. Sheikh N, Fountain J, Khurana J, *et al. Planning Drug and Alcohol Services for Adults from Black and Minority Ethnic Communities in Waltham Forest and Redbridge*. Final report on a needs assessment for Waltham Forest and Redbridge Drug Action Teams. Preston: Centre for Ethnicity and Health, Faculty of Health, University of Central Lancashire, 2002.

5. Bentley C, Hanton A. *A Study to Investigate the Extent to which there is a Drug Problem amongst Young Asian People in Nottingham. How Effective are Drugs Services in Providing Assistance for such Minority Ethnic Groups?* Nottingham: ADAPT, 1997.

6. The Bridge Project. *A Report of a Survey of Asian women aged 14–25*. Bradford: The Bridge Project, 1996.

7. National Treatment Agency. *Black and Minority Ethnic Communities in England: A Review of the Literature on Drug Use and Related Service Provision*. London: NTA, 2003.

8. Patel K, Wibberley C. Young Asians and drug use. *Journal of Child Health Care* 2002; **5(1)**: 53–61.

9. Haw S. *Drug problems in Greater Glasgow*. London: Standing Committee on Drug Abuse (SCODA), 1985.

10. Peck D F, Plant M A. Unemployment and illegal drug use: concordant evidence from a perspective study and national trends. *BMJ* 1986; **293**: 929–32.

11. Social Exclusion Unit. *Bringing Britain Together: a National Strategy for Neighborhood Renewal*. London: HMSO, 1998.

12. Commission for Racial Equality. *Census Data*. London: CRE, 1995.

13. Jones T. *Britain's Ethnic Minorities*. London: Policy Studies Institute, 1996.

14. Home Office. *Statistics on Race and the Criminal Justice System*. Home Office publication under section 95 of the Criminal Justice Act 1991. London: HMSO, 1998.

15. Mental Health Act Commission. *9th Biennial Report*. London: HMSO, 2001.

16. Erens B, Primatesta P, Prior G. (Eds). *Health Survey for England: The Health of Minority Ethnic Groups 1999*. London: Stationery Office, 2001.

17. Social Exclusion Unit. *Report of Policy Action Team 12: Young People*. London: HMSO, 2000.

18. Chahal K. *Ethnic Diversity, Neighborhoods and Housing*. Foundations Series No. 110. York: Joseph Rowntree Foundation, 2000.

19. Pearson G, Patel K. Drugs, deprivation, and ethnicity: outreach among Asian drug users in a northern English city. *Journal of Drug Issues* 1998; **28(1)**: 199–224.

20. Singh G, Passi P. *Drug Use in the South Asian Community*. Report to North West Lancashire Health Promotion Unit. Manchester: North West Lancashire Health Promotion Unit, 1997.

21. Sangster D, Shiner M, Sheikh N, Patel K. *Delivering Drug Services to Black and Minority Ethnic Communities*. DPAS/P16. London: Home Office, 2002 (available at: www.drugs.gov.uk).

22. Chantler K. *An Analysis of Present Drug Service Delivery to Black Communities in Greater Manchester*. Manchester: Black Drug Workers Forum North West and Greater Manchester Drug Action Partnership (SRB Initiative), 1998.

23. Ramsey M, Baker P, Goulden C, *et al. Drug Misuse Declared in 2000: Results from the British Crime Survey*. Home Office Research Study 224. Home Office Research, Development and Statistics Directorate. London: Home Office, 2001.

24. National Treatment Agency. *Models of Care*. London: NTA, 2002.

25. Reid G, Crofts N, Beyer L. Drug treatment services for ethnic communities in Victoria, Australia: an examination of cultural and institutional barriers. *Ethnicity and Health* 2001; **6**: 1.

26. National Treatment Agency. The black and ethnic community drugs misuse needs assessment project. In: *Black and Minority Ethnic Communities in England: A Review of the Literature on Drug Use and Related Service Provision*. London: NTA, 2003.

27. Patel K. Using qualitative research to examine the nature of drug use among minority ethnic communities in the UK. In: Fountain J. (Ed). *Understanding and Responding to Drug Use: the Role of Qualitative Research*. Lisbon: European Monitoring Centre for Drugs and Drug Addiction (EMCDDA), 2000.

28. Johnson M R D, Carroll M. *Dealing with Diversity: Good Practice in Drug Prevention Work with Racially and Culturally Diverse Communities*. Paper 5, Drugs Prevention Initiative. London: Home Office, 1995.

29. Southhall Community Drug Education Project. Conference report (unpublished but available at: www.daap.org.uk/pdfs/southall/report.pdf).

CHAPTER 21

Drug use and housing issues

Nat Wright

What is homelessness? Challenging the myth of migrancy

Having a home has been defined as 'having an adequate dwelling (or space) over which a person and his/her family can exercise exclusive possession, being able to maintain privacy and enjoy social relations, and having a legal title to occupy'.[1]

Often both professionals and homeless people can adopt a narrow definition of 'homelessness' as rough sleeping.[2] The popular stereotype of the 'tramp' or 'drifter' remains. However, at the start of the 21st century, such a stereotype could not be further from the reality of the lives of the UK homeless drug-using populations who access primary care services daily.

Many homeless drug users reside in their place of birth. Research in Leeds demonstrated that, regardless of age, homeless drug users were more likely than homeless people with alcohol dependence or mental ill health to access primary care in their city of birth.[3] For general practices working with homeless drug users, it will often entail working with people who have grown up in their practice area or locality; whereas the housing situation of some can change frequently, often such change is within the same local geographical area.

It is important for primary health care practitioners to realise that health, housing, and social needs are interlinked. Provision of effective primary health care provision can help break the cycle of chronic homelessness. Adequate housing can provide the homeless drug user with the stability required to facilitate access to primary health care. Chronic homelessness can include movement into or between any of the following housing states:[1, 4–6]

▶ 'Roofless' describes rough sleepers, newly arrived immigrants, and victims of fire, flood, or severe harassment or violence.

▶ 'Houseless' describes those living in temporary or emergency accommodation (for example night shelters, hostels, or refuges) and those released from long-term institutions (for example psychiatric hospitals, prisons, detention centres, or community or foster homes with nowhere to go upon release).

▶ 'Living in insecure accommodation' includes individuals who are staying with friends or relatives on a temporary or involuntary basis, tenants under notice to quit, those whose security is threatened by violence or threats of violence, or squatters.

▶ 'Living in inadequate accommodation' includes overcrowded or substandard accommodation. Such homeless people are often 'concealed' (also described as 'hidden') as people involuntarily share accommodation on a long-term basis because they cannot secure or afford separate housing.

The relationship between housing status and drug use

The link between poor housing and ill health has been recognised for well over a century. In the Victorian era, environmental health activists were instrumental in developing housing policy that sought to address the impact of urban slums upon poor health.[7,8]

Since that time the challenge has been to marry the medical intervention centred upon the individual with wider public health interventions to provide healthy housing. This challenge remains today in the health care of homeless drug users.

There is an emerging evidence base describing the relationship between housing status and problematic drug use. Qualitative research has documented a tendency for many drug users to increase drug use when in the hostel environment. This appears to be owing in part to being surrounded by drug using peers.[9] For some, drug use is reduced when rough sleeping owing to reduced financial means. Initiation into injecting heroin instead of smoking it because of the practical difficulties of smoking outdoors in a windy environment has also been described. Some homeless drug users describe a progression to injecting alone once they have acquired stable accommodation. As injecting alone is a risk factor for drug related death, the move to solitary accommodation as a drug career progresses could in part explain the findings of an increase in the mean age of heroin related death despite a reduction in the average age of initiation into heroin use.[10,11]

Quantitative surveys amongst UK homeless drug users have described the drugs commonly used by homeless people. They include heroin and crack cocaine, and polydrug use is common. However, owing to either unsafe injecting practices or a lifestyle that is not conducive towards maintaining adequate personal hygiene, many drug users have multiple health morbidity. Such morbidity includes:

▸ ileo–femoral deep vein thrombosis due to persistent injecting into the femoral vein

▸ pulmonary embolus

▸ blood-borne viruses – hepatitis B, hepatitis C, or HIV

▸ bacterial infections – septicaemia, cerebral abscess, spinal cord abscess, endocarditis, cellulitis and skin abscesses

▸ also difficulty of many homeless drug users in successfully carrying out routine daily living skills causing common chronic diseases (e.g. epilepsy, diabetes, asthma), which are often more challenging to manage.

Where will homeless drug users access primary care?

Homeless drug users will access primary care in a variety of settings. In part this is a response to barriers towards homeless people accessing mainstream primary care services. Such barriers include practice opening times, appointment procedures, and financial disincentives for general practitioners to work with this patient group.[12]

Discrimination against homeless people can also be a barrier to primary care access and includes inaccurate generalisations that they are violent, antisocial, or 'undeserving' of support.[13,14]

Some homeless people face a double risk of discrimination due to age, gender, ethnic background, or sexual orientation.[9, 15–17] To address such stigma and aid integration of homeless drug users into primary care treatment provision, both legislation and local innovation have helped by providing a variety of effective frameworks for delivering health care to homeless populations.[1,18] Such models entail providing primary care to homeless drug users in the following settings:

▸ mainstream general practice

▸ mainstream general practice with a special interest in homelessness

▸ specialised general practice for homeless people

▸ provision of primary health care within the secondary care hospital setting.

Mainstream general practice, defined as provision of care through normal registration in a primary care practice, remains the ideal setting for primary care provision for homeless people. It normalises primary care for homeless drug users. Its wide coverage means there is ease of access for homeless drug users, particularly in rural areas.

Because it is often a difficult setting to access for many homeless drug users, particularly when presenting with acute illness, and also for roofless people with uncontrolled problematic drug use, many such drug users present to 'specialised' general practices. These have become more common with primary medical service legislation permitting trusts or independent contractor practices to appoint salaried general practitioners and other health staff not normally employed in the primary care setting (for example community psychiatric services or client support workers). The strength of such practices is that they can provide more focused and intensive care for large numbers of homeless drug users who have complex multiple morbidity. The centres, however, are concentrated in urban areas and therefore are not a solution to the problem of rural homelessness.

Theoretical arguments against specialised practices for homeless people are that they ghettoise primary care provision and therefore further marginalise homeless people. Current thinking would therefore encourage registration with the specialised general practice at times of health and social crisis to provide early treatment and rehabilitation. Once the acute condition has stabilised and the user is familiar with the primary care setting, registration with mainstream primary care should be encouraged. Often the drug user will require support to attend the new general practice and there is a role for patient/client support workers, or receptionists from the specialised general practice to provide such support. Many of these practices now provide services commissioned by the primary care trust through enhanced services.

Planned primary care provision in the hospital setting is not a common model in the UK. It is more commonly found in Europe, and models vary from a single centralised unit to all hospital departments offering care. Key to the success of such models appears to be social worker support for the homeless person. Such primary care programmes for homeless people have led to a reduction in hospital admissions.[19]

Structured counselling to address problematic drug use

There appears to be a paucity of UK research evaluating the impact of structured counselling approaches to address problematic drug use by homeless people. US research has evaluated behavioural and empowerment drugs health promotion approaches. Common findings are that assertive community treatments retain users in services but do not yield high rates of abstinence,[20] and residential therapeutic communities for those with dual diagnoses result in greater reductions in drug use than community interventions. Both modalities reduce drug use.[21–23]

Limiting disability payments to homeless persons with a dual diagnosis of drug misuse and mental ill health in an effort to reduce drug use does not lead to a reduction in number of substance using days per month.[24]

Compared with those receiving typical day care programmes, homeless crack cocaine abusers who were randomised to an enhanced day treatment programme, plus abstinent contingent work therapy and housing, had fewer positive cocaine toxicologies, fewer days homeless, and more days employed.[25] Behavioural approaches amongst homeless drug users should therefore seek to adopt a non-coercive, harm reduction approach. Where drug users express a wish to achieve abstinence, this is best achieved in a therapeutic community/residential setting.

Key issues in safe prescribing for homeless drug users

Best practice guidelines for professionals working with drug users, which are applicable to homeless drug using communities, include GPs only prescribing with the support of a drugs nurse/therapist. The drugs nurse/therapist should offer an adequate assessment to inform an agreed treatment plan prior to initiating substitute opioid medication.[26]

It is important to avoid pressure to prescribe opiates for maintenance other than buprenorphine or methadone maintenance medication, as these are the only opiates that have demonstrated reduced crime and reduced drug use.[27] Prescribing of other opiates should take place only in a research setting.

Some homeless drug users move areas and present to primary care requesting immediate continuation of the prescription prior to assessment. The prescriber should agree to this only once the history has been confirmed with the previous prescriber to minimise the risk of duplicate prescribing. Homeless drug users are at increased risk of drug related death.[28] Prescribing practice that has the potential to increase the risk of either unintentional or intentional death should be avoided. Such practice would include concomitant prescription of methadone and benzodiazepines; prescribing without good reason for less frequently than daily pick-up from the pharmacist; not undertaking supervised dispensing of maintenance opiates for at least three months.

Many homeless drug users spend periods of time in prison. Amounts of heroin consumed are usually much lower in the custodial setting than in the community. Many drug users are therefore able to remain abstinent in the prison environment. For those entering on maintenance medication, there is still not an established evidence base demonstrating the effectiveness of maintenance opiate therapy. In part this is because the trials have not yet been completed.

The main positive outcomes of opiate replacement therapy (namely a reduction in both illicit drug use and acquisitive crime) are common occurrences in the prison custodial setting. Where maintenance medication is initiated in the prison setting, there is a need to first ensure that there is a community prescriber willing to continue prescribing the medication upon release.

Drug users often spend a period of time in the inpatient hospital setting. This can present a dilemma for hospital clinicians, many of whom have limited experience working with drug users. This dilemma is demonstrated by the case study in Box 21.1. It shows that many drug users present with unusual symptoms as a consequence of injecting. This often necessitates hospital admission. It demonstrates a training need for many hospital colleagues on aspects of drug misuse.

In this case, the patient was discharged on a cocktail of dihydrocodeine and diazepam, a combination for which there is no evidence of effectiveness as maintenance medication.

Clearly there is a need for close communication between GPs and hospital doctors. Despite having serious health problems, many homeless drug users will discharge themselves so as to access drugs to mitigate acute opiate withdrawal symptoms. One of the major positive benefits of replacement opiate maintenance therapy is retention in service provision. Ideally such users should be considered for opiate maintenance therapy. We would argue that the primary goal of such treatment should be retention on the ward until the acute medical condition is controlled.

At the time of writing, there appears to be a dearth of best practice care pathways for transfer of care between hospital and primary care drug treatment services. It could be argued that hospital addiction clinicians should prioritise the initiation of opiate maintenance therapy for those with acute or multiple medical morbidity. Community addiction clinicians should prioritise such referrals into their services owing to the high level of complex physical morbidity.

Developing integrated working – key principles

In whatever setting homeless drug users receive drug treatment, care will need to be integrated with partner organisations. Key stakeholders include housing, social service, hospital, and prison providers. There have been historical barriers to integrated working. Although in some areas collaboration between health and social care organisations has been reasonably good, often housing agencies have been omitted from collaborative working.[29] The following have been described as common threats to collaborative working:

▸ lack of understanding of other agencies, their roles and responsibilities, boundaries between them, and the constraints that others are working under

▸ uncertainty of the services provided by, and personnel within, other agencies

▸ collaboration at strategic level not being implemented or mirrored at service delivery level

Box 21.1 **Case study of care of a homeless drug user whilst in hospital**

A male resident in a homeless hostel, who has been homeless for 32 years, registered for a new appointment with his general practitioner. He had an 8-year history of intravenous heroin use and was currently injecting into his groin. He presented to his GP with a one-week history of tiredness, malaise and difficulty walking. Examination revealed low-grade pyrexia, reduced power in the lower limbs, associated with paraesthesia to light touch, but no other neurological abnormality. There was evidence of groin injecting but no evidence of infection at the injecting sites. The GP was unable to make a definitive diagnosis but referred the patient to the local hospital as an emergency medical admission with a diagnosis of possible Guillain-Barré syndrome. Hospital baseline investigations revealed a raised white cell count and a raised plasma viscosity. A CT scan revealed an extradural thoracic abscess. This was evacuated leaving residual weakness in the lower limbs. Whilst on the ward, he also received a positive diagnosis for hepatitis C. He was discharged on 14×30 mg dihydrocodeine per day and 9×5 mg diazepam tablets per day. The discharge summary to the general practitioner stated that he had been referred for physiotherapy. However, he never received an appointment and when the GP tried to re-refer the patient he was informed that the referral needed to come from the consultant. The GP phoned the consultant's secretary who agreed to raise the matter with the consultant. The secretary phoned the GP the following day and informed him that the consultant did not feel that physiotherapy was necessary. The patient still complained of residual weakness and reduced proprioception in the lower limbs so the GP persisted with a request for physiotherapy. Two weeks later the physiotherapy department accepted the referral.

▸ difficulties in communication and sharing information between agencies, including false expectations and mistrust of other professional groups

▸ unsuccessful user involvement at strategic level.

Clearly primary care clinical staff taking on roles as board members of primary care organisations, housing, social service, or prison agencies can seed significant opportunities for effective partnership working.

Within the confines of the consulting room there is much that the general practitioner or practice team member can do to aid partnership working. One key area is in providing meaningful letters of support for housing. This should take place only when first requested by the housing department. Patient-led requests for housing letters tend not to aid integrated working. Where the patient presents a request to the GP, they should be directed to the housing department so that the need for a GP support letter can be assessed. If such a letter is deemed appropriate, the content of the letter can significantly help the homeless drug user.

In England, under the Homeless Act 2002, drug dependence by itself does not qualify as a medical condition granting 'medical priority' for rehousing. Priority can be granted if the drug user is vulnerable as a result of: old age; mental illness or handicap; physical disability or other special reason; fleeing violence (including domestic violence); having spent time in the armed forces, prison, or remanded in custody; age 16–17 (unless social services have a responsibility for accommodating); care leavers under the age of 21 who were looked after by social services when they were 16 or 17 (with some limited, uncommon exceptions). Many drug users will be experiencing one or more of these conditions; it is important to highlight this in the medical letter. It is also important to be explicit about the user's drug habit. Being explicit also entails highlighting that you would expect a diagnosis of 'drug dependence' not to be a diagnosis of 'exclusion' from adequate housing.

Many housing departments, housing associations, and private landlords are now able to provide all kinds of different supported housing options. This ranges from frequent visits from a client support worker, to shared housing, to semi-independent hostel accommodation. Being explicit in the support letter regarding the drug user's level of competence in carrying out daily living skills can help housing agencies find the most appropriate accommodation to support rehousing of homeless drug users.

At a policy level such work is supported by the recent introduction of a government framework for housing related support services. This entails local authorities taking over the funding, governance, and monitoring of such support services. It is the largest wholesale change to the housing sector in recent years. The ethos is one of a constantly evolving programme, building new partnerships across probation, health, and social services. Such programmes at local level will have a great potential to provide an integrated approach to meeting the full range of homeless drug users' basic needs as they seek rehousing.

Further reading

Wright N. *Homelessness: A Primary Care Response.* London: Royal College of General Practitioners, 2002.

References

1. Edgar B, Doherty J, Meert H. *Review of Statistics on Homelessness in Europe.* Brussels: European Federation of National Organisations Working with the Homeless, 2003 (available a: www.feantsa.org).

2. Hutson S, Liddiard M. *Youth Homelessness: The Construction of a Social Issue.* London: Macmillan, 1994.

3. Tompkins C N, Wright N M J, Sheard L, Allgar V L. Associations between migrancy, health and homelessness: a cross-sectional study. *Health & Social Care in the Community* 2003; **11(5)**: 446–52.

4. Bramley G, Doogan K, Leather P, *et al.* (Eds). *Homelessness and the London Housing Market.* Bristol: School for Advanced Urban Studies, 1988.

5. Connelly J, Crown J. *Homelessness and Ill Health.* Report of a Working party of the Royal College of Physicians. London: Royal College of Physicians, 1994.

6. Fitzpatrick S, Kemp P, Klinker S. *Single homelessness: An Overview of Research in Britain.* Bristol: Policy Press, 2000.

7. Wright N. *Homelessness: A Primary Care Response.* London: Royal College of General Practitioners, 2002.

8. Hawtin M. Collaboration for meeting housing needs. In: Gill P, de Wildt G. (Eds). *Housing and Health, the Role of Primary Care.* Oxford: Radcliffe Medical Press, 2003.

9. Wright N, Oldham N, Jones L. Homelessness and heroin related death – a qualitative study exploring associations. *Drug and Alcohol Review* (in press).

10. Darke S, Ross J. Heroin-related deaths in Southern Western Sydney, Australia 1992–1996. *Drug and Alcohol Review* 1999; **18**: 39–45.

11. Hall W, Darke S. Trends in opiate overdose deaths in Australia 1979–1995. *Drug and Alcohol Dependence* 1998; **52(1)**: 71–7.

12. Griffiths S. *Addressing the Health Needs of Rough Sleepers.* A Paper to the Homelessness Directorate. London: HMSO, 2002.

13. Riley A J, Harding G, Underwood M R, Carter Y H. Homelessness: a problem for primary care? *Br J Gen Pract* 2003; **53(491)**: 473–9.

14. Lester H, Bradley C. Barriers to primary healthcare for the homeless: the general practitioners perspective. *Eur J Gen Pract* 2001; **7**: 6–12.

15. Crane M. The associations between mental illness and homelessness among older people: an exploratory study. *Ageing and Mental Health* 1998; **2(3)**: 171–80.

16. Edgar B, Doherty J, Mina-Coull A. *Women and Homelessness in Europe.* Bristol: Policy Press, 2001.

17. Kruks G. Gay and lesbian homeless/street youth: special issues and concerns. *Journal of Adolescent Health* 1991; **12(7)**: 515–18.

18. Crane M, Warnes A M. Primary health care services for single homeless people: defects and opportunities. *Family Practice* 2001; **18(3)**: 272–6.

19. Doering T J, Hermes E, Konitzer M, Fischer G C, Steuernagel B. Health situation of homeless in a health care home in Hannover. [German]. *Gesundheitswesen* 2002; **64(6)**: 375–82.

20. Meisler N, Blankertz L, Santos A B, McKay C. Impact of assertive community treatment on homeless persons with co-occurring severe psychiatric and substance use disorders. *Community Mental Health Journal* 1997; **33(2)**: 113–22.

21. Conrad K J, Hultman C I, Pope A R, *et al*. Case managed residential care for homeless addicted veterans. Results of a true experiment. *Medical Care* 1998; **36(1)**: 40–53.

22. De Leon G, Sacks S, Staines G, McKendrick K. Modified therapeutic community for homeless mentally ill chemical abusers: treatment outcomes. *Am J Drug Alcohol Abuse* 2000; **26(3)**: 461–80.

23. Nuttbrock L A, Rahav M, Rivera J J, Ng-Mak D S, Link B G. Outcomes of homeless mentally ill chemical abusers in community residences and a therapeutic community. *Psychiatric Services* 1998; **49(1)**: 68–76.

24. Frisman L K, Rosenheck R. The relationship of public support payments to substance abuse among homeless veterans with mental illness. *Psychiatric Services* 1997; **48(6)**: 792–5.

25. Milby J B, Schumacher J E, Raczynski J M, *et al*. Sufficient conditions for effective treatment of substance abusing homeless persons. *Drug and Alcohol Dependence* 1996; **43(1–2)**: 39–47.

26. The National Treatment Agency for Substance Misuse. *Models of Care for Treatment of Adult Drug Misusers*. London: National Treatment Agency for Substance Misuse, 2002.

27. Mattick R P, Kimber J, Breen C, Davoli M . Buprenorphine maintenance versus placebo or methadone maintenance for opioid dependence. In: The Cochrane Library, Issue 2. Chichester: John Wiley, 2003.

28. Home Office. *Reducing Drug Related Deaths*. A report by the Advisory Council on Misuse of Drugs. London: HMSO, 2000.

29. Arblaster L, Conway J, Foreman A, Hawtin M. *Asking the impossible: inter-agency working to address the housing, health and social care needs of people in ordinary housing*. Bristol: Policy Press/ Joseph Rowntree, 1996.

CHAPTER 22

Drug misuse and co-morbid illness: 'dual diagnosis'

Clare Gerada

Definition

The term dual diagnosis, or co-morbidity, has risen to higher prominence in recent years. The definition tends to be applied to people with a diagnosed mental illness, usually psychotic illness, who also experience difficulties with alcohol and/or drug use, as well as to people with problematic alcohol and drug use who develop symptoms of mental illness, perhaps as a result of their substance use.

Unfortunately the term is imprecise, as these patients seldom have just two problems. The combination of psychiatric and drug/alcohol problems means that individuals are at risk from a number of problems, ranging from physical ill heath, homelessness, unemployment, social exclusion, and so on. The term 'multiple morbidity', suggested by Wright and colleagues,[1] might more accurately describe the common predicament of patients who have more than one health problem. For the sake of brevity the term dual diagnosis will be used in this chapter.

Relationship between addiction and mental health problems

The relationship between those with addiction and mental health problems is complex with possibilities for the interrelationships including:[2]

▶ a primary psychiatric illness precipitating or leading to substance use

▶ substance use worsening or altering the course of a psychiatric illness, for example intoxication and/or substance dependence leading to psychological symptoms

▶ substance use and/or withdrawal leading to psychiatric symptoms or illnesses

▶ substances, particularly alcohol, cannabinoids, hallucinogens, and stimulants (especially amfetamines and cocaine) that can produce psychotic symptoms directly without mental illness.

What is the role of the primary care practitioner?

Why should the primary care practitioner need to know anything about patients with dual diagnosis? After all, these patients have complex needs that should place their management outside the normal confines of general practice. It is the author's belief that the more complex the patients' problems the greater their need for well organised primary care services to coordinate care.

Good primary care services are vital to make sure that these patients do not slip through the net of multiple carers and services. It is the very complexity of their problems, requiring many contacts with health and social care professionals, that makes primary care such an important part of their overall management, able to provide continuity throughout their care. This does not negate the key working role undertaken by specialist mental health or dual diagnosis services, or the importance of other services in providing valuable input, as ultimately it is through effective shared care that these patients are best served.

What primary care can offer patients with complex co-morbidities

▶ continuity of care

▶ general medical services

▶ enhanced services for coexisting physical problems

▶ coordination between services

▶ crisis intervention

▶ containment

▶ care to the family

▶ advocacy

▶ medication review

▶ help with housing and benefits issues.

Prevalence

The prevalence of dual diagnosis has increased over the past decade. This may be owing to two factors. First, the general increase in substance use across the United Kingdom means that patients with mental health problems are as likely (if not more so) to be caught up in the general increase in prevalence. Secondly, since the advent of care in the community in the latter 1970s, patients with mental health problems are more exposed to drugs and hence more likely to use them than when incarcerated within long-stay asylums. See Table 22.1.

Important epidemiological work has been conducted in the United States. The American Epidemiological Catchments Area (ECA) study surveyed over 20,000 people living in both community and psychiatric settings.[3] Substance use problems were more prevalent among individuals with mental illness than among the general population, with mental illness, on average, doubling the chance of a coexistent substance use problem. The ECA study also reported the chances of lifetime substance use by diagnosis as follows:

▶ schizophrenia, 47%

▶ any bipolar disorder, 56%

▶ any affective disorder, 32%

▶ any anxiety disorder, 24%.

On this basis it appears that approximately half of those who experience serious mental illness will have a positive history of substance use.[4]

A smaller scale study of 171 people with psychosis in south London found that the one-year prevalence rate for any substance problem was 36.3%.[5] Broken down further, 31.6% had alcohol problems, while 15.8% had drug problems. Young males were identified as being more likely to have substance use problems and were found to have spent almost twice as long in hospital as those without such problems in the two-year period preceding the study. Significant mental health problems were identified in opiate dependent patients and amfetamine users in a south Wales drug dependence clinic.[6]

Table 22.1   **The proportion of drug users with specific psychiatric
conditions found in NTORS study**[7]

Psychiatric disorder	Females (%)	Males (%)
Anxiety disorder	32	17
Depression	30	15
Paranoia	27	17
Psychotic illness	33	20

Using the General Practice Research Database in work commissioned by the
Department of Health, Frischer *et al*. looked at the prevalence of dual diagnosis in
primary care in England and Wales from 1993 to 1998. The database recorded 1.4
million patient contacts with 230 practices. They checked for recorded individuals
with both substance misuse and a psychiatric disorder and found that the rate for
dual diagnosis increased by 62% during this period, with significant increases in
schizophrenic disorder (128%), paranoia (144%), and psychotic disorder (147%).
The authors also noted a regional variation, with a 300% increase in the Northern
and Yorkshire district and a slow increase in London.[8] This study identified
alcohol and cannabis to be the drugs most frequently used by individuals with
schizophrenia, and smaller UK studies have reported the same.[9,10]

Patterns of drug and alcohol use

Research findings concerning the substances preferred by people with mental
illness are equivocal. An early study reviewed patterns of drug use among people
with schizophrenia. A propensity to use stimulants as a possible mechanism for alle-
viating negative symptoms was reported.[11] Currently cannabis appears to be the
illicit substance most commonly used by people with mental illness in the United
Kingdom mirroring the high use by those without mental health problems.

Amongst the general population there is an increase in the availability of
cocaine and a resurgence in heroin use in some cities.[12–14]

As any drug becomes more readily available we should expect their increasing
use to permeate many existing drug cultures including those with which
psychiatric patients have contact.

Patients with schizophrenia have a threefold greater risk of developing alcohol
dependence than individuals without a mental illness.[15] The most common
psychiatric disorder amongst injecting drug users is antisocial personality
disorder.[16]

Co-morbid mental health and substance use problems are especially prevalent in the homeless and rough sleepers and offenders, including prisoners. There are significant differences between men and women in their patterns of substance use and psychiatric co-morbidity.[17] For example:

▸ Women who use substances are significantly more likely than other women or men to have experienced sexual, physical, and/or emotional abuse as children.

▸ Substance use lifestyles can impact on women's sexual health and establish a pattern of 're-victimisation', for example, women are more likely to fund their habit through prostitution and hence are more likely to place themselves at risk of violence, assault, and abuse.

▸ Women are more likely to present at mental health or primary care services for psychological difficulties rather than for any associated substance use problem.

▸ Women tend to access alcohol and drug services later than men and this may explain their more severe presentation.

▸ Women may have children, or want children, and this can deter them from contact with statutory services for fear that their children will be removed from them, thus they are likely to present later for care at a time when their use has become more problematic.

Clinical implications

Box 22.1 **Case study**

Charlie was 35 years old, living with his brother. Charlie had been diagnosed as having schizophrenia and had been started on antipsychotic medication by the mental health services. Both he and his brother used heroin – smoking – and cannabis. Recently both had started to use crack cocaine. Both came to you requesting help: they felt that life as a user was getting dangerous, Charlie had been assaulted several times and he found that the 'crack' was 'getting to his head'. Their housing situation was relatively stable though they often had unwelcome guests.

✓ Where do you start?

✓ Who should be involved in the care of Charlie and his brother?

✓ What risks does Charlie face?

The implications for people with mental health problems who also misuse drugs and/or alcohol can be serious and it is important that the primary care practitioner is aware of them. Substance use by individuals with psychiatric disorders is associated with significantly poorer outcomes, including:[18–20]

▶ worsening psychiatric symptoms

▶ increased rates of suicidal behaviour

▶ increased rates of violence[21]

▶ poor medication adherence

▶ increased risk of HIV infection

▶ higher service use

▶ higher rates of homelessness.

Both mental health problems and substance use are associated with higher rates of physical illness, including complications related to cigarette smoking, poor nutrition, and infections, including tuberculosis. The primary care practitioner has an invaluable role in making sure that none of these problems is ignored.

Reasons for substance use

People with mental illness are more likely to be misusing drugs and/or alcohol than people without (Table 22.2). Several theories have been proposed to explain the high rates of substance use among people with schizophrenia.[22]

Table 22.2 **Possible reasons for misusing drugs and/or alcohol**

Reason	Comments
People with schizophrenia often use drugs and/or alcohol to self-medicate and to alleviate the side effects of drugs	Research evidence does not strongly support this view. For example, problematic alcohol use often precedes schizophrenia; specific drugs are not selected in relation to specific symptoms; importantly, various substances of use produce a range of different effects but generally exacerbate rather than relieve symptoms of schizophrenia[23]
Underlying neuropathological abnormalities caused by schizophrenia facilitate the positive reinforcing effects of substance use and hence may predispose people to both conditions	This may explain why people with schizophrenia prefer drugs such as cocaine and nicotine

Reason	Comments
People with schizophrenia are especially vulnerable to the negative psychosocial effects of substance use because it impairs thinking and social judgement and induces poor impulse control	This would explain why even when using small amounts of drugs and/or alcohol people with schizophrenia are prone to develop significant substance-related problems[24]
People with antisocial personality disorder are at risk of developing substance use problems	
The increased availability and acceptance of many substances in society means that people with schizophrenia are more likely to come into contact with drugs and/or alcohol	People with schizophrenia use substances for the same reasons as the general population, namely to enjoy the experience of intoxication, to escape from emotional distress, and as a social activity.[25] Drug dealers can exploit people with an obvious vulnerability

Assessment of co-morbidity

It is important to distinguish between substance-induced and substance-related psychiatric disorders. It is advisable to allow three to four weeks of abstinence before making a diagnosis of mental health disorder, but this is often impractical. A complete substance history should be obtained, with urinalysis and blood tests if possible.

The assessment should elucidate the individual's pattern of substance use, its context, severity, risk, and associated needs. These aspects of use can be obtained by history taking in the following areas:

▶ **Patterns of use** – the amounts of each substance used, frequency of use, length of time used, and by which route of administration.

▶ **Context of use** – personal and environmental factors that may be associated with an individual's drug use, including peer group attachments, positive and negative expectations of use, and experiences of physical and/or psychological dependence.

▶ **Severity of use** – patterns of use can give some indication of severity of dependence. This can be specified with instruments designed to gauge severity of alcohol use,[26] drug use,[27, 28] and more appropriately, substance use among individuals with serious mental illness.[29]

▶ **Assessment of risks** – including suicidal behaviour, aggressive or antisocial behaviour,[32] blood-borne infections from sharing injecting equipment, and an increased risk of accidents. The safety of prescribing a particular medication must be determined with regard to drug–drug interactions and how the medication is delivered or monitored.

Treatment approaches

Practitioners need to have a realistic and long-term view of treatment and be aware of the different approaches that may be necessary during different stages of treatment. The following stages of treatment have been described:

▶ engagement

▶ motivation for change

▶ active treatment

▶ relapse prevention.

Which do you treat first?

Management should involve the two problematic elements: treating the substance misuse and treating any coexisting mental health problem.

Three approaches are currently used for delivering services to patients and the choice of course depends on local circumstances. The general practitioner with special interest may have an important role in determining which service is commissioned. Whatever model is used, a most important aspect of any service is the ability to be flexible and to offer services that meet the needs of that individual patient, at the time they present.

Sequential treatment

This addresses the more acute problem first, the other problem receiving greater attention later. This model is commonly used in acute hospitals, where, for example, little attention would be paid to substance use in a patient exhibiting florid psychosis.

Parallel treatment

This addresses both disorders simultaneously but in different settings and often by different services.

Integrated treatment

Both problems are dealt with together, in the same setting. This method of service delivery is reported to be associated with the best outcome. Different models exist that vary according to the psychiatric disorder.[30]

A Cochrane review of different interventions found little evidence to support the effectiveness of any particular treatment, or to recommend one approach over any other.[31] The research suggests a growing agreement that integrated mental health and substance use services offer a more tolerant, non-confrontational approach for patients and are probably the best and most appropriate way forward.[20]

Champney-Smith makes the point that whatever the model of service provided, there are a number of steps that should be considered in order to maximise the effectiveness of treatment:[32]

▸ comprehensive assessments of both mental health and substance use problems

▸ training for mental health workers in the recognition and management of substance use problems

▸ training for substance use workers in the recognition and management of mental health problems

▸ services that are non-judgmental, flexible, and take account of the principles of harm minimisation

▸ assertive outreach with appropriate case loads

▸ clear understanding of roles and responsibilities

▸ good liaison between agencies, clearly identifying who has the lead

▸ development of care pathways

▸ evaluation of new services using a range of outcome measures.

Whatever model of care is used to deliver services, close communication and effective shared care between all those involved is important. Practitioners with special clinical interest may have a role in supporting patients with dual diagnosis, helping them move across the many interfaces of care, but all primary care practitioners will play an important role.

Depression with alcohol misuse or dependence

Alcohol dependency and depression often coexist. Clinicians are often in a dilemma as to which to treat first; it is not always simple or obvious. In this situation it is good practice that the first line of treatment is to assist the patient to withdraw from alcohol and then to reassess mental state. It is difficult to assess their mental state accurately when they are drinking heavily. Alcohol can both cause and mask underlying mental health problems. It is likely that alcohol misuse has contributed to the depressive features and once abstinence has been achieved that the depressive symptoms will significantly reduce.

Antidepressants may improve mood but not necessarily alcohol drinking behaviour in depressed alcohol-dependent patients. The prescribing of anti-depressants for patients who continue to drink needs to be done with caution. Tricyclic antidepressants (TCA) are best avoided completely owing to potentially serious interactions with alcohol, including cardiotoxicity and death in overdose. Selective serotonin reuptake inhibitors (SSRIs) appear to be effective in improving drinking behaviour and depression only in severely depressed patients.

Depression with opioid dependence

As with alcohol dependence, opioid use is a significant risk factor for the develop-ment of depression and may persist even when the patient is abstinent. Patients withdrawing from opioids, especially methadone, often report dysthymia and depressed mood, as do patients on buprenorphine.

For long-term users, the loss of not only the drug but also of the lifestyle involved in taking drugs (which can be a full-time occupation) leaves them empty and deflated. Coming off drugs also exposes the losses associated with a lifetime of drug taking: the years spent seeking and using illicit substances rather than pursuing relationships, education, and employment.

There are limited studies from which to derive recommendations: antidepressants may improve mood but not necessarily drug behaviour in depressed opioid addicts. Perhaps the most important impact the primary care practitioner can make is 'being there' and continuing to provide regular support, certainly for the first six months following abstinence.

Where patients continue to use opioids (prescribed or otherwise) as with concurrent alcohol misuse, TCAs are not recommended owing to potentially serious interactions including cardiotoxicity and death in overdose.

Cocaine and depression

As Chapter 11 dealing with cocaine addiction discussed, depression is a common feature of cocaine use and can be so severe as to risk deliberate self-harm.

As with other drugs of abuse, achieving abstinence or minimising misuse is critical in trying to improve mood. Antidepressants may directly compensate for cocaine-related reduction in neurotransmitters such as dopamine, serotonin, and noradrenaline.

In all pharmacological studies, the importance of psychosocial interventions has been emphasised and should be addressed since there is no robust evidence showing pharmacotherapy is effective. Desipramine and fluoexetine show no significant advantage over placebo in cocaine dependence alone or in cocaine misusing methadone maintained opioids addicts. TCAs are not recommended owing to potentially serious interactions including cardiotoxicity and death in overdose.

Anxiety and alcohol/drug dependence

Because anxiety is a feature of alcohol withdrawal, waiting until the acute withdrawal period is over for a clearer assessment is critical. There is limited knowledge about treating this co-morbid condition. Prescribing benzodiazepines for anxiety in patients who currently misuse alcohol, or have done so previously, is not generally recommended. Abstinent alcohol dependent patients may be at greater risk of benzodiazepine abuse and dependence owing to greater rewarding effects.

Those patients who are severely dependent, with antisocial personality disorder or with polysusbtance abuse, are most at risk of abusing benzodiazepines. There is evidence to suggest that for those who are less severely dependent, benzodiazepine prescribing may not result in abuse.[33]

How then should you treat anxiety in substance-abusing patients: deny them benzodiazepines and risk under-treatment, or prescribe benzodiazepines for the anxiolytic effect and risk contributing to addiction? There is no definitive answer and although most benzodiazepine prescriptions are not abused,[34] a history of alcohol and drug abuse suggests high potential for benzodiazepine abuse.

Alcohol and substance abusers tend to ingest benzodiazepines for recreational purposes. Thirty to 50% of alcoholics undergoing detoxification and 44% of intravenous drug abusers may also be abusing benzodiazepines.[35] Benzodiazepines are cross-tolerant with alcohol, and alcoholics may use them with alcohol or as a substitute when alcohol is unavailable. They may also self-medicate with benzodiazepines to ease alcohol's withdrawal symptoms.

Opiate, amfetamine, and cocaine misusers may use benzodiazepines with their drugs of choice, as may younger abusers of MDMA ('ecstasy') and LSD.

Even patients who begin taking benzodiazepines for legitimate reasons may end up misusing them. In one study of 2,600 patients prescribed diazepam, up to 60% had misused and/or become dependent.[36] Long-term users of prescribed benzodiazepines often develop tolerance and may escalate their doses to get the same desired effects. If their supply is threatened, these patients may seek benzodiazepines illicitly.

Benzodiazepines may enhance or prolong the elation ('high') associated with other drugs or mitigate the depression ('crash') that follows a stimulant 'high'. Sometimes benzodiazepines are the drug of choice, as high doses of potent, short-acting agents may provide a stimulant 'high'.

Prescribing benzodiazepines to substance abusers is not absolutely contrain-dicated, despite an elevated relative risk of misuse or dependence. In the absence of convincing data, physicians must decide on their own, usually case by case, the merits of using benzodiazepines to treat anxiety in substance abusers.

An American group has developed a treatment algorithm for benzodiazepine substance abusers presenting with anxiety.[37] This information is based on clinical experience, more than 200 relevant articles, and the consensus of psychiatrists trained and certified by the American Board of Psychiatry and Neurology and the American Society of Addiction Medicine. This can be found on the following web address: www.currentpsychiatry.com/2003_05/0503_benzodiazepines.asp.

Non-pharmacological treatments have been shown to reduce substance use and control anxiety in some studies. These include cognitive-behavioural therapy, motivational enhancement therapy, interpersonal therapy, and brief dynamic therapy, among others. Their use requires specific training or referral to more experienced colleagues. For information on these treatments, consult the web-sites of the National Institute on Drug Abuse and National Institute on Alcohol Abuse and Alcoholism. Group and self-help therapies such as Alcoholics Anony-mous or Narcotics Anonymous have also been shown to reduce substance use.

Conclusion

Patients with coexisting serious mental/physical problems and substance use problems place great challenges on treatment services, including primary care services. As a group they are more difficult to treat and manage because of their higher level of physical, social, and psychological impairment. Gaining compli-ance with taking medication can also be a problem and reduce the chance of improvement. Keeping these patients engaged is perhaps the greatest impact that primary care can make, so that primary care practitioners, in partnership with their specialist colleagues, can provide these patients with effective care. Too many dual diagnosis patients fall through the net as treatment services pass responsibility to each other. A primary care practitioner is in the obvious position to prevent that.

Further Reading

Banerjee, Clancy, Crome, 2002 • www.rcpsych.ac.uk/cru/complete/ddipPracManual.pdf

Crawford V. Co-existing problems of mental disorder and substance misuse. A review of relevant literature. Crome I. (Ed). London: RCP, 2001 • www.rcpsych.ac.uk/cru/complete/literature%20Review.pdf

Rassool H. *Dual Diagnosis: Substance Use and Psychiatric Disorders.* Oxford: Blackwell, 2001.

National Treatment Agency. *Models of Care for the Treatment of Drug Misusers.* London: NTA, 2002 • http://www.nta.nhs.uk/

Health Advisory Service Substance. *Misuse and Mental Health Co-morbidity (dual diagnosis). Standards for Mental Health Services.* London: Health Advisory Service, 2001.

References

1. Wright N, Smeeth, Heath I. Moving beyond single and dual diagnosis in general practice. *BMJ* 2003; **326**: 512–14.

2. Crome I. *Psychiatric Disorder and Psychoactive Substance use Disorder: Towards Improved Service Provision.* London: Centre for Research into Drugs and Health Behaviour, 1996.

3. Regier D, Farmer M, Rae D, *et al.* Comorbidity of mental disorders with alcohol and other drug use. *JAMA* 1990; **264**: 2511–18.

4. Mueser K, Bennett M, Kushner M. Epidemiology of substance use disorders among persons with chronic mental illness. In: Lehman A, Dixon L. (Eds). *Double Jeopardy: Chronic mental illness and Substance use Disorders.* Chur, Switzerland: Harwood Academic, 1995.

5. Menezes P, Johnson S, Thornicroft G, *et al.* Drug and alcohol problems among individuals with severe mental illnesses in South London. *Br J Psy* 1996; **168**: 612–19.

6. Barrowcliff A, Champney-Smith J, McBride A. The opiate treatment index OTI. Treatment assessment with Welsh Samples of opiate prescribed or amphetamine prescribed clients. *Journal of Substance Use* 1999; **4(4)**: 98–103.

7. Marsden J, Gossop J, Stewart D, Rolfe A, *et al.* Psychiatric symptoms amongst clients seeking treatment for drug dependent: intake data from the National Treatment Outcome Research Study. *Br J Psy* 2000; **176**: 285–89.

8. Frischer M, Hickman M, Kraus L, Mariani F, *et al.* A comparison of the different methadones for estimating problematic drug use in Great Britain. *Addiction* 2000; **96**: 1465–76.

9. McKeown M, Liebling H. Staff perceptions of illicit drug use within a special hospital. *Journal of Psychiatric and Mental Health Nursing* 1995; **2**: 343–50.

10. Ryrie I, McGowan J. Staff perceptions of substance use among acute psychiatric in-patients. *Journal of Psychiatric and Mental Health Nursing* 1998; **5**: 137–42.

11. Schneier F, Siris S. A review of psychoactive substance use and abuse in schizophrenia: patterns of drug choice. *Journal of Nervous and Mental Disease* 1987; **175**: 641–52.

12. Corkery J. *Drug Seizure and Offender Statistics, United Kingdom 1998.* Home Office statistical bulletin 3/00. London: Home Office Research Development and Statistics Directorate, 2000.

13. Boys A, Marsden J, Griffiths P. Reading between the lines: Is cocaine becoming the stimulant of choice for urban youth? *Druglink* 1999; **14(1)**: 20–3.

14. Eggington R, Parker H, Bury C. Heroin still screws you up: responding to new heroin outbreaks. *Druglink* 1998; **13(5)**: 17–20.

15. Crawford V. Comorbidity of substance use and psychiatric disorders. *Current Opinion in Psychiatry* 1996; **9**: 231–4.

16. Drake R, Noordsy D. Case management for people with co-existing severe mental disorder and substance abuse disorder. *Psychiatric Annals* 1994; **24**: 427–31.

17. Department of Health. *Mental Health Policy Implementation Guide: Dual Diagnosis Good Practice Guide*. London: HMSO, 2002.

18. Carey M, Carey K, Meisler A. Psychiatric symptoms in mentally ill chemical abusers. *Journal of Nervous and Mental Disease* 1991; **179**: 136–8.

19. Drake R, Wallach M. Substance abuse among the chronic mentally ill. *Hospital and Community Psychiatry* 1989; **40**: 1041–6.

20. Kelly J, Heckman T, Helfrich S, *et al*. HIV risk factors and behaviours among men in a Milwaukee homeless shelter. *American Journal of Public Health* 1995; **85**: 465–8.

21. Smith J, Frazer S, Boer H. Dangerous dual diagnosis patients. *Hospital and Community Psychiatry* 1994; **45**: 280–1.

22. Siegfried N. A review of comorbidity: major mental illness and problematic substance use. *Australian and New Zealand Journal of Psychiatry* 1998; **32**: 707–17.

23. Chambers A, Krystal J H, Self D W. A neurobiological basis for substance abuse comorbidity in schizophrenia. *Biological Psychiatry* 2001; **50**: 71–83.

24. Mueser K T, Drake R E, Wallach M A. Dual diagnosis: A review of etiological theories. *Addictive Behaviours* 1998; **23**: 717–34.

25. Lamb H R, Bachrach L. Some perspectives on deinstituisation. *Psychiatric Services* 2001; **52**; 1039–45.

26. Selzer M. The Michigan Alcoholism Screening Test: the quest for a new diagnostic instrument. *American Journal of Psychiatry* 1971; **127**: 1653–58.

27. Raistrick D, Bradshaw J, Tober G, *et al*. Development of the Leeds Dependence Questionnaire (LDQ): a questionnaire to measure alcohol and opiate dependence in the context of a treatment evaluation package. *Addiction* 1994; **89**: 563–72.

28. Marsden J, Gossop M, Stewart D. The Maudsley Addiction Profile (MAP): a brief instrument for assessing treatment outcomes. *Addiction* 1997; **93**: 1857–68.

29. Drake R, Osher F, Noordsy D, *et al*. Diagnosis of alcohol use disorders in schizophrenia. *Schizophrenia Bulletin* 1990; **16**: 57–67.

30. Drake R, Essock S, Shaner A, *et al*. Implementing dual diagnosis services for clients with severe mental illness. *Psychiatric Services* 2001; **52**: 469–76.

31. Ley A, Jeffrey D P, McLaren S, Siegfried N. Treatment programmes for people with both severe mental illness and substance use. In: Cochrane Collaboration. *Cochrane Library*. Issue 1. Oxford: Update Software, 2000.

32. Champney-Smith J. Dual Diagnosis. In: Petersen T, McBride A. (Eds). *Working with Substance Users: a Guide to Theory and Practice*. London: Routledge, 2002; 267–274.

33. Ciraulo D A, Sands B K, Shader R I. Critical review of liability for benzodiazepine abuse among alcoholics. *Am J Psychiatry* 1988; **145(12)**: 1501–6.

34. Woods J H, Katz J L, Winger G. Use and abuse of benzodiazepines. Issues relevant to prescribing. *JAMA* 1988; **260(23)**: 3476–80.

35. Shaw M, Brabbins C, Ruben S. Misuse of benzodiazepines. Specify the formulation when prescribing. *BMJ* 1994; **308(6945)**: 1709.

36. Woody G E, O'Brien C P, Greenstein R. Misuse and abuse of diazepam: an increasingly common medical problem. *Int J Addict* 1975; **10**(5): 843–8.

37. Sattar S P, Bhatia S. Benzodiazepines for substance abusers: Yes or no? Do addiction worries outweigh the need for effective anxiety treatment? A sobriety-based algorithm addresses both concerns. *Current Psychiatry on Line* 2003; **(2)**: 5
(available at: www.currentpsychiatry.com/2003_05/0503_benzodiazepines.asp).

CHAPTER 23

Clinical management of substance misuse in prisons

David Marteau and Michael Farrell

IN THIS CHAPTER

The size of the problem || *Health and prisoners* || *Suicide and drug withdrawal* || *Fatal overdose* || *The treatment journey through prison*

The size of the problem

The prison service of England and Wales has a current population of 75,000 offenders in 138 prisons. The average stay in prison is a little over six months; 140,000–150,000 people enter prison each year, which affects an estimated 1.5 million relatives and friends.[1]

The prison population is largely young and male, although there are growing numbers of women and older people. About 20% of prisoners are from black and ethnic minority groups.[2] The prevalence of drug and alcohol problems is far higher among offenders than it is among the general population with approximately 60% of male prisoners and 90% of female prisoners having a history of problematic use. More than half of these prisoners will be dependent on alcohol and/or street drugs on the day of their arrival in prison.

Health and prisoners

Prisoners tend to have poor health: 90% of prisoners have a mental health problem (including personality disorder) and/or substance misuse problem, more than 80% of prisoners smoke, and 24% report having injected drugs.[3] There are also relatively high rates of HIV and hepatitis. Prisoners consult healthcare staff much more often than their peers in the community; this demand may not reflect healthcare needs. Healthcare in prisons (especially mental health provision) is often much poorer than in the community. Opportunities for informal care and self-care are limited.[4,5]

In England and Wales the responsibility for the health care of prisoners has moved from the Home Office to the NHS with primary care trusts (PCTs) now responsible for commissioning health care of prisoners within their boundaries (England), and local health boards providing a similar function in Wales. By April 2006, service commissioning will lie with PCTs; 18 PCTs started as trailblazers in April 2004.[1]

Prison Health aims to improve the health of prisoners, to tackle health inequalities, and to provide prisoners with access to the same quality and range of healthcare services as the public gets from the NHS by:

▸ improving the standard of prison health services through greater integration with the wider NHS

▸ reducing or mitigating the effects of unhealthy or high-risk behaviours

▸ promoting effective links with health and related services in the community to improve throughcare.

Primary care trusts are increasingly using the flexibilities of the new NHS to deliver innovative primary care services to prisoners, for example using Personal Medical Services practices or by commissioning specialist community services to provide drug and/or alcohol services. Both of these systems often use the skills of general practitioners with special clinical interest and clinician nurse specialists. As general practitioners and primary care nurses are becoming more involved with these patients they are coming face to face with the constraints of delivering high quality care in a custodial setting (Box 23.1).

Clinicians working in prisons are often the subjects of criticism from their colleagues who practice in non-custodial settings. Of the more persistent complaints made by community practitioners are that prison doctors and nurses are poor at communicating treatment information about their prisoner patients, often providing the outside general practitioner with little or no information about the treatment given whilst in custody. Another common criticism is that prisons do not provide continuation of methadone or buprenorphine programmes to patients who are subsequently incarcerated. These complaints are born from frustration and are also wholly understandable.

To remedy the problems, however, is no mean feat. Prison health care has for decades been underfunded, a Cinderella among healthcare services, with the clinicians often as demoralised and disillusioned as the patients they care for.

Lack of modern information technology compounds the problems faced by clinicians treating this large, transient group of patients. The sheer numbers of prisoners with drug and/or alcohol dependence puts an enormous burden on prison healthcare services and on the clinical staff providing treatment.

In 2003/04, 57,893 alcohol and drug detoxification regimens were prescribed. The busier prisons (for example, Her Majesty's Prisons Leeds, Pentonville, and Holloway) will each provide clinical management to around 2,500 patients per annum.

Extended in-depth assessments may be wholly impractical in a service that has to screen, assess, and initiate treatment plans for as many as 20 new drug-dependent patients each day. Of male prisoners, 45% will be regular injecting drug users, of whom many will have other complex physical, psychological, and social needs. Some of these needs will be substantial (for example, deep vein thromboses, severe depression, Type 1 diabetes, special learning needs, history of serious self-harm, or withdrawal seizures). Severity of dependence runs higher still among female prisoners, where 80% of drug-dependent patients are injecting users.

Clinicians treating prisoners are often unable to choose the most effective treatment for their patients, with each prison dictating its own policy, based in part on cost rather than clinical need. In the treatment of opioid dependence, for example, there has been a policy of automatic detoxification. This practice has, in recent years, been brought into question. In 2002, for example, the Home Affairs Select Committee made the following recommendation:

> We recommend that appropriate treatment forms a mandatory part of custodial sentences and that offenders have access to consistent treatment approaches within the prison estate as well as outside it. This should include strictly supervised methadone treatment in the first instance, as the most effective treatment available.[6]

As a consequence of this, and informed by evidence of effectiveness drawn from clinical prison research in Australia and France, the practice of automatic detoxification has now been replaced by clinical guidance that facilitates far greater access to extended substitution prescribing.

International evidence suggests that this intervention can have a beneficial impact on both health and offending. A retrospective study of over 3,000 offenders in nine prisons in France found that for over three and a half years, from 1997, there was a highly significant difference in the reincarceration rates between those heroin-dependent prisoners who were prescribed maintenance treatments (methadone or buprenorphine) and those who were not.[7] Those on maintenance treatments were reportedly reimprisoned at half the rate of the non-maintenance group (19% *vs.* 39%).

Further evidence of the effectiveness of maintenance treatment programmes in prisons has come from a long-term research study of methadone maintenance conducted in New South Wales prisons between 1997 and 2003.[8] This study found those offenders who received methadone maintenance during their imprisonment spent, after release, over a third (38.8%) less time in custody over the course of the following four years than those who did not receive maintenance treatment. The 'maintained' group returned to prison for an average of 41 weeks compared with 67 weeks for prisoners receiving no treatment or those who dropped out of treatment (four weeks per annum).

Studies from the Spanish prisons maintenance programme have shown substantial reductions in the transmission of both HIV and viral hepatitis.[9]

Box 23.1 **Problems working in custodial settings**

✓ Large turnover of prisoners with the additional work this causes to clinical staff

✓ Arrival of prisoners en-masse and the need to 'process' these arrivals within severe time constraints

✓ Lack of information technology

✓ Lack of treatment flexibilities normally available in community settings

✓ Poor communication between courts, police, and prison staff

✓ Inability to plan treatment: often prisoners released or transferred with no or little notice

✓ Clinical decisions often based on prison policy rather than individual need

✓ Professional isolation of staff

✓ Poor continuity of clinical substance misuse management for prisoners as they enter and leave prison

---

Perhaps the biggest challenges facing clinicians working in secure environments are:

▶ the growing rate of suicide in prison with an apparent correlation between suicidal intent and drug withdrawal

▶ the high rate of fatal overdose in the first week of release from prison.

Both of these worrying problems present opportunities for beneficial clinical intervention.

Suicide and drug withdrawal

The greatest risk to a prisoner's wellbeing occurs in the first few weeks of custody. This is the time of highest vulnerability regarding self-harm and suicide. It is also a period when many prisoners are withdrawing from a variety of street drugs. The experience of capture and incarceration can lead to profound regret and anxiety. When these uncomfortable emotions are coupled with the negative psychological effects of drug and alcohol withdrawal, the risk of impulsive self-harm grows.

Evidence gained from a retrospective study of the 172 self-inflicted deaths in prisons in the years 1999–2000 revealed that a third of all these deaths occurred in the first week of imprisonment.[10] The most common clinical diagnosis of those who died was drug dependence. Forty-six (32%) of those who died had an additional mental health ('dual') diagnosis. This figure indicates that prisoners with a combination of drug dependence and a serious mental health problem are at particular risk of suicide and other self-inflicted harm.

A Prison Service internal review of prevention of suicide and self-harm in prisons published the previous year also identified drug withdrawal as a factor that contributed to risk of self-destructive actions. The review included the recommendation that 'the Prison Service should pay special attention to the safe management of prisoners in the early stages of custody in a prison, with a focus on excellence of care for all prisoners in reception, first night, induction and detoxification units'.[11]

Experience gained from professional practice in individual prisons supports the notion that there is a correlation between drug withdrawal and suicide in the early days of custody. In more recent years, stimulant withdrawal (often from crack cocaine) is a growing part of this problem. To reduce these risks there needs to be a more coordinated approach to services for drug-using offenders entering prison. Innovative services piloted in a number of prisons include specialist 'first night' centres, rapid assessment for drug problems, and referral to residential clinical management units. These units provide active withdrawal management with prescribing that accords with national and international best practice, and a varied range of harm minimisation and psychosocial interventions for up to and beyond 28 days.

The prisons piloting this safer custody approach include Birmingham, Eastwood Park, Feltham, Leeds, Wandsworth, and Winchester. The results of the pilot schemes will inform future developments in this critical area of drug treatment.

As a separate but related initiative, the Prison Health department has drafted a document that gives guidance on the management of patients with both substance misuse and serious mental health problems. This dual diagnosis guidance will be issued as a companion to a new best practice guide to clinical substance misuse management in prisons. These documents will make provision for extended opioid prescribing regimes for this vulnerable patient group, in line with approaches recommended by the Department of Health for England and the Royal College of Psychiatrists.[12, 13]

Figure 23.1   **Excess mortality ratio for different time periods post-release by cause of death**

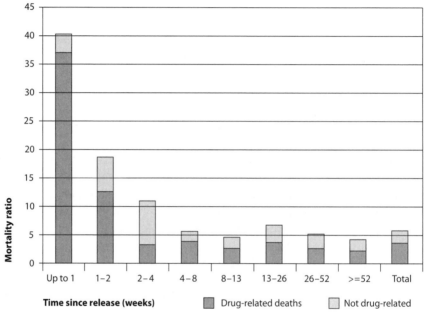

Fatal overdose

With regard to the risks of fatal overdose within the first few days of freedom, in a Home Office study of 12,438 prisoners discharged in June and December 1999, 79 drug-related deaths were recorded in the study period up to 31 January 2001.[14] Thirteen of these deaths occurred in the first week after release (55 deaths/ thousand per annum), at a ratio eight times greater than the annual mean average, and 40 times greater than the mortality rate for the general population. Six more deaths occurred in the second week and three to four a week in the following third and fourth week. Thus significant numbers of prisoners die within the first month of freedom, with loss of tolerance to opioids following withdrawal in prison appearing to be a major contributing factor; other risk factors include the use of multiple drugs and/or alcohol.

The study's authors recommended that methadone maintenance should undergo clinical trials in prisons as a means of preserving opioid tolerance and thereby lowering overdose risk following release. Additionally, the option of the initiation of naltrexone treatment prior to discharge from prison represents a potential protection for those patients who have become heroin-free in prison and would like clinical assistance in remaining so as they face up to life on the outside.

Methadone or buprenorphine maintenance treatment is still rarely available in prisons, although there is a greater provision of methadone maintenance in women's prisons.[15]

The treatment journey through prison

Arrival

Working in prison health care is never dull and has been well described by some as the substance misuse equivalent of a Saturday night accident and emergency shift. Such a blur of faces, files, and urgent health problems makes the loss of vital clinical information or the mistaking of identities a risk with potentially tragic implications. So the clinical imperative to do no harm is paramount, and the maxim adopted by clinical teams working in prison settings.

Working in prisons is not simple, beginning at the moment of arrival where most prisoners are taken into prisons at the end of the day, either on remand or under sentence from the courts. Times vary, but as a rule prisoners arrive between 4.00 pm and 8.00 pm. At this point they are seen by a team of prison officers who provide clothing and personal effects, search for forbidden articles, and make a risk assessment, which informs a decision as to the type of cell in which they should be accommodated.

The prisoner is invariably seen on this first evening by a member of the health-care team who completes a healthcare screen, designed to reveal a need for more in-depth assessment. It is important that this happens on the first night. Prison is a demoralising place to be in and the young or first-time prisoner is often disorientated and very frightened. Dealing with the symptoms of withdrawal can tip the balance of their mental state and could result in suicidal behaviour.

Immediate treatment of dependence

During the initial assessment a urine test will help to establish whether the prisoner has used opioids or other drugs. Presence of a positive urine test does not necessarily mean the person is dependent. They may have been administered opioids or benzodiazepines whilst in police custody; they may use only intermittently and not be dependent at all. Alcohol dependence can only be established through a careful history, aiming to establish, often in a matter of minutes, how much and how often they drink and whether or not they have a history of withdrawal complications. Even if they have been receiving opioid substitution treatment it is virtually impossible to determine how much they have been receiving; prisoners rarely arrive with clinical notes and information technology within prisons is rudimentary with no linkage at present with NHS medical records. The clinician has to proceed with caution. Too little treatment risks the prisoner having withdrawal problems, too much and there is a risk of overdose and death. If alcohol dependence is suspected, this is treated immediately with the initiation of a chlordiazepoxide detoxification regime.

Detoxification

For the other two dependencies for which medicated management is indicated, (opioid and benzodiazepines), the current practice is to commence a detoxification programme, starting on the first night or following morning of incarceration. In the case of benzodiazepine dependence, particularly where there is no physical health reason for continuing treatment, detoxification is almost always the best policy.

For opioid dependence, once an adequate assessment has been undertaken, prescribed management begins. Prisons aim to initiate treatment at the earliest opportunity to restrict the development of withdrawal symptoms, this being a greater imperative in prisons as supply of heroin is generally less available than outside prison.

To treat so many new patients safely doctors working in prisons have devised a number of interventions, which have been regulated under a prison standard for the clinical management of substance misuse.[16] This standard authorised the use of methadone, lofexidine, and dihydrocodeine for the provision of detoxification. It also approved maintenance methadone prescribing, but within a set of very strict criteria. Since its issue, buprenorphine has emerged as a viable treatment option. A number of prisons have now linked with outside NHS specialists to provide buprenorphine detoxification.

A standard opiate detoxification programme lasts for ten days, but this is set to be increased to a minimum of 14 days to accord with the National Treatment Agency's Models of Care.

Additional medication is prescribed to manage residual withdrawal symptoms.

Location

Until recently patients undergoing clinical withdrawal management have ordinarily been accommodated in cells throughout the landings and wings of a remand prison. More recently there has been a move towards the opening of residential withdrawal management units. These are prison landings of between 10 and 100 cells that have been converted to assist the safer management of drug-dependent patients. The cells have improved observation through the fitting of larger hatches and, for patients who are assessed upon arrival as being of greater risk of self-harm or suicide, furniture and fittings that have been specifically designed to limit the opportunity for self-injury.

Withdrawal management units have a blend of clinical and non-clinical drug workers and prison officers; many of these officers work in these extremely busy units as a matter of personal and professional preference.

Psychosocial programmes

Offenders in all of the 138 prisons in England and Wales have access to the Counselling Assessment Referral Advice and Through Care (CARAT) service, which acts as a case management service, providing entry to a range of structured treatment interventions. These services can be summarised as:

▶ CARAT support – group work and individual counselling

▶ short-duration intensive treatment programmes for individuals who are in prison only for a brief time

▶ intensive rehabilitation programmes for those able to participate actively in longer-term abstinence-based treatment

▶ close coordination with any continuing clinical treatment

▶ harm minimisation advice prior to release

▶ input to release planning, including through care to criminal justice integrated teams (CJIT) service on release, for individuals who require it.

The journey continues

The most clinically significant of these approaches involves methadone. Doses tend to be lower than in the community, and prescribing protocols are rigid. Stabilisation is by a conservatively paced dose induction in increments of 10 mg with at least six hours between each dose. The Prison Health department recommend ceiling doses of 40 mg per day, an amount that would prove inadequate for the same patient in the community but – as a consequence of the diminished appetite for heroin many offenders experience in prisons – it is effective in this environment.

Injecting drug users serving a custodial sentence often report that they reduce or discontinue drug use during their stay in prison, taking the opportunity to give their bodies (and minds) a break from the punishing ordeal of maintaining a serious drug habit.

The reasons why so many do reduce are unclear: the reduced availability of drugs in prison is an important factor as is the more structured regimen and greater scrutiny of prisons. This reduction in drug use goes some way to explaining the low HIV rate (0.5%) among injecting drug users in British prisons.[17] Sharing injecting equipment, however, represents a risk to those prisoners who do continue their habit, evident from the results of a large Public Health Laboratory Service screening study. This research indicated a strong correlation between injecting drug users who had been in prison and infection with hepatitis B and hepatitis C.[18] See Table 23.1

Table 23.1   **Prevalence of hepatitis B and C and self-report injecting drug use in England and Wales[19]**

N = 2839	Been to prison 1,740 (61%)	Not been to prison 1,099 (39%)
Hepatitis B + ve	24%	17%
Hepatitis C + ve	39%	28%
Injected while in prison (self-report)	17%	N/A

The relationship between incarceration and hepatitis infection cannot necessarily be attributed to needle sharing while in prison. Prisoners tend to be more severely dependent drug users, and, as offenders, are also more prone to risk taking. It is plausible therefore that a sizeable proportion of these additional infections were contracted outside prison.

In response to the high prevalence of blood-borne viruses, the Prison Health department has instigated a programme that will make sterilising tablets available across all prisons, the function of which will be to facilitate the cleansing by prisoners of illicit injecting equipment.

Needle exchange is not currently available in any prison in England and Wales. In 1996 the Advisory Council on Drug Misuse concluded that needle exchange in prisons was not a practical proposition.[20] The council subsequently adjusted its position by stating: 'If studies currently underway demonstrate a high rate of hepatitis C transmission in prison, a fresh initiative may be needed in this area.'[21]

Prisons present a unique opportunity for further clinical work with this hard-to-reach group.

A prison hepatitis B vaccination programme, which began in 2001, was expanded to include all prisons accepting prisoners directly from court. Sixty-five prisons are currently participating in the programme with increasing success. Between April 2003 and May 2004, over 16,300 prisoners received one or more doses of hepatitis B vaccine and over 30,800 doses of vaccine were administered;

7,684 prisoners completed the vaccination programme by receiving a third dose of vaccine. The number of prisoners vaccinated continued to increase throughout the year. Each month, an average of 1,892 prisoners received at least one dose of vaccine. This increased from 1,369 prisoners in May 2003 to 2,480 in March 2004.

Blood-borne virus testing is also available in many prisons, either offered by the in-house staff or by visiting genitourinary or primary care clinicians.

Naltrexone is available in over a third of prisons in England and Wales. As many prisoners take the opportunity to largely abstain from drugs while they are behind bars, the approach of liberty can cause anxieties about a relapse to heroin dependence. Many prisoners regard naltrexone as a means to protection against this susceptibility. The drug alone cannot keep a person safe from further destructive use,[22] but when used as part of a supportive resettlement plan, involving specialist help, it is a useful clinical option for the days or weeks that precede release. Urine or oral fluid drug screens and liver functioning tests are a prelude to any initiation of treatment.

References

1. Department of Health, HM Prison Service. *Prison Health Handbook*. London: DoH and HM Prison Service, 2003.

2. Social Exclusion Unit. *Mental Health and Social Exclusion*. London: Office of the Deputy Prime Minister, 2004.

3. Department of Health, HM Prison Service, *Health Promoting Prisons: a Shared Approach*. London: DoH and HM Prison Service, 2002.

4. Department of Health, HM Prison Service. *Changing The Outlook: A Strategy for Developing and Modernising Mental Health Services in Prisons*. London: DoH and HM Prison Service, 2001.

5. Marshall T, Simpson S, Stevens A. *Health Care In Prisons: A Health Care Needs Assessment*. Birmingham: University of Birmingham, 2000.

6. House of Commons Home Affairs Select Committee. *Review of Drug Policy, May 2002*. London: HMSO, 2002.

7. Levasseur L, Marzo J-N, Ross N, Blathier C. Frequency of re-incarceration in the same detention centre: role of substitution therapy. A preliminary retrospective analysis. *Ann Med Interna* 2002; **153** (Suppl. to No. 3): 1S14–1S19.

8. Dolan K A, Shearer J, MacDonald M, *et al*. A randomised controlled trial of methadone maintenance treatment versus wait-list control in an Australian prison system. *Journal of Drug & Alcohol Dependence* 2003; **72**: 59–65.

9. Pallas J R, Lopez A. Modificación de las prácticas de riesgo tras la inclusión en un programa de mantenimiento con metadona. Barcelona: II Congreso de Sanidad Penitenciaria, 1998.

10. Shaw J, Appleby L, Baker D. Safer Prisons – A National Study of Prison Suicides 1999–2000 by the National Confidential Inquiry into Suicides and Homicides by People with Mental Illness. London: DoH, 2003.

11. HM Prison Service. Prevention of suicide and self-harm in the Prison Service, an internal review. 2001.

12. Department of Health. *Dual Diagnosis Good Practice Guide*. Mental Health Policy Guide. London: DoH, 2002.

13. Royal College of Psychiatrists. *Co-existing Problems of Mental Disorder and Substance Misuse (dual diagnosis): an Information Manual*. London: RCP, 2002.

14. Singleton N, Pendry E, Taylor C, Farrell M, Marsden J. *Findings 187, Drug-related Mortality among Newly Released Offenders*. HOORS (Home Office Online Report Series), 2003 (available at: www.homeoffice.gov.uk/rds/pdfs2/r187.pdf).

15. Palmer J. Detoxification in prison. *Nurse to Nurse* 2002; **3**: 2.

16. HM Prison Service. PSO 3550. Standard for the clinical management of substance misuse. 2000.

17. Weild A R, Gill O N, Bennett D, *et al*. Prevalence of HIV, hepatitis B and hepatitis C antibodies in prisoners in England & Wales: a national survey. *Commun Dis Public Health* 2000; **3**: 121–6.

18. Department of Health. *Annual Report of the Unlinked Anonymous Prevalence Monitoring Programme: Prevalence of HIV and Hepatitis Infections in the United Kingdom 2001*. London: DoH, 2001.

19. Department of Health. Unlinked Anonymous Prevalence Monitoring Programme. London: DoH, 2001.

20. Advisory Council on the Misuse of Drugs. *Drug Misusers and the Prison Service – an Integrated Approach*. London: HMSO, 1996.

21. Advisory Council on the Misuse of Drugs. *Reducing Drug-Related Deaths*. London: Home Office, 2000.

22. Tucker T K, Ritter A J. Naltrexone in the treatment of heroin dependence: a literature review. *Drug & Alcohol Review* 2000; **19 (1)**: 73–82.

CHAPTER 24

Drugs, doctors, and the GMC

Clare Gerada

IN THIS CHAPTER

Problems with controlled drugs || *Doctors and the General Medical Council* ||
Addicted professionals || *Why do health professionals become addicted?* ||
Treating dependent health professionals || *Controlled drugs and problem doctors* ||
The 'irresponsible' doctor || *What is irresponsible prescribing* || *Common themes* ||
How to prevent trouble || *Issues raised by the Shipman case* || *Conclusion*

Problems with controlled drugs

The relative autonomy of doctors in prescribing controlled drugs reflects the desired principle for them to enjoy clinical autonomy over the way they treat their patients. When this applies to the treatment of drug use this is commonly referred to as the the 'British System', as described in Chapter 1. Whereas most doctors behave honestly and appropriately in their dealings with controlled drugs there are a few who do not. Though the actions of the former general practitioner Harold Shipman has recently placed the spotlight on problems associated with controlled drugs, ever since controlled drugs have been used there have been problems with their misuse and as long as doctors have been able to prescribe them there have been problems with some who abuse their position of trust.

Doctors and the General Medical Council

It is a sad fact that drugs and/or alcohol are often implicated when doctors appear in front of the General Medical Council (GMC) either as the doctors' own addiction has caused them to run into problems, or their management (or strictly speaking, mismanagement) of drug users has been deemed as seriously irresponsible or inappropriate.

More than two-thirds of the cases considered by the GMC's Health Committee in 2002 involved the misuse of drugs or alcohol.[1] Most of these appearances should never have seen the light of day at a GMC hearing. Often tell-tale signs that a doctor is running into problems have been ignored and the doctor is forced to continue digging deeper and deeper holes with sometimes tragic consequences. Lack of training plays its part: often doctors have a blind spot in their training and do not even know what they do not know and hence the idea of engaging in training never crosses their mind. This chapter will discuss where doctors can go wrong and ways in which these errors can be prevented. See Box 24.1.

Box 24.1   **Examples where health professionals have problems with aspects of controlled drugs**

✓ Doctors addicted to drugs and/or alcohol where use interferes with their clinical practice or where they obtain their drug through self-prescribing, from 'returns' from patients, or stolen from wards or general practice stock

✓ Doctors who self-medicate for their anxiety, depression, or physical pain

✓ Doctors who prescribe in an irresponsible or inappropriate manner, usually in the context of the management of drug-using patients

✓ Doctors who treat family with controlled drugs

✓ Criminal doctors who exchange prescriptions for money

✓ Shipman who used controlled drugs to murder

Addicted professionals

It is estimated that as many as one doctor in fifteen may be affected by drug or alcohol dependence problems at some point during their professional life.[2,3] The work of healthcare professionals places them at risk of mental health problems,[4] and they are more likely to develop problems associated with the misuse of drugs and alcohol. It is common for doctors to drink heavily at an early stage of their careers, especially during training and as medical students.

One study found that about two-thirds of recently qualified doctors exceeded recommended safe drinking limits, and 10% were drinking at hazardous levels. A quarter of the doctors in this sample were using cannabis, and 10% were using hallucinogens.[5] Doctors who misuse alcohol are often also taking other drugs, most commonly benzodiazepines, and may switch from one substance to another over time.

346

Frequently the primary problem of the doctor in this category appears to be alcohol, but on closer scrutiny it is often found that they are dabbling in other substances such as opioids, amfetamines, and other controlled drugs. Junior doctors and nurses may be among the first to recognise such problems in senior colleagues, but may be reluctant to take action for fear of damaging their career or because of the sense of loyalty owed to a mentor or senior colleague; it is difficult to 'shop' a senior.

Why do health professionals become addicted?

There are several reasons why doctors and other healthcare professionals may be at increased risk of drug and alcohol misuse.[6-8] The relative ease of obtaining medication is a major risk for all health professionals,[3] and something that should be partly remedied if the recommendations from the fourth report of the Shipman Inquiry are enacted (see Chapter 25). But ease of obtaining drugs only explains the means by which doctors feed their addiction; it does not explain why they start using them in the first place.

Doctors, pharmacists, and nurses are not an obvious high-risk group. They tend to be successful, intelligent, committed, and economically stable individuals. Yet, as discussed, a significant minority run into problems. For doctors, the long years of medical training are characterised by intense competition, excessive workload, and fear of failure, and few occupations face the intense stresses experienced in the daily practice of medicine.

Misuse of drugs by healthcare professionals may begin with a 'legitimate' reason such as insomnia, depression, or back pain, particularly when these professionals choose to diagnose and treat themselves, usually inappropriately.[9] The most frequent pathways into substance use are personality difficulties and anxiety or depression.[8]

Seeking medical advice

Doctors' and nurses' drug or alcohol problems often lead them into their disciplinary procedures implying that, more often than not, matters reach crisis point before action is taken.[10] This is partly because health professionals are reluctant to seek help owing to the stigma attached to psychological illness, in particular substance misuse, and the professional risks associated with acknowledgement of this.

This is reinforced by a study in south London where a service dedicated to providing confidential and specialised help to addicted health professionals found that fewer than 10% were self-referrals, most having been referred by senior colleagues or occupational health only once their problem had been discovered.

Delay in attendance may be linked to the natural embarrassment at seeing a colleague as a patient, with the issues of confidentiality that this entails, as well as concern for their careers. Hospital doctors and general practitioners hold these beliefs to equal degree.

A study of 144 doctors who had received treatment for substance misuse in a specialist treatment service showed that there was no difference between general practitioners and hospital doctors in terms of their substance misuse histories and problems they incurred. Differences did emerge between the consultant and the non-consultant grades of hospital doctor. The consultants were older at onset of problematic use (42.6 +/− 8.6 vs. 29.9 +/− 9.8 years); they suffered fewer career problems and used fewer substances.

Treating dependent health professionals

As health professionals often try to avoid detection and do not seek help until late on in their problem it is important to find ways of attracting them into treatment programmes by making sure that they have access to high quality, confidential, and sensitive treatment, preferably with the option of care being provided outside their immediate geographical area.

In the United States, every state has an 'impaired physicians' programme that provides support for addicted professionals.[11] Unfortunately, elsewhere, including in the United Kingdom, awareness of the problems of healthcare professionals has been slower to develop and the NHS provides few specialist services for such professionals.[12] When drug and/or alcohol problems are identified, there are rarely any therapeutic or rehabilitative structures in place to promote return to work under supervision or to ensure safe clinical practice.

The BMA has suggested that procedures should be in place to allow early recognition and management of substance use problems among healthcare professionals, and that even those who have had serious problems can be helped to return to productive professional engagement.

When engaged in treatment health professionals do remarkably well. A 21-year follow up of 100 alcohol-dependent doctors found a unique recovery rate of at least 73% over an average interval of 17.3 years within a range of 12–38 years.[13] The medical and dental professions have established their own self-support groups, including the Sick Doctors Trust and the British Doctors and Dentists Group (see Conclusion).

Controlled drugs and problem doctors

In 2001, of 51 practitioners found guilty of serious professional misconduct by the General Medical Council, 21 were for offences relating to prescription of controlled drugs; 16 were unable to practise, following erasure of their name from the Medical Register, or imposition of suspension or conditions of their practice, including an inability to prescribe controlled drugs. In recent years there has been a steady increase in the numbers of general practitioners and other doctors, in particular private psychiatrists, who have come to the attention of the General Medical Council accused of irresponsible and inappropriate prescribing to drug users.

The 'irresponsible' doctor

What is an irresponsible doctor? In its simplest term it is a doctor who fails to fulfil the criteria set out in the General Medical Council's *Good Medical Practice*.[10] These are that every doctor must:

- ▸ be professionally competent
- ▸ perform consistently well
- ▸ practise ethically
- ▸ do patients no harm
- ▸ be an effective team player
- ▸ take action if poor practice places patients at unnecessary risk.

What is irresponsible prescribing?

This is a deceptively easy question to ask but a very difficult one to answer. In most circumstances it represents prescribing that falls well short of established good practice – either in the type of drug, including combinations and formulations, the quantities prescribed on single prescriptions, or the means by which the doctor makes a decision to issue certain drugs.

What consititutes good practice changes. For example, the 1991 National Clinical Guidelines placed great emphasis on methadone detoxification, to be carried out over days or weeks. Maintenance prescribing, especially by general practitioners, might have been deemed irresponsible and inappropriate. Times change, and with the increasing evidence base recommending maintenance prescribing, it would now be considered irresponsible to stop a methadone prescription merely because of an arbitrary timescale. Similarly with dose: experts in the past may well have condemned doses of much more than 100 mg/day. Now, the National Treatment Agency's advice is that doses should be between 60 and 120 mg.

It seems that one generation's irresponsible prescribing has become another's good practice.

Prescribing alone must not be taken in isolation and separated from the overall care that the practitioner provides the patient. Perhaps the best definition of irresponsible prescribing is practice that places either the public or the patient at risk, whereby the doctor fails to take necessary precautions to ensure that the right drug is being administered in the correct dose, to the right patient, for the right indication, and in a manner that reduces the risk of diversion.

Common themes

So are there any common themes that cause a doctor to digress from good practice to such an extent that they are censured by the GMC? It may be useful first to examine some high profile cases, beginning perhaps with the case of Dr A, in the 1980s, who the GMC found guilty of serious professional misconduct as she had 'irresponsibly treated addicts privately by providing methadone in the long term without reasonable medical care'. Some saw this as punishment by the medical establishment for her policy of maintenance prescribing and prescribing of injectables as part of private practice and it led many to regard her as a cause célèbre.[14]

In early 2000, Dr B, a London general practitioner, was sanctioned by the General Medical Council after more than 25 years treating hundreds of long-term users. Both in the NHS and at his busy private clinic, he prescribed patients maintenance amfetamines, methadone ampoules, and other opiates, all in very high doses to patients from all over the London area. This doctor gave patients combinations of different drugs with few checks to ensure that they were not diverted onto the illicit market. Despite an appeal to the Privy Council, the decision of the GMC to erase his name from the medical register was upheld, stating that: 'The Committee heard evidence that your policy of giving patients what they asked for may have been accompanied by social and health benefits and that it helped to shield some from impure street drugs ... however that the risks to your patients and the public as a whole far outweighed any benefits.'[15]

A psychiatrist, Dr C, prescribed a concoction of the sedatives morphine and methadone combined with dexedrine from his private clinic in south London. This doctor was found to prescribe before drug dependence had been confirmed in the patient. The General Medical Council heard that the drugs ended up fuelling a black market and two patients died of overdoses. Dr C was found guilty of serious professional misconduct relating to charges involving 31 patients who travelled from far and wide to get drugs. One witness stated: 'Your routine practice was to prescribe a range of controlled drugs in exceptionally large quantities, which displayed a reckless disregard for the safety of your patients and your responsibility to public health. A doctor who decides to depart from established guidelines must clearly record his reasons for doing so. This you failed to do. You were apparently oblivious to and unconcerned about the inherent dangers of over-prescribing.'[16]

Less high profile cases

Below are other less high profile cases of doctors appearing before the GMC in recent years.

Box 24.2 **Case history**

Doctor X, male single-handed GP. In addition to NHS service, provided private care to drug users from a caravan in his garden. He prescribed usually on first consultation, without waiting for any confirmatory results of urine or other tests. Prescriptions to most of his 'list' of well over 100 patients would be very similar, namely 200 mg methadone ampoules, 20 mg diazepam ampoules, flunitrazepam 2 mg, temazepam 20 mg × 4 all prescribed for monthly prescriptions. The patients were then reissued prescriptions when medication was inevitably 'lost, stolen, damaged' etc. The patients were not expected to undergo any urine or other tests and their registered general practitioners were not contacted at any time to inform them of the prescription(s) that were being issued.

Box 24.3 **Case history**

Dr Y, single-handed doctor who had a number of patients whom he treated with dihydrocodeine and various benzodiazepines for drug dependence. One of his patients, new to the practice, came to see him asking for dihydrocodeine. The patient was 16 years old at the time. Dr Y prescribed this patient, on the first occasion, with 84 diazepam 20 mg tablets and 100 dihydrocodeine 60 mg tablets. The patient was admitted to hospital that night with an overdose and re-presented to Dr Y three days later. Dr Y had been made aware of the admission by the admitting doctor and a discharge letter was faxed directly to the GP. Dr Y reissued the same prescription to the patient on re-presentation. This was just one case amongst 10 others that was considered by the GMC to be irresponsible and inappropriate care.

Box 24.4   **Case history**

> Dr Z, male, who was part of a large group practice. He saw drug users, though
> none of his other partners did. He had well over 150 patients and saw them at
> an annex at the back of the surgery. Drug-using patients were expected to be
> segregated from other 'normal' patients. This doctor felt it his duty to care for
> these patients, which extended to providing them with money and to taking
> them to appointments. He carried out few checks on the patients' compliance
> and would often leave three-month repeat prescriptions at reception for
> collection. Despite help from the local drug service he continued to feel he
> knew the only way to manage drug users was to offer them what they wanted.
> He began to drink heavily to deal with the stress that the job was creating and
> would arrive in the surgery smelling of alcohol. The doctor began to have
> a sexual relationship with a patient, who then blackmailed him. The case
> eventually was discovered and the doctor retired.

Themes emerging from the doctors who have appeared in front of the GMC

In general terms what themes are emerging? It is difficult without conducting a large case controlled study to pull out common themes, though in the author's experience, there are in general three types of doctor who run into problems. (See Box 24.5.)

The first of these is the *naive doctor,* one who feels that they have a mission to treat drug users, that if they do not, no one else will. These doctors tend to work in an isolated manner, perhaps single-handed or, if part of a group practice, as the only doctor that cares for drug users. They may start off by seeing only a few drug users, but soon become identified either as a 'soft touch' or as the kindly doctor that looks after them. Unsupported, and often not working in shared care, these doctors soon take on more and more patients inevitably leading them to take short cuts in treatment.

It is not unknown for these doctors, for example, to post prescriptions to the patient's home for many months' treatment, rarely seeing the patient and certainly not carrying out any tests of compliance. Often this doctor tries to adhere to clinical guidelines but rarely succeeds, prescribing more erratically to larger and larger numbers of patients. Unless helped and supported this doctor is likely either to become 'burnt out' or to end up before the GMC, accused of irresponsible or inappropriate prescribing. This doctor tends to have no formal training in drug misuse, learning on the job and hence unaware of serious gaps in their knowledge base.

The second type of doctor likely to run into problems with the GMC over management of drug users is the *'maverick'* doctor. These doctors believe themselves to be right, believing that they 'know best' and that guidelines or protocols are for others. They tend to have some training in drug misuse, and perhaps have worked in the addiction field either as a clinical assistant or associate specialist.

They frequently prescribe drugs that are not licensed for use in addiction treatment, such as dihydrocodeine, methadone tablets, amfetamines, injectable preparations, or naltrexone implants. They usually ignore the advice from others practising in the area and continue to provide treatment that is outside the mainstream. When challenged they recourse to using the media to fight their cause.

These doctors rarely use urine or other tests of compliance, and if they do the results are usually ignored. Often different patients receive the same repertoire of treatment, with little adaptation for the individual needs of the patient. These doctors are likely to come to the attention of the GMC when the volume and type of medication prescribed is discovered, usually because of a patient's death or serious overdose or through chemist inspections.

Although it is perfectly acceptable to prescribe treatment outside standard practice, it must be in the context of well thought out treatment plans. The greater a doctor deviates from standard practice the more the onus is on the doctor to justify this, to his patients, his peers, and, when necessary, to the GMC.

The third type of doctor likely to come to the attention of the GMC is the doctor who practices in a *criminal* manner. This group of doctors is fortunately rare though a steady stream of doctors do appear in front of the criminal justice system for offences related to the misuse of drugs. Shipman is probably the most notorious of these doctors, although during the Shipman Inquiry Dame Janet Smith heard evidence of doctors (see Box 24.5) who had supplied drugs for monetary gain and of doctors obtaining controlled drugs to feed their own addiction.

Box 24.5 **Examples from the Shipman Inquiry**

In 2002, Dr A was convicted of the unlawful supply of controlled drugs, including diazepam, Rohypnol and Dexedrine. He issued private prescriptions on the payment of £30, often issuing prescriptions in false names to make detection less likely. He was also prepared to sell controlled drugs from his own supply to callers on demand.

In 1996, Dr C supplemented his living by selling temazepam capsules which he obtained from writing prescriptions for patients who were exempt from NHS charges. He would instruct the patients to go to the pharmacy and to bring back the medication for him to check. He would then remove and keep the temazepam and sell them for £3–4 each.

This type of doctor frequently prescribes drugs that have a high resale value if diverted onto the illicit market, such as amfetamines, methadone, diazepam ampoules, morphine sulphate, Palfium, and flunitrazepam. These doctors can be responsible for a thriving illicit market in drugs and users flock to them in the knowledge that few questions will be asked. In all three cases, it is not unknown for the local illicit market to be fuelled by prescriptions generated from these doctors.

At this stage it is worth mentioning the doctor who falls foul of the GMC by prescribing to themselves (ostensibly for pain or other physical reasons but more probably to feed their own addiction) or to members of their immediate family. Though not strictly against the 1971 Misuse of Drugs Act, the GMC, the British Medical Association, and the Royal College of General Practitioners all agree that self-prescribing or prescribing to family or close friends constitutes poor practice. One of Dame Janet Smith's recommendations in the fourth report of the Shipman Inquiry is to restrict this right and to make such action a GMC offence.

Box 24.6   **Characteristics of doctors who run into trouble with the GMC around managing drug users**

✓ Male

✓ Single-handed

✓ Managing large numbers of drug users

✓ Managing drug users not in the context of shared care

✓ Providing care within a private rather than NHS setting

✓ Doctor with an addiction problem

✓ Prescribing for self or family

How to prevent trouble

Lack of training and support are common features of doctors who run into problems in the management of drug users. It is important that doctors do not feel under any pressure to practise care beyond their level of competence. Doctors often feel that they are obliged to care for drug users, especially if other doctors in the area are unwilling.

They also seem to forget simple rules learnt at medical school and reach for the prescription pad too early. It is amazing that when given a new patient with, for example hypertension, a doctor will assess, investigate, and plan care before resorting to the prescription pad, and on the other hand, the same doctor, given a complex intravenous heroin user will carry out a cursory history, carry out no examination or investigations, and prescribe dangerous drugs in high doses before even confirming the diagnosis of dependence.

To prevent these cases coming before the GMC it is important that doctors have the opportunity to attend training, preferably before they start to manage drug users, are supported through clinical guidelines, shared care, and a peer network, and are able to gain the confidence to say 'no' to patients that they do not feel able to manage. Clinical governance emphasises a team approach to developing high quality care within a service and the importance of reflective practice within the organisation. A well organised practice, with systems in place for audit, continual professional development, significant event analysis, and learning from patients would prevent many of the problems discussed in this chapter, and, it is hoped, would reduce the numbers of doctors facing disciplinary action by the GMC.

Issues raised by the Shipman case

'None of your victims realised that yours was not a healing touch. None of them knew that in truth you had brought her death, death which was disguised as the caring attention of a good doctor.'[17]

The Honourable Mr Justice Forbes when sentencing Shipman on 31st January 2000.

Shipman perhaps deserves his own entry into this chapter. Doctors who commit murder are fortunately very rare, though history is interspersed with high profile cases of doctors (and nurses) who murder, some using controlled drugs.

One of the first recorded medical practitioners to kill using morphine was Dr Robert Buchanan, who was executed for the murder of his second wife in 1895. Carlyle Harris, a medical student, was convicted of a similar crime the same year.

Doctors who use their expertise to kill seem especially heinous as their motive for becoming doctors seems to be more about power, control, and gain rather than about healing and helping. Victims are readily available and it is easier to cover up certain types of murder in a major hospital, especially if the patients are elderly or have a serious illness. Even if the person dies, the doctor will have appeared to try as hard as possible to be the rescuer, which wins accolades from colleagues and staff. For example, Dr John Bodkins Adams was charged with 21 counts of murder in 1957 when it was found that some 40 of his elderly female patients had died under mysterious circumstances. Although Adams was acquitted, it was clear that he had built up severe dependency in his patients of morphine or barbiturates as a way to 'ease' the passage. He did not consider this to be murder.

On January 2000 Harold Shipman was found guilty of 15 counts of murder and one of forgery of a will. He is thought to have murdered as many as 400, mainly elderly women, over the course of 20 years, as a general practitioner and a clinical assistant.

The subsequent inquiry (Smith Inquiry) tried to establish how he had killed these people and what could be learnt to prevent any recurrence. Shipman probably killed his patients by lethal injections of diamorphine obtained by writing prescriptions for dead or non-existent patients or by obtaining controlled drugs from patients' homes. Although he was not the highest prescriber of controlled drugs (including diamorphine) in his area, he did have an extraordinary pattern of prescribing. For example, whereas most doctors have a saw-tooth pattern of prescribing of high dose diamorphine (for example 100 mg and 500 mg sizes) reflecting the rare patient with, for example, carcinoma head of pancreas requiring these drugs for palliative care, Shipman had a more even pattern of these medicines, prescribing large numbers year on year. He also had a habit of obtaining single ampoules of diamorphine 30 mg from his local pharmacist, ostensibly for the emergency treatment of a patient in acute distress.

He claimed in his trial that he had fallen into the habit of asking for this ampoule size instead of the more obvious 5 or 10 mg one, and would discard any unused drug. The inquiry postulated that he must have used other ruses to obtain controlled drugs, so that he would prescribe for patients and present the prescription himself to the pharmacist for dispensing claiming that he would deliver the drug when he conducted a home visit – in many cases it was found that the patient never received the medication.

There were cases where he would prescribe for patients who had died. He would also collect unused controlled drugs from deceased patients' homes. What the Shipman case has uncovered is the relative ease with which unscrupulous doctors can obtain controlled drugs and the relative lack of monitoring at any stage in the process from prescribing to administering to collection and disposal of unused medication.

Conclusion

Doctors who transgress the law with respect to controlled drugs are fortunately rare. Considering their position of trust, the impact they have when they do transgress can be significant – both in terms of the pain caused to themselves, to their patients, and to those closest to them.

It is important that doctors do not translate clinical freedom to prescribe with the right to prescribe as they wish and to ignore the basic principle of being a doctor, that is 'first to do no harm'. Clinical governance structures, appraisal and revalidation, and better routine monitoring of use of controlled drugs will, it is hoped, prevent problems before they happen, though it is probably impossible to stop a doctor hell-bent on abusing their responsibilities.

Information   **Details where advice or help may be obtained for doctors with addiction problems**

Sick Doctors Trust · www.sick-doctors-trust.co.uk/ | Help line 0870 4445163

The British Doctors and Dentists Group · Tel: 020 7487 4445 | Fax: 01252 350242
The British Doctors and Dentists Group have local groups in most regions of the UK and a group in Eire. These self-help groups offer support and advice to doctors recovering from alcohol or drug dependency. A list of local groups, times of meetings, and contact names and addresses can be obtained online at: www.medicouncilalcol.demon.co.uk/bddg.htm.

References

1. General Medical Council. Fitness to practise statistics for 2002 [Council paper]. Annex E.

2. British Dental Association. The dependent professional. *Br Dent J* 1989; **166**: 315.

3. British Medical Association. *The Misuse of Alcohol and Other Drugs by Doctors*. London: BMA, 1988.

4. Higgs, R. Doctors in crisis: creating a strategy for mental health in health care work. In: Litchfield P. (Ed). *Health Risks to the Health Care Professional*. London: Royal College of Physicians, 1995; 113–31.

5. Birch D. Ashton H, Kamali S. Alcohol, drinking, illicit drug use, and stress in junior house officers in North East England. *Lancet* 1998; **352**: 785.

6. Vaillant G E, Brighton J R, McArthur C. Physicians' use of mood-altering drugs: a twenty-year follow-up report. *N Engl J Med* 1970; **282**: 365–70.

7. McAuliffe W E. Nontherapeutic opiate addiction in health professionals: a new form of impairment. *Am J Drug Alcohol Abuse* 1984; **10**: 1–22.

8. Brooke D, Edwards G, Andrews T. Doctors and substance misuse: types of doctor, types of problem. *Addiction* 1993; **88**(5): 655–63.

9. Winick C. A theory of drug dependence based on role, access to, and attitudes towards drugs. In: Lettieri D J, Sayers M, Pearson H. (Eds). *Theories on Drug Abuse: Selected Contemporary Perspectives*. Rockville, Maryland: National Institute on Drug Abuse, 1980.

10. General Medical Council. The duties of a doctor registered with the General Medical Council. In: *Good Medical Practice*. London: GMC, 2001.

11. Hankes L. Bissell L C. Health Professionals. In: Lowinson J H, Ruiz P, Millman R B. (Eds). *Substance Abuse: A Comprehensive Textbook*. Baltimore: Lippincott, Williams & Wilkins, 1992; 897–908.

12. Strang J, Wilks M, Wells B, Marshall J. Missed problems and missed opportunities for addicted doctors. *BMJ* 1998; **316**: 405–6.

13. Lloyd G. One hundred alcoholic doctors: A 21–year follow-up. *Alcohol* 2002; **37 (4)**: 370–4.

14. Dally A. *A doctor's story*. London: MacMillan, 1990.

15. www.privy-council.org.uk/files/other/garfoot.%20%20%20%20%20(No.%2035%20rtf).rtf

16. www.thisisbrightonandhove.co.uk/brighton__hove/archive/2001/08/15/NEWS475ZM.html

17. Shipman Inquiry. Vol 1. Final Report. London: HMSO, 2004.

CHAPTER 25

Controlled drugs, regulations, controls, and diversion

Clare Gerada

IN THIS CHAPTER

Introduction ‖ *Brief history of regulation of controlled drugs* ‖
Misuse of Drugs Act 1971 ‖ *Drug diversion* ‖ *2004 Shipman Inquiry* ‖
Conclusion

Introduction

The main aim of laws governing controlled or dangerous drugs must be to minimise the serious harms that these drugs can do to the individual and to society. At
the same time, any law must enable the United Kingdom to fulfil its international
obligations. For the general practitioner and other members of the primary care
team, drug laws should be understood in so far as transgressing such laws would
cause serious problems to the clinician or to the patient. This chapter gives the
clinician information about laws relevant to their day-to-day practice and places
the current Misuse of Drugs Act (MDA) in a historical context.

The main instrument for drugs control in the United Kingdom is the Misuse of
Drugs Act 1971, which is now nearly four decades old. This act should be seen in
context of other acts of parliament and United Nations conventions on drugs. A
review of the MDA by an independent inquiry, chaired by Viscountess Runciman
was undertaken in 1997. The task of the inquiry was to consider the changes that
had taken place in society since the MDA was first enacted and to assess whether
the law as it currently stands needed to be revised to make it both more effective
and responsive to these changes. In all, the committee made 81 recommendations, in which the reclassification of cannabis from Class B to C is perhaps the
best known.[1]

Drug diversion

In modern times the biggest problem with controlled drugs is that of drug diversion, where the drug prescribed is not used in the manner or by the patient that it was initially prescribed or dispensed for. Shipman killed his patients by diverting diamorphine, using different ruses to obtain drugs from patients (alive and dead). Fortunately the cases of doctors diverting drugs in order to harm their patients are very rare, the commoner problem being drug users who divert their prescribed drugs for resale on the illicit market to be used by others.

Diverted drugs generally form part of a polydrug-using repertoire of heavy drug users. There have been few UK studies dealing solely with prescription drug diversion; perhaps the best of those that have been published is a qualitative study of users in different settings by Fountain et al.[4] She and her colleagues found that factors influencing the risk of drugs being diverted included doctors prescribing large amounts on single prescriptions and lack of identity checks on patients requesting medication from general practitioners.

It is possible that these forms of diversion have been made easier since the discontinuation of the Home Office Addicts Index. Patients may now 'shop around' until they find a naive practitioner who is willing to prescribe controlled drugs to them.

Techniques used to dupe prescribers include:

- exaggerating the amount of drugs used in order to obtain a larger prescription of substitute medication than needed

- claiming to be addicted to alcohol in order to obtain benzodiazepines

- professing to be trying to reduce opiate use and asking for benzodiazepines to alleviate withdrawal symptoms

- claiming insomnia/stress in order to obtain drugs

- giving false identities in order to obtain multiple prescriptions

- claiming to be a temporary resident

- exploiting prescribers who are judged to be sympathetic

- claiming to be an injector by displaying false injecting marks

- claiming drugs have been stolen/spilt/lost etc.

- forging prescriptions.

In some cases, the names of 'sympathetic' private doctors or pharmacists are sold.

The two main reasons why drug users in treatment sell their prescribed drugs are to raise money to buy drugs and/or formulations preferred to those prescribed, or to pay for a private prescription.

It is generally accepted that some diversion of controlled drugs is unavoidable and the price to pay for attracting and retaining large numbers of drug users in treatment. The right balance needs to be achieved between a doctor's freedom to prescribe and attract and maintain patients in treatment on the one hand, and on the other the need to minimise the risk of diversion by instituting safe, effective practices, such as those outlined in the clinical guidelines.

Brief history of legislation of controlled drugs

Pharmacy Act 1868

The Pharmaceutical Society of Great Britain was established in 1841 and granted a Royal Charter in 1843 (it was to become the Royal Pharmaceutical Society of Great Britain in 1988). Soon after the original formation of the society, there were calls to restrict the right to practice pharmacy to those who were licensed to do so; the aim was to promote and maintain professional standards and to establish control on the sale of drugs.

Until the second half of the nineteenth century, apothecaries, chemists, and druggists, as well as medical practitioners, supplied medicinal drugs. Any general dealer, equivalent to grocers of today, could also sell them. To prevent the unregulated sale by 'quacks' of dubious potions, tonics, and remedies (some of which contained opium) restrictions were placed on who could sell medicines and hence the Pharmacy Act 1868 was introduced. The Pharmacy Act outlined a number of drugs, including opium, that could be sold only by 'pharmaceutical chemists'.

In 1916, a regulation was passed, under the Defence of The Realm Act, to curb the use of cocaine and opium by soldiers in London on leave from war service – the effect of the drug being to encourage rampant sexual activity with prostitutes. The Americans had their own legislation enacted a few years earlier with the Harrison Act 1914, which banned heroin prescriptions, whether for addicts or for more orthodox requirements. To this day heroin cannot be prescribed in the United States.

Dangerous Drugs Act 1920

This prohibited the importation and exportation of certain dangerous drugs, including opium, cocaine, morphine, and diamorphine except under special licence granted by the secretary of state. It also created an offence of being an occupier of premises that permitted the smoking of prepared opium.

Dangerous Drugs Regulations 1921

This legislation laid down the formal obligations of doctors and pharmacists with regard to prescribing and dispensing dangerous drugs. Many of these obligations still exist today. The regulations stipulated that these drugs had to be dispensed only from written prescriptions when issuing publicly funded prescriptions for dangerous drugs and that doctors should use the same prescription form as for other medicines. This new 'official' form would be used for the private prescribing of dangerous drugs. It is ironic that the recommendation to reinstitute an 'official form' should be made nearly 80 years later by Dame Janet Smith in her fourth report on the Shipman Inquiry. The regulations also required a pharmacist to record relevant transactions in a register and imposed an obligation of record keeping on a doctor supplying dangerous drugs to a patient. This obligation persists to this day.

Rolleston Report 1926

A committee, chaired by the president of the Royal College of Physicians, Sir Humphrey Rolleston, was commissioned by the Ministry of Health as a result of concerns from the Home Office of doctors prescribing dangerous drugs to addicts. His task was to assess the extent of the opioid problem on the United Kingdom and to make recommendations.

At this time the Home Office opposed the treatment of addiction and the prescribing of maintenance prescribing. The committee, made up mainly of doctors, recommended that in most cases the steady prescription of the drug of addiction was appropriate. The committee set the scene for what is now called maintenance prescribing in that it recommended, for patients where it was impossible to wean them away from a long-standing addiction, the issuing of a small maintenance dose of their drug of addiction and that addiction should be regarded as an illness and not as a 'mere form of vicious indulgence'.

In the report, Rolleston identified many of the same problems seen today: some doctors were prescribing large amounts of dangerous drugs to patients on an open ended basis with no obvious treatment plan; some doctors were seeing their patients too infrequently – in some cases the prescriptions were sent by post; and some doctors had supplied dangerous drugs or had issued prescriptions to people unknown to them and without making any attempt to contact the patients' normal medical practitioners. There were even cases where the person had obtained drugs from different medical practitioners at the same time. Finally, the committee found that in some cases supplies had been purchased or prescribed by practitioners for self-administration. The Rolleston Report set the United Kingdom apart from many other countries in that treatment (at this time heroin) could be given for medical reasons. Consequently, this treatment philosophy was termed the 'British System'.

Brain Committees

In the years that followed the Rolleston Committee, far from containment of the addiction problem to a few 'respectable' iatrogenic addicts, the heroin problem expanded into new, young users, with a burgeoning black market of diverted prescribed heroin. Again at the instigation of the Home Office, the Brain Committee was set up; this time the remit was to review the policy of using dangerous drugs for the treatment of addiction. The stimulus for the First Brain Report was the manufacture and use of new synthetic opioids, which were being used by doctors for therapeutic reasons yet were causing addiction in large numbers of individuals.

The First Brain Report in 1961 endorsed many of the conclusions of the Rolleston Committee, in particular that there was no need to change existing British legislation governing dangerous drugs and the view that addiction should be regarded as an expression of mental disorder rather than a form of criminal behaviour and that the satisfactory treatment of addiction was possible only in 'suitable institutions'. This report was, however, criticised for failing to acknowledge the emerging and serious drugs problem in the United Kingdom and the committee was asked to reconvene in 1964 to examine the growing heroin problem in the United Kingdom (the Second Brain Committee). At this time the type of addict was changing from the 'typical', predominantly health professional, stable addict, using mainly prescribed heroin, to the younger, more chaotic person using 'diverted' illicitly obtained pharmaceutical heroin. The total number of drug addicts in 1967 was reported as 1,299 and by 1967 there were 381 heroin addicts under the age of 20.

The committee concluded, in its second report that the main new source of heroin on the illicit market was over prescribing by a very small number of general practitioners. The committee heard evidence of apparent indiscriminate prescribing by general practitioners where large amounts of heroin were being prescribed by a small number of doctors, especially general practitioners working in London. The committee concluded that there were serious problems with the unrestricted practice of these doctors and recommended that the prescribing of certain drugs to addicts, in particular heroin and cocaine, should be restricted to doctors with special Home Office licences.

The committee also recommended that the treatment of addiction should take place in specialised clinics (these became the precursors of drug dependency units) and that the clinics should be run by specialists, thus taking care away from the generalist and untrained general practitioners.

It also recommended sanctions, in the form of referral to the General Medical Council, for doctors who were thought to be prescribing in an irresponsible or inappropriate manner.

Finally, the committee recommended the formation of a central register for drug addicts; this was to become the Home Office Addicts Index until its demise in 1997. In reaching the conclusions, the Brain Committee considered the dilemma facing authorities responsible for the control of dangerous drugs in this country: 'if there is insufficient control it may lead to the spread of addiction – as is happening at present. If, on the other hand, the restrictions are so severe as to seriously discourage the addict from obtaining any supplies from legitimate sources it may lead to the development of an organised illicit traffic', this dilemma persists today with the current debate of expanding the number of patients being treated with prescribed heroin.

The dangerous drug legislation of 1967 and 1968 implemented some of the recommendations of the second Brain Committee. Under the 1968 act practitioners were prohibited from prescribing, supplying, or administering heroin or cocaine to addicts, except in the treatment of organic disease or injury, unless they were specially authorised to do so by the Home Secretary. In practice these doctors were granted authorisation only if they worked in the newly created specialist drug dependency clinics.

Misuse of Drugs Act 1971

The Misuse of Drugs Act 1971 (the act) replaced the Drugs (Prevention of Misuse) Act 1964 and the Dangerous Drugs Acts of 1965 and 1967. It thus brought controlled drugs under the same statutory framework and in doing so incorporated the following:

▸ the relatively new system of licensing doctors to prescribe heroin and cocaine to addicts

▸ the requirements for all doctors to notify addicts to the Home Office

▸ regulations on safe custody of drugs and national stop and search powers for the police.

The act also set up the Advisory Council on the Misuse of Drugs (ACMD), whose main duty was (and is still) to keep under review:

the situation in the United Kingdom with respect to drugs which are being or appear to them likely to be misused and of which the misuse is having or appears to them capable of having harmful effects sufficient to constitute a social problem

and to give:

advice on measures (whether or not involving alteration of the law) which in the opinion of the Council ought to be taken for preventing the misuse of such drugs or dealing with social problems connected with their misuse, and in particular on measures which in the opinion of the Council ought to be taken.

The act's system of classification was also new. It divided drugs in three classes, A, B, and C listed in schedule 2 of the act, and penalties for offences were related to the class of drug involved in the offence. Confusingly the drugs are sometimes described as being schedule 1, 2, 3, 4, or 5 drugs; such references are not to the classes in schedule 2 to the act but to the schedules to the related Misuse of Drugs Regulations 1985.

Class A drugs are those that are considered to be the most harmful if misused (e.g. morphine, cocaine, diamorphine) and as such offences in relation to class A drugs include the more severe punishment of penalties. Class C drugs such as anabolic steroids and benzodiazepines are considered to be less harmful and hence carry lower tariffs for offences.

Class of the drug relates to the different penalties for offences under the act. The class reflects the level of potential harm inherent in the drug.

Section 8 of the MDA made it an offence for the occupier or someone concerned with the management of premises knowingly to permit those premises to be used for:

▸ production

▸ supply of any controlled drugs

▸ preparation of opium for smoking

▸ smoking cannabis.

It is this section that the 'Cambridge Two', Ruth Wyner and John Brock, who ran a hostel for homeless people fell foul of. These two were sentenced to five years imprisonment in 1999 for 'allowing' illicit drugs to be used at the hostel and set in train debate to try to clarify the legal obligations of those running institutions where drug taking may be taking place and the dilemmas of having to weigh up the needs of the individuals using these premises against the rigorous interpretation of the law.

Section 9A makes it an offence to supply or offer to supply any article (except a hypodermic syringe) which the supplier believes to be used or adapted to be used in the unlawful administration (including self-administration) of drugs. The purpose of this section of the act, which was inserted in 1986, was to outlaw the supply of cocaine kits, which contained items for facilitating drug use, such as razor blades, foil, and lemon juice. An exception was made for sterile syringes and needles to permit the supply of clean injecting equipment to reduce sharing of injection equipment.

Despite this legislation many pharmacists and needle exchange schemes did provide drug users with swabs and sterile water and hence were technically in breach of the act and theoretically risked prosecution, although the police and the Crown Prosecution Service took the view that prosecution in such cases was not in the public interest.

In August 2003, after a review by the ACMD, an amendment was made to section 9 of the MDA that now allowed medical practitioners, pharmacists, and drug workers (including nurses and employees of needle exchange schemes) to supply certain items for drug injecting:[2] swabs, utensils for the preparation of a controlled drug, citric acid, and filters. The supply of ampoules of water for injection is also allowed, but only when supplied or offered for supply in accordance with the Medicines Act 1968, which means supply to an individual 'in accordance with a prescription' or when supplied to an individual under a patient group direction. The change in the law above applies in the first instance only to England, Wales, and Scotland. The Northern Ireland administration has subsequently amended its legislation to allow the same dispensations to apply in the province.

Section 10 gives powers to the secretary of state to make regulations around safe custody, documentation of transactions, record keeping, packaging and labelling, methods of destruction, and so on.

Misuse of Drugs Regulations 1973 and 2001 (The 'Main Regulations')

The regulations under the MDA specify the requirements for handling controlled drugs by certain authorised persons, including who can produce, supply, prescribe, or administer controlled drugs in the practice of their work. They also apply selective controls to groups of drugs, which are defined in the five schedules of the current (2001) regulations.[3] The schedules correspond to the therapeutic usefulness and misuse potential of the drugs.

The schedules under the Misuse of Drugs Regulations (MDR) are to ensure that practitioners are appropriately exempt from offences under the act while undertaking their lawful practice and include issues around supply, recording, storage, and destruction.

Summary of the Misuse of Drugs Act and its Regulations

This is not comprehensive guidance; the reader is advised to consult the 'further reading' texts recommended at the end of this chapter for specific details pertaining to their requirements under the MDR.

The Misuse of Drugs (Safe Custody) Regulations 1973

Retail pharmacists, private hospitals, and nursing homes must store schedule 2 and some schedule 3 controlled drugs in a receptacle that complies with the requirements of these regulations.

Table 25.1   **Misuse of Drugs Regulations 2001 (several amendments have been made since first iteration in 1973)**

Schedule 1 (controlled drug licence)	This contains the most strictly controlled drugs of all, and includes those that have no therapeutic use in standard practice. A Home Office licence is required to possess, produce, supply, or administer drugs in this schedule: cannabis in its various forms, hallucinogens such as LSD, ecstasy, and other drugs such as raw opium
Schedule 2	For medical practitioners this is the most relevant schedule as it includes pharmaceutical opioid and amfetamines used in clinical practice. Over 100 drugs are in this schedule. Schedule 2 drugs are subject to safe custody requirements, dispensing, and recording and destruction requirements
Schedule 3	Includes a small number of minor stimulants and other drugs not thought so likely to be misused and not as harmful if misused. Most are exempt from safe custody requirements, except drugs such as flunitrazepam, temazepam, and buprenorphine
Schedule 4	Part 1 includes most of the benzodiazepines and eight other drugs, including zolpidem but excluding zopiclone and zaleplon. Possession of a drug in schedule 4 part 1 is an offence without the authority of a prescription
	Part 2 includes anabolic steroids. There is no restriction on the possession of a part 2 schedule 4 drug when contained in a medicinal product
Schedule 5	Drugs included in this schedule are exempt from most controls, primarily those prohibiting possession, importation, and exportation, which apply to drugs in schedules 2 and 3. It does not contain any preparations intended for injection. The drugs in this schedule include preparations, often in minute quantities, that contain codeine, dihydrocodeine, and medicinal opium, dextropropoxyphene. The schedule contains both prescription [POM] and pharmacy [P] medicines. The latter can be sold over the counter (OTC) under the supervision of a pharmacist

The Misuse of Drugs (Supply to Addicts) Regulations 1997

These regulations prohibit doctors prescribing or administering heroin, cocaine, and dipipanone for the treatment of addiction unless the doctor has the necessary Home Office licence.

Misuse of Drugs Act Regulations 2001

Purchasing (requisition)

A requisition is required before any schedule 2 (or 3) drug can be supplied to medical or dental practitioners or a person in charge of a nursing home (unless on a prescription or by way of administration). The supplier must be reasonably satisfied that the signature on the requisition is genuine and the signatory is engaged in the profession or occupation stated. There are no limits on the amount of controlled drugs that can be held in a general practice surgery and it is entirely dependent on the dictate of the practitioner/s. In an emergency, practitioners may personally obtain from a supplier a schedule 2 or 3 drug if, for some reason, they cannot immediately supply a signed requisition. However, they must provide the supplier with the necessary requisition within 24 hours.

Prescriptions

All prescriptions for schedule 2 and 3 drugs must comply with the detailed requirements of the regulations. This is the requirement that causes most problems for the dispensing pharmacist. Not infrequently, controlled drug prescriptions contain minor errors, for example the date is omitted, the total quantity is added up incorrectly, or the doctor has forgotten to comply fully with the requirement to write this in both words and figures. The pharmacist is then faced with an irate patient – as it is a criminal offence to dispense the medication before the prescriber rectifies these errors. At the time of writing, prescriptions should contain the following information, written in indelible ink by the prescriber in his/her own handwriting – or computerised prescription (only doctors with a handwriting exemption from the Home Office are able to prescribe controlled drugs on a computer generated prescription):

▸ patient's name, address, age (where appropriate)

▸ name and form of the drug even if only one form exists

▸ strength of the preparation where appropriate

▸ dose to be taken

▸ total quantity, or total number of dosage units, to be supplied in both words and figures.

The prescription must be signed by the prescriber with his or her usual signature and be dated by the prescriber. For computerised prescriptions, the date and signature must be handwritten, but it is acceptable for the prescription to be dated using a rubber stamp.

From October 2003, extended nurse prescribers have been permitted to prescribe independently any of the following six controlled drugs:

▸ diazepam, lorazepam, midazolam (for palliative care only)

- co-phenotrope

- dihydrocodeine

- codeine.

From October 2003, the supply and administration of the following controlled drugs has been allowed under patient group directions:

- diamorphine – for the treatment of cardiac pain by nurses working in coronary care units or hospital accident and emergency departments

- all drugs, in any situations, except injectable formats, for the purpose of treatment of a person who is addicted to a drug in schedule 4 except anabolic steroids

- all drugs in schedule 5, at any time.

Prescribing in instalments (FP10 [MDA (blue)])

In England, these instalment prescriptions can be used only for schedule 2 drugs and buprenorphine. The prescriber needs to specify the number of instalments, intervals to be observed between instalments, and the quantity to be prescribed at each time. The situation in Wales and Scotland differs. In Wales, buprenorphine is not included in the drugs that can be dispensed in instalments and in Scotland any medicine, controlled or otherwise, can be issued for instalment dispensing.

Administration

Doctors may administer or direct any other person to administer these drugs to patients for whom the drug is properly prescribed. In most cases doctors delegate this task to a primary care or palliative care nurse who administers controlled drugs that have been prescribed by a general practitioner in accordance with their directions. Community midwives can possess and administer pethidine and pentazocine.

No entry needs to be made by a doctor or dentist for any drug supplied to a patient on prescription and dispensed by a pharmacist even if it is then administered by the doctor or dentist. It is, however, considered good practice that full and robust records are kept in the patient's records of all drugs for personal administration (i.e. given by the doctor/nurse to the patient from requisitioned stock). These records should make clear the details of the date, approximate time of administration, strength, presentation, and form. A record of the batch number and expiry date would also be considered good practice.

Registers and other record keeping

This is the area that is perhaps least complied with and understood by general practitioners. It relates to drugs kept personally by the doctor in the surgery (or bag) and not to those prescribed to the patient by way of a prescription. The MDA dictates that all registers must be kept for recording transactions in all drugs specified in schedule 2. Regulations govern the details of how entries are to be made in the record book and the form of book that can be used; for instance, the register must be in a bound book, loose-leaf formats are not permissible. Doctors working in groups or partnerships in shared premises may keep a joint register, or individual registers, but not both.

An area of confusion exists about record keeping of personally administered items from the doctor's bag. This is perhaps the most confusing and contentious area and causes more problems to prescribing and dispensing practices than any other aspect of compliance with controlled drug regulations and legislation. The doctor's bag and the central stock must be considered to be one and the same, with one controlled drugs register. Confusion arises where different doctors use the same bag, with the inevitable failure in the audit trail where drugs are then used and not recorded. In all cases, doctors are not precluded from making informal notes about drugs supplied or administered to patients they attend away from their surgery, but this must be entered in the central register later.

Disposal

Once prescribed, controlled drugs become the property of the patient, who can destroy them if they are no longer required. If they are returned to a doctor or pharmacist, there is currently no legal requirement to make a record of their destruction. It is good practice to dispose of such returns in the presence of a witness so that proof of their fate can be documented, and ensuring that they do not fall into unauthorised hands. The witness should sign the record of destruction. Stock controlled drugs may need to be destroyed if they are out of date. Schedule 2 drugs can be destroyed only in the presence of an authorised person. A record of their destruction must be made detailing date, strength, and quantity of the drug destroyed. Returned drugs cannot be recycled for further use. Persons authorised to witness destruction are any serving police officer, Home Office inspectors, other persons authorised by the secretary of state, and Royal Pharmaceutical Society inspectors.

2004 Shipman Inquiry

The activities of Harold Shipman and general issues of irresponsible prescribing are discussed in greater detail in Chapter 24. In July 2004 Dame Janet Smith published, in her fourth report, recommendations for the regulation of controlled drugs in the community.

These recommendations include:

▸ the formation of a controlled drugs inspectorate comprising small multidisciplinary teams

▸ placing restrictions on doctors prescribing to themselves or to close members of their family

▸ ensuring that doctors who have been convicted or cautioned in connection with a controlled drug offence should be under a professional duty to report the conviction or caution to the GMC

▸ introducing a special printed form for use when prescribing a controlled drug, whether within the NHS or on a private basis, and that such forms should be supplied only to doctors who need to prescribe such drugs in the course of their 'actual clinical practice'

▸ limiting the amount of a controlled drug that can be dispensed on a single prescription to a supply sufficient to last 28 days

▸ limiting the validity of a prescription for controlled drugs to 28 days.

With respect to pharmacists, the report has recommended that where the prescriber's intentions are clear, there should be some relaxation of the strict requirement that a pharmacist is not permitted to dispense a controlled drug prescription unless there is full compliance with every technical requirement of the MDR 2001. There are many other recommendations made in the fourth report and the reader is encouraged to read these *in full* and to follow the debates to consider which recommendations are implemented in full or in part or not at all (available at: www.the-shipman-inquiry.org.uk/4r_page.asp).

Conclusion

Controlled drugs are an important part of the armamentarium for the treatment of patients with a number of clinical conditions. As the number and range of practitioners able to prescribe them increases, and as the volume of controlled drugs prescribed increases, so too will the associated problems. The fourth report of the Shipman Inquiry recommended more controls to try to reduce the problems associated with their use and misuse. How many of these recommendations will be implemented still needs to be determined and whether, if implemented, they would prevent another doctor determined on criminal activity is another matter.

Further reading

A guide to good practice in the management of controlled drugs in primary care. National Prescribing Centre. NHS, 2004 (available at: www.npc.co.uk/background_for_cd.htm).

BMA and RPSGB. Controlled drugs and drug dependence. In: *British National Formulary*. London: BMA and RPSG, 2004 (available at: www.BNF.org).

Department of Health. *Drug Misuse and Dependence: Guidelines on Clinical Management*. London: HMSO, 1999.

Police Foundation. *Drugs and the Law*. Report of the Independent Inquiry into the Misuse of Drugs Act 1971. London: Police Foundation, 2000.

Royal Pharmaceutical Society of Great Britain. *Medicines, Ethics and Practice: A Guide for Pharmacists*. London: RPSGB, 2004.

Release: www.release.org.uk/html/~The_Law/~Legal_History/1900_to_1939.php

The Shipman Inquiry. Fourth Report. *The Regulation of Controlled Drugs in the Community*. London: HMSO, 2004.

References

1. Police Foundation. *Drugs and the Law*. Report of the Independent Inquiry into the Misuse of Drugs Act 1971. London: Police Foundation, 2000.

2. Statutory instrument 2003 No. 1653 Dangerous drugs. The Misuse of Drugs (Amendment) (No. 2) Regulations 2003 (available at: www.hmso.gov.uk/).

3. Dangerous Drugs The Misuse of Drugs Regulations 2001 No 3998 (available at: www.hmso.gov.uk).

4. Fountain J, Griffiths P, Farrell M, *et al*. Diversion tactics: how a sample of drug misusers in treatment obtained surplus drugs to sell on the illicit market. *Int J Drug Pol* 1997; **9**: 159–67.

Index